BASIC NEPHROLOGY AND ACUTE KIDNEY INJURY

Edited by **Manisha Sahay**

Basic Nephrology and Acute Kidney Injury
Edited by Manisha Sahay

Published by InTech
Janeza Trdine 9, 51000 Rijeka, Croatia

Publishing Process Manager Adriana Pecar

Technical Editor Teodora Smiljanic

Cover Designer InTech Design Team

Additional hard copies can be obtained from orders@intechopen.com

Basic Nephrology and Acute Kidney Injury, Edited by Manisha Sahay
p. cm.
ISBN 978-953-51-0139-0

For EU product safety concerns:
IN TECH d.o.o., Prolaz Marije Krucifikse Kozulić 3, 51000 Rijeka, Croatia,
info@intechopen.com or visit our website at intechopen.com.

Meet the editor

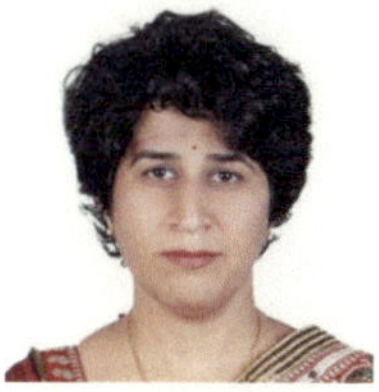

Dr Manisha Sahay is currently the Professor and Head, Department of Nephrology, Osmania General Hospital & Osmania Medical College and Consultant Nephrologist, Aditya Hospital, Hyderabad, Andhra Pradesh, India. She did her DNB in Nephrology in 2003 under National Board of Examinations, National Academy of Medical Sciences, India in which she secured first rank and gold medal. She acquired her MD in 1998 from Osmania Medical College, Hyderabad and MBBS from SMS Medical College, Jaipur, Rajasthan. She was State topper in 10th Board Examination and has been awarded 12 gold medals till date. She has received the "Tanker – Young Investigator Award" of Indian Society of Nephrology. She has many publications to her credit both in national and international journals. She is the executive committee member of Young nephrologists' committee of International society of nephrology. She is also the governing body member of Indian society of nephrology. She has contributed to several textbooks and is the reviewer for Indian and international journals. She is the Associate editor of Journal of Academy of Medical Sciences and Guest Editor for Indian journal of endocrinology and metabolism - Renal endocrinology.

Contents

Preface XI

Part 1 Basics of Nephrology 1

Chapter 1 **Is Body Surface Area the Appropriate Index for Glomerular Filtration Rate? 3**
Liesbeth Hoste and Hans Pottel

Chapter 2 **How Measuring Glomerular Filtration Rate? Comparison of Reference Methods 21**
Pierre Delanaye

Chapter 3 **Effects of Preterm Birth on the Kidney 61**
Mary Jane Black, Megan R. Sutherland and Lina Gubhaju

Chapter 4 **Renal Potassium Handling and Associated Inherited Tubulopathies Leading to Hypokalemia 89**
Jelena Stojanovic and John Sayer

Chapter 5 **Variability of Biological Parameters in Blood Samples Between Two Consecutive Schedules of Hemodialysis 105**
Aurelian Udristioiu, Manole Cojocaru, Alexandra Dana Maria Panait, Radu Iliescu, Victor Dumitrascu and Daliborca Cristina Vlad

Part 2 Acute Kidney Injury 123

Chapter 6 **The Metamorphosis of Acute Renal Failure to Acute Kidney Injury 125**
John W. Pickering and Zoltán H. Endre

Chapter 7 **Acute Kidney Injury in Pregnancy 151**
Manisha Sahay

Chapter 8 **Evaluation of Acute Kidney Injury in Intensive Care Unit 173**
Itir Yegenaga

Chapter 9 **Vancomycin-Induced Nephrotoxicity 183**
Ahmad Bilal, Omar Abu-Romeh, Talla A. Rousan and Kai Lau

Preface

Nephrology is an ever expanding and dynamic field of medicine. It is important to have a clear understanding of basic concepts for proper evaluation and management of renal diseases. Our book aims to fulfill this objective. The first section deals with basic nephrology. It describes the methods of estimation of glomerular filtration rate which is the basic test for renal function. The second section of the book deals with acute kidney injury. Acute kidney injury is an important preventable and treatable form of renal damage. The etiology of AKI varies in different parts of the world. AKI may occur in various clinical settings e.g. in an intensive care unit or in the community where it may occur as a result of adverse reaction to drugs or infections. The incidence of AKI in pregnancy in the developed world has fallen dramatically over the past 40 years, however it continues to be an important cause of maternal and fetal mortality in developing countries. The various causes of Pregnancy AKI are discussed in the chapter on acute kidney injury in pregnancy. Exhaustive reviews, pioneering original articles and interesting case reports showcase the wide spectrum and challenging vistas of nephrology. The editors hope that this will encourage more original researchers in this field across the globe.

Dr. Manisha Sahay
Professor and Head, Dept. of Nephrology
Osmania General Hospital / Osmania Medical College, Hyderabad
Consultant Nephrologist, Aditya Hospital, Tilak Road, Abids
Member of Young Nephrologists Committee - International Society of Nephrology
Executive Committee Member - Indian Society of Nephrology (Central)
Executive Committee Member - Southern Chapter of Indian Society of Nephrology
Ameerpet, Hyderabad
India

Part 1

Basics of Nephrology

1

Is Body Surface Area the Appropriate Index for Glomerular Filtration Rate?

Liesbeth Hoste and Hans Pottel
Katholieke Universiteit Leuven Campus Kortrijk
Belgium

1. Introduction

Indexing glomerular filtration rate (GFR) for body surface area (BSA) is routine practice, but criticism has been raised on indexing GFR for BSA in children, obese and anorectic patients. Over the years other ways of indexing GFR have been proposed, including height, lean body mass, body weight, ideal weight, plasma volume, total body water and especially extracellular volume (ECV). Based on a literature review and on statistical analyses of GFR data of children, we consider the following main questions: Why do we normalize GFR for BSA? Is it really necessary to index GFR? And if so, are there other or better ways to normalize GFR?

2. History of BSA formulas

In the late 19th century, Max Rubner introduced the 'surface' hypothesis that the metabolic rate of any animal is closely related to BSA. (Rubner, 1883) Although we know today that this assertion is not correct, the surface hypothesis was well embraced at that time and considered as a law. Since measuring heat production with direct calorimety is rather complex, BSA was seen as an alternative for reflecting the metabolic rate. The question then became how to measure BSA?

2.1 The formula of Meeh (1879)

In 1879, Meeh published a formula to estimate BSA from body weight. (Meeh, 1879) Meeh derived his formula in 6 adults and 10 children, using a variety of methods. Some parts of the body were marked out in geometrical patterns, which were then traced on transparent paper. Next, the surface of these areas was determined by geometry, or if the pieces of paper were very irregular, by weighing. Some of the cylindrical parts of the body were wound with strips of millimeter paper like a bandage. The widely used formula proposed by Meeh was based on the fundamental mathematical law which states that similar solids have a surface area proportional to the 2/3 power of their volumes. He used body weight to represent volume, and derived the following equation, based on dimensional analysis: $BSA = 0.1053 \text{ weight}^{2/3}$.

2.2 The formula of DuBois & DuBois (1916)

Meeh's formula remained standard until 1916 when the DuBois brothers published several manuscripts exploring different formulas to measure the BSA. To determine the surface area of the various parts of the body, the brothers tightly covered patients' bodies with manila paper molds. The area of the mold was determined by cutting it in pieces and placing the pieces flat on photographic film which was exposed to sunlight. The unexposed paper was then cut and weighed. The BSA was derived from the weight divided by the average density of the photographic paper. The brothers used 19 detailed measurements from 7 different body parts of 5 patients to derive a geometric formula to predict BSA that had an acceptably limited error compared with the true BSA. (DuBois & DuBois, 1915) One year later, DuBois & DuBois added 4 patients to their 5 initial patients and they derived, by iteration, a 'height-weight' formula from this dataset. Among the 9 patients, there was a child of 2 suffering from rickets, an obese adult female, a 36 year old adult with mental and physical development of an 8 year old and a diabetic patient of 18 with a very low body mass index. (DuBois & DuBois, 1916)

In order to construct their formula, the brothers concluded that the error in Meeh's formula could be reduced by also taking height into consideration, since adding height made the formula more applicable for patients of the same general shape but differing somewhat in relative dimensions. DuBois & DuBois assumed that area could be estimated from the formula $BSA = CW^aH^b$, with C a constant, W = weight in kg and H = height in cm. As the left side in this equation has the dimensions of an area (squared length L^2), the right side needs to have the same dimensionality. As weight is considered proportional to a volume (L^3) when mass density is considered constant, the following dimensionality condition is obtained: $2 = 3a + b$. This constraint reduces the complexity of the problem, as only two parameters (the constant C and a or b) have to be obtained from the data. Logarithmic transformation of both sides of the equation reduces the problem even further to a simple linear regression fit. With the aid of a computer this is easily performed with modern statistical methodology, but back in 1916, DuBois & DuBois had to use repetitive combinations for a and b to arrive at their final and today's well known DuBois & DuBois formula: $BSA = 0.007184 * W^{0.425} * H^{0.725}$.

2.3 The search for a better formula (1935-2010)

In the following years, several authors have proposed other formulas using more sophisticated statistical techniques and studying larger populations. In 1935, Boyd listed 401 direct measurements of surface area obtained by direct coating, triangulation or surface integrator methods. (Boyd, 1935) Boyd recommended 2 formulas for calculating surface area, one based on height and weight and one based on weight only. The formula involving height and weight was superior to that based on weight alone. In 1970, Gehan & George used Boyd's database to refine the exponents in the equation proposed by DuBois & DuBois. (Gehan & George, 1970) Although Gehan & George did find that their equation failed for small children and obese subjects, no further attempt was made to assess other models relating height and weight to BSA. In 1978, Haycock et al. started calculating BSA by using a geometric method with schematic reduction of body segments to cylinders and a sphere. (Haycock et al., 1978) Validation in 81 persons, from premature infants to adults, was done by comparison with the DuBois & DuBois formula (DuBois & DuBois, 1916) for adults and with the Faber & Melcher formula (Faber & Melcher, 1921) for infants. The formulas of Boyd, Gehan & George and Haycock rely on linear regression of logarithmically transformed weight and height measurements. The authors published equations of the type of DuBois & DuBois, in which different values for the constants a, b and C were obtained. Although the constraint $3a + b = 2$ was not used in the construction of these formulas, one may notice that the dimensionality condition is nearly always fulfilled. For Boyd's formula

3a + b gives a value of 1.95, the formula of Gehan & George gives a value of 1.97 and Haycock's equation gives 2.01. In 1987, Mosteller also used dimension analysis to derive a simplified formula from that of Gehan & George, which is easier to remember. (Mosteller, 1987) In 2000, Shuter & Aslani presented the original results of the DuBois & DuBois formula on a more robust statistical footing (non-linear regression), yielding values for the model constants that would have been obtained if the brothers had had access to modern statistical methods and modern computers. (Shuter & Aslani, 2000) Since fitting BSA estimates directly by non-linear regression is more accurate, this was the technique Livingston & Lee preferred in 2001 to derive their formula which, like Meeh's formula, only relies on body weight. Based on the data of 47 patients, they developed an equation, which is especially useful to predict BSA in obese patients. (Livingston & Lee, 2001)

In general, the correlation between all these formulas is high (Verbraecken et al., 2006), but there are no clear advantages of the others over the DuBois formula, which remains the best known and most used formula today. Although, it is unrealistic to expect that one single height-weight formula predicts BSA with the same accuracy in all people, since humans change shape as they grow and age. Errors in height-weight formulas will be exaggerated in very small people like children or in obese patients. It has been shown that for children weighing below 10 kg and in the obese population, the DuBois formula does not give the best results. For children with a weight below 10 kg the formulas of Haycock or Mosteller are preferred (van der Sijs & Guchelaar, 2002), for obese persons the formula of Livingston & Lee is advised. (Livingston & Lee, 2001) A simulation with virtual data showed us that the formulas of Boyd, Gehan & George, Haycock and Mosteller overestimate the BSA as compared to the BSA calculated with the DuBois & DuBois formula. In Figure 1 one may observe an elliptical shape of the data in the plot of the BSA calculated with the Gehan & George equation against the DuBois & DuBois calculated BSA. The graph also illustrates that a BSA of 1.73m² calculated by DuBois & DuBois can vary between 1.65m² and 2.15m² if calculated by the Gehan & George equation. This elliptical shape is also seen when plotting the formulas of Boyd, Gehan & George, Haycock et al. and Mosteller against the DuBois & DuBois formula (graphs are not shown).

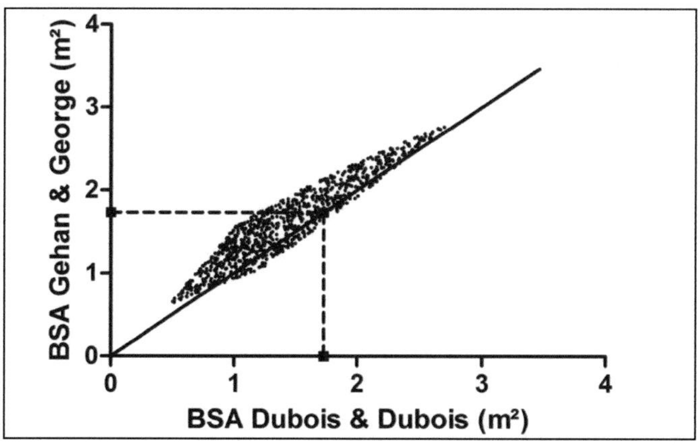

Fig. 1. BSA calculated with the formula of Gehan & George plotted against the DuBois & DuBois calculated BSA. The solid line is the identity line. The dotted lines indicate a body surface area of 1.73m².

For the determination of the body surface area of Indians, Banerjee et al. updated the constant C of the formula of DuBois & DuBois. (Banerjee & Bhattacharya, 1961; Banerjee & Sen, 1955) Nwoye et al. computed new variables for height and weight formulas that accurately predict the surface area of Africans and Saudi males. (Nwoye, 1989; Nwoye & Al-Shehri, 2003) The formula of Fujimoto et al. was developed to calculate the BSA in the Japanese population (Fujimoto et al., 1968), while Stevenson developed a formula to estimate the BSA in Chinese people. (Stevenson, 1937) Interesting is that recently, a new 3D-scanning method for measuring BSA is introduced and used to propose new BSA formulas. (Tikuisis et al., 2001; Yu et al., 2010) An overview of a non exhaustive list of BSA formulas is given in Table 1.

AUTHOR	FORMULA
Meeh (1879)	BSA = 0.1053 weight $^{2/3}$
DuBois & DuBois (1916)	BSA = 0.007184 * weight $^{0.425}$ * height $^{0.725}$
Faber & Melcher (1921)	BSA = 0.007850 * weight $^{0.425}$ * height $^{0.725}$
Boyd (1935)	BSA = 0.017827 * weight $^{0.4838}$ * height $^{0.5}$
Stevenson (1937)	BSA = 0.0128 * weight + 0.0061 * height - 0.1529
Banerjee & Sen (1955)	BSA = 0.007466 * weight $^{0.425}$ * height $^{0.725}$
Banerjee & Bhattacharya (1961)	BSA = 0.0070 * weight $^{0.425}$ * height $^{0.725}$
Fujimoto et al. (1968)	BSA = 0.008883 * weight $^{0.444}$ * height $^{0.663}$
Gehan & George (1970)	BSA = 0.0235 * weight $^{0.51456}$ * height $^{0.42246}$
Haycock et al. (1978)	BSA = 0.02465 * weight $^{0.5378}$ * height $^{0.3964}$
Mosteller (1987)	BSA = (weight $^{0.5}$ * height $^{0.5}$)/60
Nwoye (1989)	BSA = 0.001315 * weight $^{0.2620}$ * height $^{1.2139}$
Shuter & Aslani (2000)	BSA = 0.00949 * weight $^{0.441}$ * height $^{0.655}$
Livingston & Lee (2001)	BSA = 0.1173 * weight $^{0.6466}$
Tikuisis for men (2001)	BSA = 0.01281* weight $^{0.44}$ * height $^{0.60}$
Tikuisis for women (2001)	BSA = 0.01474 * weight $^{0.47}$ * height $^{0.55}$
Nwoye & Al-Sheri (2003)	BSA = 0.02036 * weight $^{0.427}$ * height $^{0.516}$
Yu et al. (2010)	BSA = 0.00713989 * weight $^{0.4040}$ * height $^{0.7437}$

Table 1. Overview of BSA formulas. BSA is expressed in m^2, weight in kg, height in cm.

3. Indexing GFR for BSA

The GFR of a healthy person can vary from 1 ml/min for neonates to 200 ml/min for large adults. White et al. stated that this makes the interpretation of a GFR measurement not easy for the physician unless the physician is familiar with the expected normal value for the particular patient. (White & Strydom, 1991) Therefore, it would be worth considering to normalize GFR in such a way that the influence of patient variables is minimal.

In 1928, renal function was for the first time corrected for BSA by McIntosh et al. (McIntosh et al., 1928) McIntosh et al. built their indexation theory on the experience of the research of Taylor et al., which assumed a correlation between urea excretion and the weight of the kidneys in rabbits. Taylor et al. also showed that there exists a better correlation between kidney weight and BSA, than between kidney weight and animal's weight. (Taylor et al., 1923) When McIntosh et al. on their turn corrected urea clearances of 18 adults and 8 children for BSA, the data from the small children yielded the same normal values as for adults. In the footsteps of Taylor et al., MacKay illustrated a direct correlation between BSA and kidney weight and between BSA and urea excretion in humans. (MacKay, 1932). Based on these observations, the indexation of GFR for BSA became standard in the medical community.

McIntosh et al. also introduced the use of the reference surface area of $1.73m^2$, which was the average calculated BSA of 25 year old Americans at that time. The value of $1.73m^2$ has served the physiological community well for nearly 80 years, but is clearly no longer applicable to modern Western populations, as has been shown by Heaf et al. (Heaf, 2007) A value of $1.95m^2$ would probably be more appropriate for the average BSA of today's 25 year old adults in America. Switching from $1.73m^2$ to $1.95m^2$ has severe repercussions for the current classification system for Chronic Kidney Disease, which is based on fixed limits of 15, 30, 60 and 90 $ml/min/1.73m^2$. The importance of $1.73m^2$ or $1.95m^2$ is not the value as such, but the fact that it serves as a reference point. Therefore, there is no need to change the reference value.

Recently, Delanaye et al. recalculated Taylor's correlation and noted that the correlation between BSA and kidney weight was not different from that between kidney weight and body weight. (Delanaye et al., 2009a) This indicates that the BSA-indexation theory of McIntosh et al. was based on false assumptions.

4. Is it necessary to index GFR?

In 1928, McIntosh et al. already noticed that indexing is not necessary for 'normally built' people. McIntosh stated: "*The nature of the standard clearance formula is such that correction for body size in persons between 62 and 71 inches in height does not exceed 5 per cent, and in tests of renal function may be neglected.*" (McIntosh et al., 1928) It follows that in longitudinal studies, the absolute GFR should be used for evaluating the kidney function, avoiding the use of BSA-indexed GFR which is affected by weight changes. On the other hand, indexation seems to be necessary to compare different patient values and to allow comparison with fixed reference values. Three cases will here be studied to illustrate these statements: (1) the GFR of a small and heavy person will be compared with each other, (2) the GFR evolution during childhood will be presented and (3) the GFR of two adult men, one with a stable weight and one with a weight that increases with age, will be followed.

4.1 Case 1: Comparison of the GFR of a small and heavy person

Imagine the body of a small and heavy person as a small and big pond with the kidneys as a pump and filter combination to clear the dirt out of the pond. The dirt is equally present in the pond and the pump sends a constant flow through the filter which is here assumed to have the same clearing efficiency, after which the cleared water is drained off in the pond again. Repeated cycles will diminish the concentration of dirt in the water. If the small and the big pond both have an equally working pump and filter combination of 60 ml/min, it will take much longer for the big pond to be cleared than it will take for the small pond. Or the pump of the big pond will have to work at a higher rate than the pump of the small one to clear all the dirt out of the water in the same time. This indicates that the function of the pumps must be corrected for a value that describes the size of the ponds in a certain way.

If we normalize the absolute GFR of 60 ml/min of the small and heavy person for the BSA (Table 2), then we get a corrected cGFR of 73 $ml/min/1.73m^2$ for the small person as opposed to a much smaller cGFR of 46 $ml/min/1.73m^2$ for the heavy person. Once the GFR is BSA corrected, it becomes clear that the small person has a better kidney function than the heavy person. We may conclude that indexation of the GFR is necessary to allow comparison between different patients.

DATA	SMALL PERSON	HEAVY PERSON
Age (years)	55	55
Length (cm)	150	190
Weight (kg)	50	100
BSA (m²)	1.43	2.28
GFR (ml/min)	60	60
cGFR (ml/min/1.73m²)	73	46

Table 2. Data for comparison of the GFR of a small and heavy person.

4.2 Case 2: GFR evolution during childhood

In this case, we study the evolution of a healthy boy during his childhood. In Table 3 the age, length, weight, BSA, absolute GFR and cGFR of the boy at the age of 3.5, 7.5, 11 and 15 years are listed. For the average healthy boy, the corrected cGFR remains constant during childhood (from 2-3 years till 14 years) (Piepsz et al., 2008, 2009) but the absolute GFR values of the boy at different ages cannot be compared with each other. From the data in Table 3 or by inspection of Figure 2, one may observe an increasing absolute GFR, as well as an increasing BSA as a function of age because the child and his kidneys are still growing. Referring to our pond analogy, one could say that the pump and filter combination of the pond are constantly changing in order to keep the pond clearance at the same rate. Correcting GFR for BSA leads to the same clearance value, independent of age. With the corrected cGFR, the child's kidney function can be followed, regardless of his growth process.

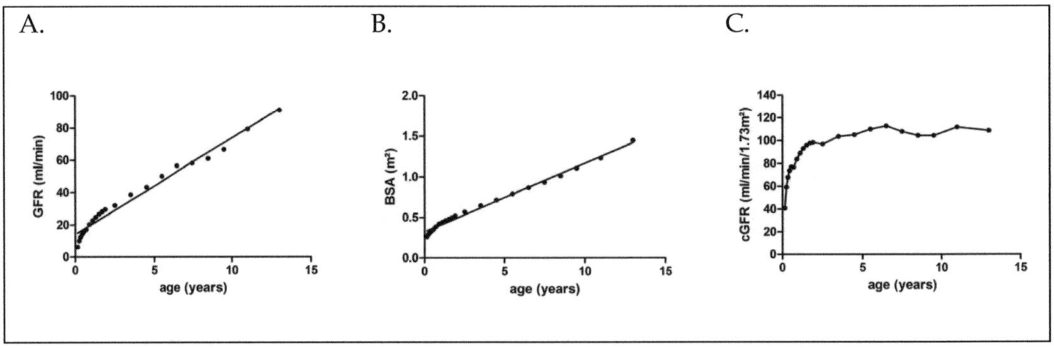

Fig. 2. (A) Absolute GFR as a function of age; (B) BSA as a function of age; (C) cGFR as a function of age.

4.3 Case 3: GFR evolution during adulthood

It is known that the GFR shows an age-dependent decline for the average healthy person, which may be considered as part of the normal biological process of senescence. The body weight is also often increasing with age. That is why in this case we study the GFR of two adult men, one with a stable weight during adulthood and one with a weight that increases with age (Table 4). The man with a stable weight has a normal age-dependent decreasing

DATA	HEALTHY BOY			
Age (years)	3.5	7.5	11	15
Length (cm)	99	126.5	146	173
Weight (kg)	15.5	25	37	58.5
BSA (m^2)	0.64	0.94	1.24	1.70
GFR (ml/min)	44.5	65.0	86.0	118.0
cGFR (ml/min/1.73m^2)	120	120	120	120

Table 3. Data for GFR evolution during childhood.

GFR. The man with the increasing weight has a GFR which is decreasing with age, but the cGFR is faster decreasing because of his increasing body surface area. There is indeed a double decreasing effect on the corrected cGFR. In Table 4, it is shown that the man with a stable weight has a cGFR of 111 ml/min/1.73m^2 at the age of 65. However, the man with the increased weight has a cGFR of 95 ml/min/1.73m^2 at the age of 65 years. This illustrates that weight-changes influence the BSA corrected GFR. Therefore one may wonder whether BSA is the appropriate index for GFR.

DATA	MAN - STABLE WEIGHT				MAN - INCREASING WEIGHT			
Age (years)	18	35	50	65	18	35	50	65
Length (cm)	180	180	180	180	180	180	180	180
Weight (kg)	70	70	70	70	70	80	90	100
BSA (m^2)	1.89	1.89	1.89	1.89	1.89	2.00	2.10	2.20
GFR (ml/min)	142	138	133	121	142	138	133	121
cGFR (ml/min/1.73m^2)	130	126	122	111	130	119	110	95

Table 4. Data of an adult man.

4.4 Conclusion

The cases described above illustrate that indexation is necessary to compare patient values with each other and with reference values. But the question remains whether BSA is the appropriate index for GFR. This has been a subject of debate during the last ten years.

5. Criticism on indexing GFR for BSA

Indexing GFR for BSA goes back to 1928 and it has become so conventional that BSA-indexing can be considered as an icon in nephrology. Nevertheless, during the last ten years there is increasing criticism on BSA indexation. According to Tanner, the dispersion of differences between data of children and adults is not a very strong argument for BSA indexing. (Tanner, 1949) Neither is the argument that BSA indexation is necessary because everybody does it and in that way results become comparable. (Kronmal, 1993) BSA indexation is also seriously questioned in populations with unusual anthropometric data such as in children, in obese or lean persons. According to Bird et al. indexing GFR for BSA does not suit children because they naturally have a relatively high BSA simply because of their small size. (Bird et al., 2003) Delanaye et al. studied obese and anorectic patients. (Delanaye et al., 2005, 2009a, 2009b) In those patients, the consequences of indexing for BSA are much more important since the cGFR is influenced by weight-variation and may obscure variations in the absolute GFR. That is why Delanaye et al. recommend using the absolute

GFR values instead of the cGFR, especially in 'abnormal' body size populations. (Delanaye, 2009a, 2009b) Geddes et al. started their article with another interesting case, in which they show that indexing for BSA can lead to a different clinical decision especially in the overweight. (Geddes et al., 2008) The case described by Geddes et al. concerns a 54 year old obese man who wants to donate a kidney to his own son. Published International guidelines and UK guidelines recommend a minimum GFR of 80 ml/min/1.73m² and 75 ml/min/1.73m² respectively for a 55 year old kidney donor. Direct measurement of the kidney function of the man resulted in an absolute GFR of 87 ml/min and in a corrected cGFR of 77.9 ml/min/1.73m². It is clear that the difference between the absolute GFR and the cGFR is of major importance in this case. Above all, we may not forget that there are several formulas to estimate the BSA. In Table 5 we illustrate that using another BSA formula can influence the decision. Since the studied man is obese (BMI of 31.5), the formula of Livingston & Lee (Livingston & Lee, 2001), which results in a negative decision towards the kidney donation, should probably be preferred.

FORMULA	BSA (m²)	cGFR (ml/min/1.73m²)
DuBois & DuBois	1.93	78
Boyd	1.98	76
Gehan & George	2.01	75
Haycock	2.05	73
Mosteller	1.99	76
Livingston & Lee	2.09	72

Table 5. BSA calculated with frequently used BSA formulas and comparative BSA indexed GFR values of a 54 year old man with a length of 165 cm, a weight of 86 kg and an absolute GFR of 87 ml/min.

6. Are there alternatives to index GFR?

One may wonder why indexing GFR for BSA is still routinely used, despite all the criticism. The fact that the frequently used estimated eGFR formulas as well as the fixed cut-off values of the current Chonic Kidney Disesase classification system are both expressed in ml/min/1.73m² might be a first and important reason why it is not obvious to stop indexing GFR for BSA. A second reason might be that indexing GFR for BSA has almost no consequences for normally built people. Questions about the effectiveness of indexing GFR for BSA only appear when 'abnormal' body size populations like children or obese patients are studied. Due to the limitations of correcting GFR for BSA in those specific populations a whole array of alternative variables for indexing GFR has been suggested.

The most evoked factor to index GFR in obese patients is height. Two studies have shown that correcting GFR for height is identical in obese and non-obese populations, whereas corrected GFR for BSA is inadequately lower in the obese population. (Anastasio et al., 2000; Schmieder et al., 1995) Delanaye et al. stated that since the range of height in the population is narrower than the range of weight (giants and dwarfs are less numerous than obese or anorectic) it is logical that indexing for height will decrease the dispersion of data in the adult population. (Delanaye, 2009a) Other height-dependent indexators that have been proposed to normalize the GFR are lean body mass (Hallynck et al., 1981; Kurtin, 1988), ideal weight (Walser, 1990) and even squared height. (Mitch & Walser, 2000) Also body weight has been indicated as a possible indexator. (Peters et al., 1994b) However, it intuitively seems better to correct GFR for body fluid, since one of the roles of the kidneys is to regulate body fluid composition. Different GFR-indexators in that area are total body water (Bird, 2003; McCance & Widdowson, 1952), plasma volume (Peters et al., 1994a) or extracellular volume (ECV) (Bird, 2003; Peters, 1992, 1994b, 2000; White & Strydom, 1991) In 1952, McCance et al claimed that total body water was the best variable to index the GFR for children. (McCance & Widdowson, 1952) But since total body water is complex to determine every time the GFR is measured, ECV became the most considered alternative to index the GFR, especially in children.

6.1 Comparison of indexing GFR for BSA, height and ECV

In this section we compare indexing GFR for BSA and for the alternatives height and ECV. True mathematical evidence for normalizing a physical quantity by any index is well-known. (Turner & Reilly, 1995) The uncorrected quantity should be a linear function of the indexator with zero intercept (Figure 3A). After indexation the relationship between the indexed quantity and the indexator then completely disappears (Figure 3B).

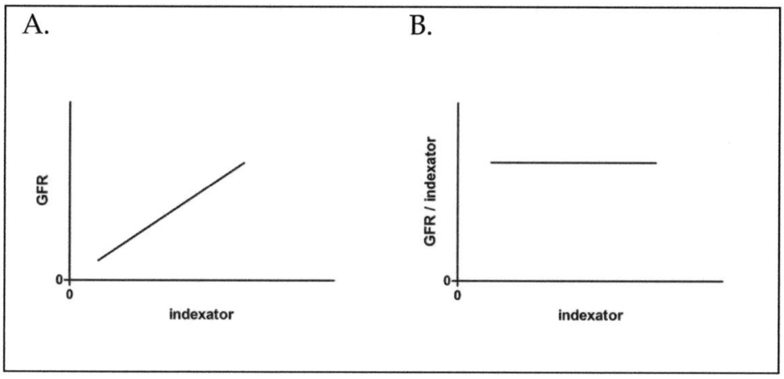

Fig. 3. (A) Linear regression of GFR versus the indexator; (B) Disappearance of the relationship indexed GFR-indexator.

Because of their rapidly increasing size and renal maturation, children may give insight into the properties of different normalization indexes. Publicly available data are used to test the mathematical requirements for the indexators BSA, height and ECV. The dataset contains data for healthy children (between 0 and 15 years) of absolute and BSA-corrected median GFR values (^{51}Cr-EDTA), median heights and weights. (Pottel et al., 2010) ECV of the children was calculated with the ECV formula of Bird et al. (Bird, 2003)

6.1.1 Indexing GFR for BSA

When considering median absolute GFR values versus BSA, one may observe a linear relationship ($y = 59.96x$ with $R^2 = 0.96$) (Figure 4A). When GFR is indexed for BSA, the relation GFR-BSA disappears once the kidneys reach maturity (Figure 4B). So, the mathematical requirement for an indexator is fulfilled.

6.1.2 Indexing GFR for height

The most evoked factor to index GFR in obese patients is height. (Anastasio, 2000; Schmieder, 1995) Again, we studied the fundamental prerequisite relationship GFR-height and the lack of relationship between GFR indexed for height and height. When the

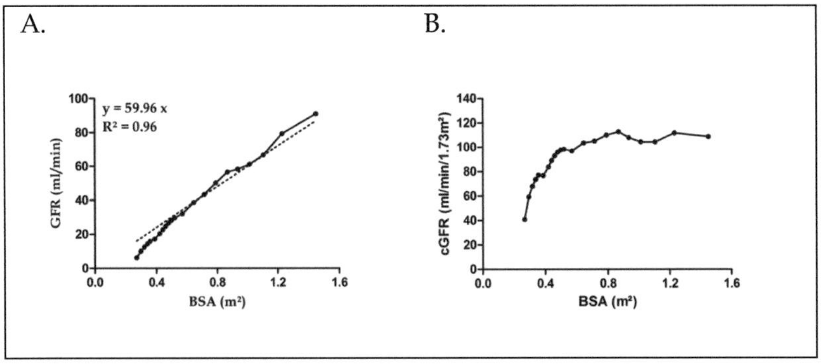

Fig. 4. (A) Linear relationship between absolute GFR and BSA; (B) Disappearance of the relationship between GFR and BSA, when GFR is corrected for BSA.

absolute median GFR values of children were plotted versus height, the results were disappointing (y = 42.01x with R^2 = 0.77) (Figure 5A). But when the absolute median GFR values of the children are plotted against the squared height, the regression is better (y = 36.89x with R^2 = 0.99) (Figure 5C) than the regression of GFR against BSA (Figure 4A).

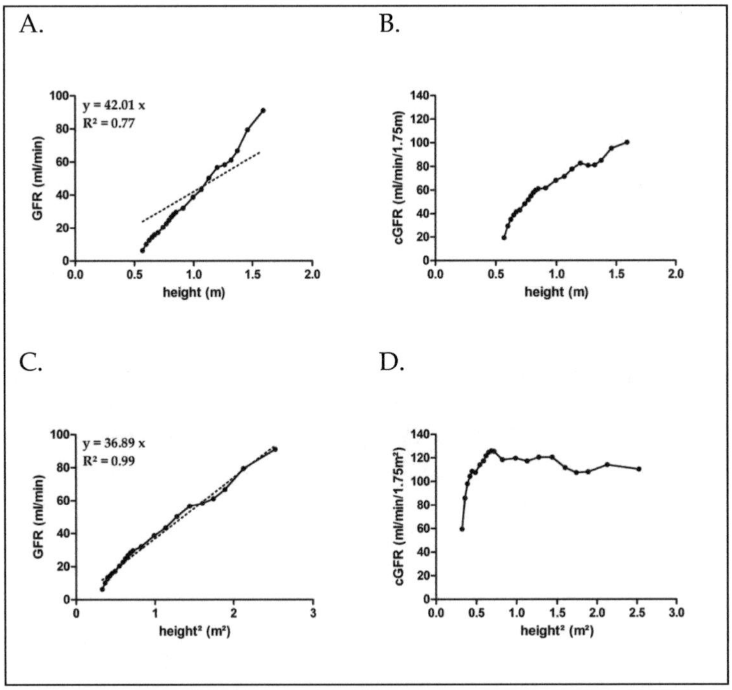

Fig. 5. (A) Linear relationship between absolute GFR and height; (B) No disappearance of the relationship between GFR and height, when GFR is indexed for height; (C) Linear relationship between absolute GFR and squared height; (D) Disappearance of the relationship between GFR and squared height, when GFR is corrected for squared height.

Although height is the most often considered index in the obese population, further research whether height or squared height may serve as a correction factor for GFR is necessary.

Delanaye et al. studied the fundamental mathematical requirement between GFR and height in a limited obese population, but did not find a satisfying linear relationship. (Delanaye, 2005) A better relationship may be found when squared height is used instead of height. It is known that correcting GFR for BSA may cause problems when considering obese or anorectic people. Indexing for height may lead to the same errors, especially in populations with extreme height.

6.1.3 Indexing GFR for ECV

The earliest study of ECV normalisation is by Newman et al., who argued that since the function of the kidneys is to sustain the chemical composition of the extracellular fluid, ECV is more closely related to kidney function than BSA. (Newman et al., 1944) Also the research group of Peters et al. intensively contemplated a change to using ECV to index the GFR. (Bird, 2003; Peters, 1992, 1994b, 2000) Furthermore, several scientists showed a high correlation between BSA and ECV. (Abraham et al., 2011; Newman, 1944; Peters, 2004; White & Strydom, 1991) One could therefore argue that since this equivalence exists, either ECV or BSA can be used to index the GFR. Various studies suggested that ECV is at least a more appropriate index for GFR in children. (Bird, 2003; Friis-Hansen, 1961; Peters, 1994b, 2000) According to Peters et al. this arises from the fact that children have a higher body surface area than adults in relation to their weight, which leads to an overcorrection of the GFR when BSA is used as an indexator. It has also been shown that humans change shape as they grow, which undermines the validity of BSA as an indexation variable. (Peters, 2004) Another argument to prefer ECV above BSA is the fact that ECV is three-dimensional wheras BSA is two-dimensional. (Peters, 2000)
Mathematical evidence for normalizing GFR for ECV based on our children's database can be found in Figure 6.

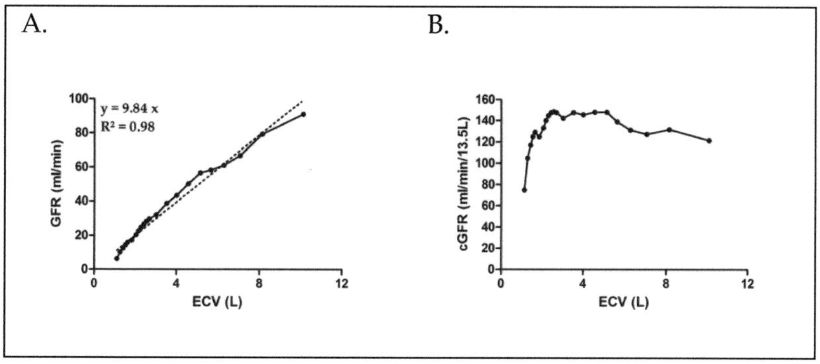

Fig. 6. (A) Linear relationship between absolute GFR and ECV; (B) Disappearance of the relationship between GFR and ECV, when GFR is corrected for ECV.

In 1961, Friis-Hansen developed a formula to estimate ECV in children. The formula is, like the DuBois & DuBois formula, of the form constant * weight^a * height^b. (Friis-Hansen, 1961) In 2003, a similar height-weight ECV equation was published by Bird et al. (Bird, 2003) In 2011, Abraham et al. found that height provided most of the information in the estimation of ECV and that ECV could be simply estimated from ECV = height * √weight. (Abraham, 2011)

AUTHOR	FORMULA
Friis-Hansen (1961)	$ECV = 0.0682 * weight^{0.400} * height^{0.633}$
Bird et al. (2003)	$ECV = 0.0215 * weight^{0.647} * height^{0.742}$
Abraham et al. (2011)	$ECV = height * \sqrt{weight}$

Table 6. Height and weight based formulas to estimate ECV. ECV is expressed in L, weight in kg and height in cm, except in the formula of Abraham et al. where height is in meter.

When considering changing GFR indexing from BSA to ECV, the reference ECV value of an average man of 1.73m^2 yields 13.5L. The ECV corrected GFR would then be expressed in ml/min/13.5L. However, one may not forget that ECV is mainly studied as an alternative index in the pediatric population. Little proof exists for application of ECV to adult or obese populations. Nevertheless, the data show that ECV might be a promising index, fulfilling both mathematical requirements. However, one may question the calculation of ECV from a height-weight equation, especially in the obese, based on the same arguments that are used to question the BSA correction.

6.2 Conclusion

When correcting for BSA, problems arise for obese or anorectic people. The data show that square height or ECV might be good alternatives to index the GFR (Figure 7). It seems more logical to index GFR with a measure of fluid volume since the purpose of GFR is to regulate body fluid composition. ECV might be a promising index, fulfilling the theoretical requirements, even in the obese.

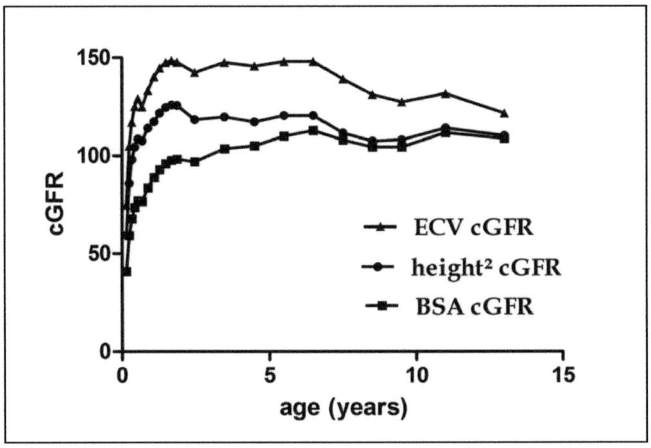

Fig. 7. Comparison of GFR indexed for BSA, squared height and ECV.

7. Using the slow rate constant or mean transit time as indicator for kidney function

In 1980, Brochner-Mortenson already pointed out that it would be more rational to express GFR in relation to ECV than in relation to BSA. (Brochner-Mortensen, 1980) He showed that the ratio GFR/ECV could easily be determined when GFR is measured as the plasma clearance of a filtration marker. This is also clearly explained in a review written by Peters. (Peters, 2004)

The glomerular filtration rate of a person can be determined accurately by measuring the plasma clearance of a filtration marker such as iohexol or ^{51}Cr-EDTA, which is generaly given by a single bolus injection. The clearance of the marker is followed from plasma sampling at multiple time points over several hours. In case the mixing is immediate, the concentration-time curve may be described as a mono-exponential decay: $c(t) = Ae^{-\alpha t}$. The distribution volume in this case is the plasma volume (PV) and the GFR equals the dose of the exogenous marker divided by the area under the concentration-time curve: GFR = Dose/(A/α). The concentration at time zero c(0) = A equals the dose divided by the distribution volume, and therefore GFR = α * PV or GFR indexed by plasma volume (GFR/PV) equals the rate constant α. As α is expressed in min^{-1}, the inverse T = 1/α expressed in minutes, is the mean transit time. T can be seen as the time needed to reduce the concentration of the filtration marker to 37% of its original value.

In case the mixing is not immediate (as is the case for iohexol and ^{51}Cr-EDTA) and not limited to the plasma volume, the concentration-time curve should be described by a bi-exponentional decay. The concentration c of the tracer at the time t can then be written as $c(t) = Ae^{-\alpha t} + Be^{-\beta t}$. The fast first exponential decay represents mixing of the tracer in the distribution volume of the body as well as filtration of the tracer by the kidneys. After the mixing is completed, the slow second exponential decay indicates that only the kidneys are responsible for the further decrease of the tracer in the plasma. The GFR is defined as the injected dose of the marker divided by the area under the plasma clearance curve. Since the area under the c(t) curve is now equal to $A/\alpha + B/\beta$, the GFR can also be written as the injected dose divided by $A/\alpha + B/\beta$. At time zero, the dose is equal to (A + B) * PV, where PV is the plasma volume, so GFR = (A + B) * PV/($A/\alpha + B/\beta$). The mean transit time $T = (A/\alpha^2 + B/\beta^2)/(A/\alpha + B/\beta)$, expressed in minutes, equals ECV/GFR, which reduces to PV/GFR in case of a mono-exponential decay (B = 0). In that case, ECV = PV mathematically. The mean transit time T or its inverse 1/T may be seen as an excellent indicator for kidney function, which is in fact the GFR indexed for ECV.

To determine T, a complex procedure with multiple blood samplings (up to 9 samples) is required to obtain the parameters A, α, B and β of the bi-exponential decay. Since it is known that the slow component has a larger contribution to the GFR, the rate constant β is by itself a close reflection of GFR/ECV = 1/T. Therefore, methods to reduce the blood sampling to only the slow exponential decay (2 or 3 samples) were proposed. This one-compartment clearance, also called the slope-intercept technique, always slightly overestimates GFR/ECV since the area under the one-compartment slope is lower than the area under the bi-exponential curve.

In 1972, Brochner-Mortensen published an equation to correct for this overestimation when a ^{51}Cr-EDTA clearance is performed in adults (GFR = 0.990778 * slowGFR - 0.001218 * slow GFR^2). (Brochner-Mortensen, 1972) Two years later, Brochner-Mortensen et al. performed the same study in children which resulted in the correction equation GFR = 1.01 * slowGFR - 0.0017 * slowGFR. (Brochner-Mortensen et al., 1974) In 1992, Peters proposed the regression equation GFR/ECV = $-0.093 + 1.06\beta + 0.009\beta^2$, relating β or the 'approximate' GFR/ECV to the 'true' GFR/ECV based on the bi-exponentional plasma clearance curve of the radio-active agent ^{99}Tc-DTPA. (Peters, 1992) Over the years, improved equations for correcting the slope-intercept measurements in different clinical populations have been published. (Brochner-Mortensen & Jodal, 2009; Fleming, 2007; Fleming et al., 2004; Jodal & Brochner-Mortensen, 2009) Although the radio-active agent ^{51}Cr-EDTA is an excellent filtration marker, it is not accepted in the USA. Lately, the constrast medium iohexol is seen

as an excellent alternative for the radio-active markers. In 2010, Schwartz et al. showed how the GFR in children could be determined from the slow component of an iohexol clearance curve according to the equation GFR = 1.0019 * slowGFR - 0.001258 * slowGFR^2. (Schwartz et al., 2010) Since the literature often cautions that the equations are only valid in the populations similar to those in which they were developed, Derek et al. recently tried to develop, based on an iohexol study, an universal formula for use in adults as well as in children. (Derek et al., 2011) The equation of Derek et al. is already expressed in ml/min/1.73m^2 and is of the form: GFR = slowGFR/[1 + 0.12 (slowGFR/100)].
The rate constant β, or even T, may be a perfect indicator for kidney function, which immediately allows comparison of the kidney function of different persons with each other. Simulations showed us that the cut-off value of 60 ml/min/1.73m^2 agreed with a β value of 0.004 min^{-1} or a transit time of 4 hours, a cut-off value of 30 ml/min/1.73m^2 agreed with a β value of 0.002 min^{-1} or a transit time of 8 hours.

8. Conclusions and perspective

GFR indexing for BSA has little influence on normal body sized people but can be misleading in people with unusual anthropometric data. GFR indexation is necessary to compare the GFR of patients with each other and with reference values. We showed that correcting for squared height or ECV are two good alternatives to normalize the GFR in children. It seems intuitively better to correct GFR for ECV than for BSA because the role of the kidneys is to regulate body fluid composition. Additional research concerning this topic is of particular interest. Also, the rate constant β or the mean transit time T is worth considering as an indicator for kidney function. It must be emphasized that it is important to examine whether other kidney function indicators lead to different clinical decisions.

9. References

Abraham, A.G.; Munoz, A.; Furth, S.L.; Warady, B. & Schwartz, G.J. (2011). Extracellular volume and glomerular filtration rate in children with chronic kidney disease. *Clinical Journal of the American Society of Nephrology*, Vol.6, No.4, (April 2011) pp.741-747, ISSN 1555-9041

Anastasio, P.; Spitali, L.; Frangiosa, A.; Molino, D.; Stellato, D.; Cirillo, E.; Pollastro, R.M.; Capodicasa, L.; Sepe, J.; Federico, P. & Gaspare De Santo, N. (2000). Glomerular filtration rate in severely overweight normotensive humans. *American Journal of Kidney Diseases*, Vol.35, No.6, (June 2000) pp.1144-1148, ISSN 0272-6386

Banerjee, S. & Bhattacharya, A.K. (1961). Determination of Body Surface Area in Indian Hindu Children. *Journal of Applied Physiology*, Vol.16, No.5, (November 1961) pp.969, ISSN 8750-7587

Banerjee, S. & Sen, R. (1955). Determination of the surface area of the body of Indians. *Journal of Applied Physiology*, Vol.7, No.6, (May 1955) pp.585-588, ISSN 0021-8987

Bird, N.J.; Henderson, B.L.; Lui, D.; Ballinger, J.R. & Peters, A.M. (2003). Indexing glomerular filtration rate to suit children. *Journal of Nuclear Medicine*, Vol.44, No.7, (July 2003) pp.1037-1043, ISSN 0161-5505

Boyd, E. (1935). *The Growth of the Surface of the Human Body*. University of Minnesota Press, Minneapolis

Brochner-Mortensen, J. (1972). A simple method for the determination of glomerular filtration rate. *Scandinavian Journal of Clinical & Laboratory Investigation,* Vol.30, No.3, (November 1972) pp.271-274, ISSN 0036-5513

Brochner-Mortensen, J. (1980). A simple single injection method for determination of the extracellular fluid volume. *Scandinavian Journal of Clinical & Laboratory Investigation,* Vol.40, No.6, (October 1980) pp.567-573, ISSN 0036-5513

Brochner-Mortensen, J.; Haahr, J. & Christoffersen, J. (1974). A simple method for accurate assessment of the glomerular filtration rate in children. *Scandinavian Journal of Clinical & Laboratory Investigation,* Vol.33, No.2, (April 1974) pp.140-143, ISSN 0036-5513

Brochner-Mortensen, J. & Jodal, L. (2009). Reassessment of a classical single injection 51Cr-EDTA clearance method for determination of renal function in children and adults. Part II: Empirically determined relationships between total and one-pool clearance. *Scandinavian Journal of Clinical & Laboratory Investigation,* Vol.69, No.3, pp.314-322, ISSN 0036-5513

Delanaye, P.; Mariat, C.; Cavalier, E. & Krzesinski, J.M. (2009a). Errors induced by indexing glomerular filtration rate for body surface area: reductio ad absurdum. *Nephrology Dialysis Transplantation,* Vol.24, No.12, (December 2009) pp.3593-3596, ISSN 0931-0509

Delanaye, P.; Mariat, C.; Cavalier, E. & Krzesinski, J.M. (2009b). Indexing glomerular filtration rate for body surface area: myth and reality. *Néphrologie & Thérapeutique,* Vol.5, No.7, (December 2009) pp.614-622, ISSN 1769-7255

Delanaye, P.; Radermecker, R.P.; Rorive, M.; Depas, G. & Krzesinski, J.M. (2005). Indexing glomerular filtration rate for body surface area in obese patients is misleading: concept and example. *Nephrology Dialysis Transplantation,* Vol.20, No.10, (October 2005) pp.2024-2028, ISSN 0931-0509

Derek, K.S. Ng; Schwartz, G.J.; Jacobson, L.P.; Palella, F.J.; Margolick, J.B.; Warady, B.A.; Furth, S.L. & Munoz, A. (2011). Universal GFR determination based on two time points during plasma iohexol disappearance. *Kidney International,* (Online June 2011), ISSN 0085-2538

DuBois, D. & DuBois, E.F. (1915). The measurement of the surface area of man. *Archives of Internal Medicine,* Vol.16, pp.868-881

DuBois, D. & DuBois, E.F. (1916). A formula to estimate the approximate surface area if height and weight be known. *Archives of Internal Medicine,* Vol.17, pp.863-871

Faber, H.K. & Melcher, M.S. (1921). A modification of the Du Bois height-weight formula for surface area of newborn infants. *Proceedings of the Society for Experimental Biology and Medicine,* Vol.19, pp.53

Fleming, J. S. (2007). An improved equation for correcting slope-intercept measurements of glomerular filtration rate for the single exponential approximation. *Nuclear Medicine Communications,* Vol.28, No.4, (April 2007) pp.315-320, ISSN 0143-3636

Fleming, J.S.; Zivanovic, M.A.; Blake, G.M.; Burniston, M. & Cosgriff, P.S. (2004). Guidelines for the measurement of glomerular filtration rate using plasma sampling. *Nuclear Medicine Communications,* Vol.25, No.8, (August 2004) pp.759-769, ISSN 0143-3636

Friis-Hansen, B. (1961). Body water compartments in children: changes during growth and related changes in body composition. *Pediatrics,* Vol.28, (August 1961) pp.169-181, ISSN 0031-4005

Fujimoto, S.; Watanabe, T.; Sakamoto, A.; Yukawa, K. & Morimoto, K. (1968). Studies on the physical surface area of Japanese. 18. Calculation formulas in three stages over all ages. *Japanese Journal of Hygiene*, Vol.23, No.5, (December 1968) pp.443-450, ISSN 0021-5082

Geddes, C.C.; Woo, Y.M. & Brady, S. (2008). Glomerular filtration rate--what is the rationale and justification of normalizing GFR for body surface area? *Nephrology Dialysis Transplantation*, Vol.23, No.1, (January 2008) pp.4-6, ISSN 0931-0509

Gehan, E.A. & George, S.L. (1970). Estimation of human body surface area from height and weight. *Cancer Chemotherapy Reports*, Vol.54, No.4, (August 1970) pp.225-235, ISSN 0069-0112

Hallynck, T.H.; Soep, H.H.; Thomis, J.A.; Boelaert, J.; Daneels, R. & Dettli, L. (1981). Should clearance be normalised to body surface or to lean body mass? *British Journal of Clinical Pharmacology*, Vol.11, No.5, (May 1981) pp.523-526, ISSN 0306-5251

Haycock, G.B.; Schwartz, G.J. & Wisotsky, D.H. (1978). Geometric method for measuring body surface area: a height-weight formula validated in infants, children, and adults. *The Journal of Pediatrics*, Vol.93, No.1, (July 1978) pp.62-66, ISSN 0022-3476

Heaf, J.G. (2007). The origin of the 1 x 73-m2 body surface area normalization: problems and implications. *Clinical Physiology and Functional Imaging*, Vol.27, No.3, (May 2007) pp.135-137, ISSN 1475-0961

Jodal, L. & Brochner-Mortensen, J. (2009). Reassessment of a classical single injection 51Cr-EDTA clearance method for determination of renal function in children and adults. Part I: Analytically correct relationship between total and one-pool clearance. *Scandinavian Journal of Clinical & Laboratory Investigation*, Vol.69, No.3, (May 2009) pp.305-313, ISSN 0036-5513

Kronmal, R.A. (1993). Spurious Correlation and the Fallacy of the Ratio Standard Revisited. *Journal of the Royal Statistical Society Series a-Statistics in Society*, Vol.156, pp.379-392, ISSN 0035-9238

Kurtin, P.S. (1988). Standardization of renal function measurements in children: kidney size versus metabolic rate. *Child Nephrology and Urology*, Vol.9, No.6, pp.337-339, ISSN 1012-6694

Livingston, E.H. & Lee, S. (2001). Body surface area prediction in normal-weight and obese patients. *American Journal of Physiology- Endocrinology and Metabolism*, Vol.281, No.3, (September 2001) pp.586-591, ISSN 0193-1849

MacKay, E.M. (1932). Kidney weight, body size and renal function. *Archives of Internal Medicine*, Vol.50, pp.590-594

McCance, R.A. & Widdowson, E.M. (1952). The correct physiological basis on which to compare infant and adult renal function. *Lancet*, Vol.2, No.6740, (November 1952) pp.860-862, ISSN 0140-6736

McIntosh, J.F.; Möller, R. & Van Slycke, D.D. (1928). Studies on urea excretions. III. The influence of body size on urea output. *The Journal of Clinical Investigation* Vol.6, (August 1928) pp.467-483

Meeh, K. (1879). Oberflächenmessungen des menschlichen Körpers. *Zeitschrift für Biologie*, Vol.15, pp.425-485

Mitch, W.E. & Walser, M. (2000). Nutritional therapy in renal disease. In: *The kidney* (6th edition), Brenner B.M., pp.2298-2340, WB Saunders, Philadelphia

Mosteller, R.D. (1987). Simplified calculation of body-surface area. *The New England Journal of Medicine*, Vol.317, No.17, (October 1987) pp.1098, ISSN 0028-4793

Newman, E.V.; Bordley, J. & Winternitz, J. (1944). The interrelationships of glomerular filtration rate (mannitol clearance), extracellular fluid volume, surface area of the body, and plasma concentration of mannitol. *Bulletin of the Johns Hopkins Hospital* Vol.75, pp.253-268

Nwoye, L.O. (1989). Body surface area of Africans: a study based on direct measurements of Nigerian males. *Human Biology*, Vol.61, No.3, (June 1989) pp.439-457, ISSN 0018-7143

Nwoye, L.O. & Al-Shehri, M.A. (2003). A formula for the estimation of the body surface area of Saudi male adults. *Saudi Medical Journal*, Vol.24, No.12, (December 2003) pp.1341-1346, ISSN 0379-5284

Peters, A.M. (1992). Expressing glomerular filtration rate in terms of extracellular fluid volume. *Nephrology Dialysis Transplantation*, Vol.7, No.3, pp.205-210, ISSN 0931-0509

Peters, A.M. (2004). The kinetic basis of glomerular filtration rate measurement and new concepts of indexation to body size. *European Journal of Nuclear Medicine and Molecular Imaging*, Vol.31, No.1, (January 2004) pp.137-149, ISSN 1619-7070

Peters, A.M.; Allison, H. & Ussov, WYu. (1994a). Measurement of the ratio of glomerular filtration rate to plasma volume from the technetium-99m diethylene triamine pentaacetic acid renogram: comparison with glomerular filtration rate in relation to extracellular fluid volume. *European Journal of Nuclear Medicine*, Vol.21, No.4, (April 1994) pp.322-327, ISSN 0340-6997

Peters, A.M.; Gordon, I. & Sixt, R. (1994b). Normalization of glomerular filtration rate in children: body surface area, body weight or extracellular fluid volume? *Journal of Nuclear Medicine*, Vol.35, No.3, (March 1994) pp.438-444, ISSN 0161-5505

Peters, A.M.; Henderson, B.L. & Lui, D. (2000). Indexed glomerular filtration rate as a function of age and body size. *Clinical Science*, Vol.98, No.4, (April 2000) pp.439-444, ISSN 0143-5221

Piepsz, A.; Tondeur, M. & Ham, H. (2008). Escaping the correction for body surface area when calculating glomerular filtration rate in children. *European Journal of Nuclear Medicine and Molecular Imaging*, Vol.35, No.9, (September 2008) pp.1669-1672, ISSN 1619-7070

Piepsz, A.; Tondeur, M. & Ham, H. (2009). Escaping the correction for body surface area when calculating glomerular filtration rate in children. *European Journal of Nuclear Medicine and Molecular Imaging*, Vol.36, No.2, (February 2009) pp.332-333, ISSN 1619-7070

Pottel, H.; Mottaghy, F.M.; Zaman, Z. & Martens, F. (2010). On the relationship between glomerular filtration rate and serum creatinine in children. *Pediatric Nephrology*, Vol.25, No.5, (May 2010) pp.927-934, ISSN 0931-041X

Rubner, M. (1883). Ueber den einfluss der korpergrosse auf stoff-und draftwechsel. *Zeitschrift für Biology*, Vol.19, pp.535-562

Schmieder, R.E.; Beil, A.H.; Weihprecht, H. & Messerli, F.H. (1995). How should renal hemodynamic data be indexed in obesity? *Journal of the American Society of Nephrology*, Vol.5, No.9, (March 1995) pp.1709-1713, ISSN 1046-6673

Schwartz, G.J.; Abraham, A. G.; Furth, S.L.; Warady, B.A. & Munoz, A. (2010). Optimizing iohexol plasma disappearance curves to measure the glomerular filtration rate in children with chronic kidney disease. *Kidney International*, Vol.77, No.1, (January 2010) pp.65-71, ISSN 0085-2538

Shuter, B. & Aslani, A. (2000). Body surface area: Du Bois and Du Bois revisited. *European Journal of Applied Pysiology*, Vol.82, No.3, (June 2000) pp.250-254, ISSN 1439-6319

Stevenson, P.H. (1937). Height-weight-surface formula for the estimation of body surface area in Chinese subjects. *The Chinese Journal of Physiology*, Vol.12, pp.327-334

Tanner, J.M. (1949). Fallacy of per-weight and per-surface area standards, and their relation to spurious correlation. *Journal of Applied Physiology*, Vol.2, No.1, (July 1949) pp.1-15, ISSN 0021-8987

Taylor, F.B.; Drury, D.R. & Addis, T. (1923). The regulation of renal activity. VIII. The relation between the rate of urea secretion and the size of the kidneys. *American Journal of Physiology*, Vol.65, pp.55-61

Tikuisis, P.; Meunier, P. & Jubenville, C.E. (2001). Human body surface area: measurement and prediction using three dimensional body scans. *European Journal of Applied Physiology*, Vol.85, No.3-4, (August 2001) pp.264-271, ISSN 1439-6319

Turner, S.T. & Reilly, S.L. (1995). Fallacy of indexing renal and systemic hemodynamic measurements for body surface area. *American Journal of Physiology*, Vol.268, No.4 Pt 2, (April 1995) pp.R978-88, ISSN 0002-9513

van der Sijs, H. & Guchelaar, H.J. (2002). Formulas for calculating body surface area. *The Annals of Pharmacotherapy*, Vol.36, No.2, (February 2002) pp.345-346, ISSN 1060-0280

Verbraecken, J.; Van de Heyning, P.; De Backer, W. & Van Gaal, L. (2006). Body surface area in normal-weight, overweight, and obese adults. A comparison study. *Metabolism*, Vol.55, No.4, (April 2006) pp.515-524, ISSN 0026-0495

Walser, M. (1990). Progression of chronic renal failure in man. *Kidney International*, Vol.37, No.5, (May 1990) pp.1195-1210, ISSN 0085-2538

White, A.J. & Strydom, W.J. (1991). Normalisation of glomerular filtration rate measurements. *European Journal of Nuclear Medicine*, Vol.18, No.6, pp.385-390, ISSN 0340-6997

Yu, C.Y.; Lin, C.H. & Yang, Y.H. (2010). Human body surface area database and estimation formula. *Journal of the International Society for Burn Injuries*, Vol.36, No.5, (August 2010) pp.616-629, ISSN 0305-4179

2

How Measuring Glomerular Filtration Rate? Comparison of Reference Methods

Pierre Delanaye
University of Liège, CHU Sart Tilman, Liège
Belgium

1. Introduction

Glomerular filtration rate (GFR) is considered as the best way to assess global renal function (Gaspari et al., 1997; Stevens & Levey, 2009). Even if GFR estimations (based on creatinine- or cystatin C-based equations) are most often used (see Table 1)(Cockcroft & Gault, 1976; Levey et al., 1999; Levey et al., 2006; Levey et al., 2009), measuring "true" GFR is still important in clinical practice, especially in particular patients (Delanaye et al., 2011a; Delanaye & Cohen, 2008; Stevens & Levey, 2009). In this chapter, we will review the different markers which can be considered as reference methods to measure GFR. Before moving to clinical trials, we have to recall the physiological characteristics of an ideal GFR marker.

2. Clearance concept and ideal marker for glomerular filtration rate

The history of the renal physiology is deeply influenced by the book published by Homer W. Smith in 1951 (Figure 1) : « The kidney: structure and function in health and disease »(Smith, 1951b). In this best-seller of nephrology, Smith compiled all the physiological data (more than 2300 references) which have been published in the scientific literature until 1951. Smith, himself, has largely contributed to the physiological knowledge of the kidney. A large part of this book is dedicated to the GFR measurement. The concept of clearance is well explicated. Actually, the Danish physiologist, Poul Brandt Rheberg was the first to use and define the concept of clearance in 1926 even if this author did not use the word "clearance". Rheberg studied on himself the urea and creatinine clearances to prove that kidney has a filtrating and not only a secreting action (Rehberg, 1926b; Rehberg, 1926a). The term clearance was used for the first time by Möller in 1929 and was then concerning the urea clearance which was proposed as the first evaluation of renal function (Möller et al., 1929). Smith has largely contributed to make popular and classical this concept of clearance to assess GFR (Smith, 1951a). Renal clearance of a substance is defined as the volume of plasma cleared from this substance per time unit (mL/min). Clearance is thus a virtual volume but will permit to apprehend GFR and renal function. However, the concept of clearance is applicable to any internal or external substances. To be considered as a reference method, a marker must have strict physiological characteristics (Smith, 1951b):

1. Marker production and marker plasma concentration must be constant if GFR does not change

2. Marker must be free in plasma (not binding to protein) and must be freely and fully filtrated through the glomerulus
3. Marker is neither secreted nor absorbed by renal tubules
4. Marker must be inert and, of course, not toxic
5. Marker excretion must be exclusively excreted by kidneys
6. Marker must be easily measured in both plasma and urine

<u>Cockcroft</u>

$$\text{GFR (mL/min)} = \frac{(140 - \text{Age}) \times \text{Weight (kg)}}{7.2 \times \text{SCr (mg/dL)}} \times 0.85 \text{ if female}$$

<u>4-variable MDRD Study equation</u>

GFR (mL/min/1.73m^2) = 175 x SCr (mg/dL)$^{-1.154}$ x Age$^{-0.203}$ x 0.742 (if female)
X 1.21 for African-American

<u>CKD-EPI study equation</u>

African-American female
Serum creatinine<0.7 mg/dL
GFR (mL/min/1.73m^2) = 166 x (SCr/0.7)$^{-0.329}$ x 0.993^{age}
Serum creatinine>0.7 mg/dL
GFR (mL/min/1.73m^2) = 166 x (SCr/0.7)$^{-1.209}$ x 0.993^{age}
African-American male
Serum creatinine<0.9 mg/dL
GFR (mL/min/1.73m^2) = 163 x (SCr/0.9)$^{-0.411}$ x 0.993^{age}
Serum creatinine>0.7 mg/dL
GFR (mL/min/1.73m^2) = 163 x (SCr/0.9)$^{-1.209}$ x 0.993^{age}
Caucasian female
Serum creatinine<0.7 mg/dL
GFR (mL/min/1.73m^2) = 144 x (SCr/0.7)$^{-0.329}$ x 0.993^{age}
Serum creatinine>0.7 mg/dL
GFR (mL/min/1.73m^2) = 144 x (SCr/0.7)$^{-1.209}$ x 0.993^{age}
Caucasian male
Serum creatinine<0.9 mg/dL
GFR (mL/min/1.73m^2) = 141 x (SCr/0.9)$^{-0.411}$ x 0.993^{age}
Serum creatinine>0.7 mg/dL
GFR (mL/min/1.73m^2) = 141 x (SCr/0.9)$^{-1.209}$ x 0.993^{age}

Table 1. Creatinine-based equations. SCr: Serum Creatinine, GFR: glomerular filtration rate, MDRD: Modified diet in renal disease, CKD-EPI: Chronic Kidney Disease-Epidemiology group.

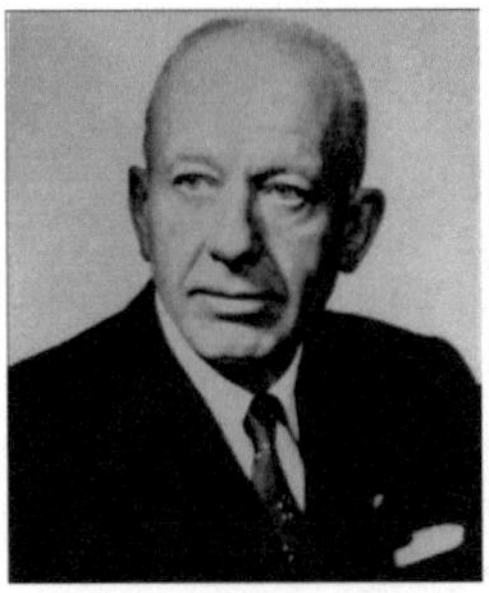

Fig. 1. Homer W. Smith

The renal clearance will be easily calculated with the following equation:

$$GFR=([U] \times V) / [P]$$

(where [U] = urinary concentration, [P] = plasma concentration, V = urinary volume)

The calculated value will be then divided by the time interval where the urine collection has been made. *Sensu strict,* the plasma concentration must be sampled from arterial blood but errors induced by venous samples are very limited (Laake, 1954; Handelsman & Sass, 1956; Nosslin, 1965). In the same view, the transit time through the urinary system should also be taken into consideration but, once again, error linked to this transit time is negligible (Ladegaard-Pedersen, 1972; Nosslin, 1965). The method originally proposed by Smith for measuring GFR is not an easy task. Actually, the marker (inulin see below) must be intravenously injected and then perfused at a constant rate to reach stable plasma concentrations. Thereafter, urine collection must be realized, which is a potential source of errors. For this reason, Smith recommended urine collection on 10 and 15 minutes with the use of urinary catheter. Smith recommended three successive collections. The patient was hydrated to assume a sufficient urinary flow though these collections. The mean of the three collection was considered as the GFR measurement (Smith, 1951a). Nowadays, the urine collections are done without urinary catheter and on a longer period of time (60 minutes) to decrease the impact of urine collection errors on the final result (Levey et al., 1991; Robson et al., 1949).
The ideal marker does not exist in the organism (or has still not been discovered if we want to be optimistic). Both urea and creatinine clearance have strong limitations, notably because creatinine is secreted and urea is absorbed by renal tubules (Dodge et al., 1967; Morgan et al., 1978). Therefore, exogenous markers are used to measure GFR. We will successively describe the markers which are still used in clinical practice in 2011: inulin, ^{51}Cr-EDTA, ^{99}Tc-DTPA, iothalamate and iohexol. For every marker, we will describe strengths and limitations both from an analytical and clinical point of view.

3. Inulin

Inulin is still considered nowadays as the gold standard to measure GFR. Smith has deeply studied this marker and makes it the most popular. Inulin is a polymer of fructose which is found in some plants which uses it as energy provider in place of amidon. Its molecular weight is 5200 Da (Gaspari et al., 1997). Some plants are especially rich in inulin: chicory, garlic, leek and Jerusalem artichoke. Humans are not able to metabolize inulin. Because inulin is the first reference method to have been used, its role in the GFR measurement has only be asserted on basis of physiological studies (because the first method is not comparable to any other !). Once again, we often refer to the studies published by Smith and Shannon (New York university)(Smith, 1951a; Smith, 1951c) and by another pioneer Richards (Philadelphia university)(Richards et al., 1934). Inulin was obviously considered as a safe product with any effect on GFR (Shannon, 1934). Inulin is freely filtrated through a semi-permeable membrane which is a strong argument for the absence of binding to protein. This has been shown by Shannon in 1934 (Shannon, 1934) and by Richards in 1937 (Hendrix et al., 1937). In the same publication, Richards proved that inulin was freely and fully filtrated through the glomerulus because he measured the same inulin concentration both in the plasma and the glomerulus of a frog and a salamander (Hendrix et al., 1937). The absence of both tubular absorption and secretion has been demonstrated by an important article published by Shannon in 1934 (Shannon, 1934). In this article, this author showed the absence of inulin excretion in two types of aglomerular fishes (goosefish, *Lophius piscatorius* and toadfish *Osteichthyes - Lophiidae*). In the same article, Shannon measured GFR by inulin clearance in another type of fish with glomerulus, the dogfish (*Chondrichthyes – Squalidae*). These fishes were then treated with phlorizin which was sensed to block all tubular activity. Although the creatinine clearance in this fish was increased, the inulin clearance was not modified by this treatment (Shannon, 1934). In the same year of 1934, inulin clearance was also measured in aglomerular fish and in dogs by Richards (Richards et al., 1934). The experimentation (measuring GFR with and without phlorizin) was then repeated in man by Smith and Shannon. The results obtained in animals were confirmed in humans. Shannon was the first human who was perfused by inulin in 1935 (Shannon & Smith, 1935; Smith, 1951c). These authors had thus suggested that inulin was not secreted by renal tubules. This assertion will be thereafter confirmed by other authors with the same type of methodology (Shannon & Smith, 1935; Alving et al., 1939; Laake, 1954). Additional arguments were developed in the sixties by animal studies using micropontions in the tubules (Gutman et al., 1965). After intravenous injection, inulin is fully excreted by kidneys in urine (Shannon & Smith, 1935), even if very low concentrations of inulin are found in bile (Höber, 1930; Schanker & Hogben, 1961).

Inulin is doubtless the marker who has been the most investigated from a physiological point of view. In this view, it is logical that inulin is still considered as the gold standard for GFR measurement. Nevertheless, there are limitations to its use in daily practice. Because its relatively high molecular weight (5200 Da), the molecule is relatively viscous and don't quickly reach its volume of distribution. Therefore, only methods using urinary clearance with constant infusion rate seem accurate for this marker. Such methods are more cumbersome. Moreover, inulin is not easily available on the market and remains relatively costly. From our point of view, the most important limitation of inulin is the difficulty linked to its measurement in urine and plasma. Actually, several methods have been proposed and these methods are probably not interchangeable. There is no standardization in inulin measurement. We have shown that GFR results could vary from -10 to +10 mL/min in the same patient only because inulin was measured by a different method (unpublished data). Moreover, most of the methods (except the enzymatic ones) are prone to interferences with glucose measurement which is a limiting factor when measuring GFR in diabetic patients (Little, 1949). Regarding the methods for measuring inulin, we can cite the "acid" methods (Kuehnle et al., 1992; Shaffer & Somogoyi, 1933; Alving et al., 1939; Corcoran, 1952; Rolf et al., 1949; Roe, 1934; Steinitz, 1938; Hubbard & Loomis, 1942; Lentjes et al., 1994; Heyrovsky, 1956; Rolf et al., 1949), the enzymatic methods (Day & Workman, 1984; Delanghe et al., 1991; Jung et al., 1990; Summerfield et al., 1993; Dubourg et al., 2010) and the new methods by high performance liquid chromatography (HPLC) (Ruo et al., 1991; Baccard et al., 1999; Dall'Amico et al., 1995; Pastore et al., 2001). Describing these methods in detail are beyond the scope of this chapter and we propose the readers the following reference if they are interested in this topic (Delanaye et al., 2011b).

4. Preliminary statistical considerations

The use of inulin as GFR marker is justified by physiologic studies. The others markers that will be proposed thereafter will be compared to inulin measurements. Therefore, the use of other markers will be justified not by physiological studies (even if some physiological studies exist for some markers) but by studies comparing these markers with inulin. Unhopefully, most of these studies comparing different GFR tests lack of strong statistical methodology. Actually, most of the authors have only shown a good correlation between the markers, which is expected but not sufficient. Ratio of new markers results on inulin results are also used (the result being considered as good if ratio is near to 1). The use of such ratio may be misleading (for example, if one method overestimates true GFR in low GFR levels but underestimates GFR in high levels, the ratio will be near to 1 although the method is actually not precise enough). To compare the performance of a new GFR measurement compared to inulin, we need to know the bias (mean difference between the two results) and the precision (standard deviation (SD) around the bias) of this new measurement. Bland and Altman analysis is thus required (Bland & Altman, 1986).

Regarding the other GFR markers, we must also stress that GFR can be measured by plasma clearance and using a bolus injection (instead of constant infusion rate) which makes the GFR measurement much more simple. Method to measure GFR by plasma clearances can be very different (number of samples, timing of samples, mathematical model used). We must keep in mind that results of plasma and urinary clearances are not strictly comparable (plasma clearances overestimate urinary clearances even if the overestimation decreases if plasma samples are drawn after 24 hours) and this must be integrated when these GFR methods are compared (Agarwal et al., 2009; Stolz et al., 2010).

5. ^{51}Cr-EDTA (Ethylenediaminetetra-acetic acid)

5.1 Physiological and analytical data

^{51}Cr-EDTA is an isotopic marker which has a low molecular weight (292 Da). Most of the authors consider that ^{51}Cr-EDTA is not binding to proteins (<0,5% (Brochner-Mortensen, 1978; Bailey et al., 1970; Garnett et al., 1967; Stacy & Thorburn, 1966; Forland et al., 1966; Kempi & Persson, 1975; Forland et al., 1966)) even if Rehling described a binding to protein of 10% (Rehling et al., 1995; Rehling et al., 2001). Due to its low molecular weight, ^{51}Cr-EDTA is freely filtrated through the glomerulus. Physiological studies about renal handling of ^{51}Cr-EDTA are few but it seems that ^{51}Cr-EDTA is neither secreted nor absorbed by renal tubules (Eide, 1970). This absence of secretion and absorption is also confirmed by Forland in dogs (Forland et al., 1966). Regarding the potential extra-renal excretion of ^{51}Cr-EDTA, Garnett described a salivary and a fecal excretion under 1% in one anephric patient (Garnett et al., 1967). Brochner-Mortensen later confirmed the poor fecal excretion (less than 0.1% of the injected dose). Studying the renal excretion and the corporal global radioactivity of 8 healthy subjects after 72 hours, Brochner-Mortensen estimated that 4.5% of the ^{51}Cr-EDTA will be retained in the body, especially in the liver and kidneys (Brochner-Mortensen et al., 1969). The difference between ^{51}Cr-EDTA total clearance and ^{51}Cr-EDTA urinary clearance corresponds to extra-renal clearance of the marker. With this methodology, the same authors estimated extra-renal clearance at 4 mL/min (and this extra-renal clearance remains stable for all GFR ranges)(Brochner-Mortensen & Rodbro, 1976). Jagenburg had also calculated an extra-renal clearance of 2 mL/min in two anuric dialysis patients (Jagenburg et al., 1978). Only, Rehling described a higher extra-renal clearance at 8.4% (Rehling et al., 1995).

Measurement of ^{51}Cr-EDTA by nuclear count is very precise and easy because ^{51}Cr-EDTA half time is long (27 days)(Chantler et al., 1969). The quantity of ^{51}Cr-EDTA injected is relatively small and therefore the irradiating dose received by the patient is very limited (absorbed dose from 0.011 to 0.0077 mSv according to the radioactive dose injected which is usually 7 MBq). This absorbed dose corresponds to the natural dose of irradiation received in one week and is much lesser than the dose received after thoracic radiography (0.02 mS). Nevertheless, we do not recommend this technique to measure GFR in pregnant women even if authors seem to use it safely (Brochner-Mortensen, 1978; Medeiros et al., 2009; Durand et al., 2006). The dose of EDTA is 1000x lesser than the dose considered as safe (Chantler et al., 1969).

5.2 Clinical data

The first studies about ^{51}Cr-EDTA have been published in the sixties, even if studies (but with questionable methodology) had been published before with EDTA marked with ^{14}Cr (Spencer et al., 1958; Foreman & Trujillo, 1954). In 1964, Downes was the first to give ^{51}Cr-EDTA to cows to study the intestinal transit (Downes & Mcdonald, 1964). In 1966, Stacy and Thorburn are the first to inject ^{51}Cr-EDTA to lambs for measuring GFR. They reported a good correlation with inulin clearance in the animal model (ratio ^{51}Cr-EDTA/inulin was 0,95)(Stacy & Thorburn, 1966). The first scientists who will be interested in GFR measurement by ^{51}Cr-EDTA in humans are English (Garnett et al., 1967; Favre & Wing, 1968; Garnett et al., 1967; Heath et al., 1968; Lavender et al., 1969). It must be underlined that nearly all studies published on this marker are coming from Europe because ^{51}Cr-EDTA is not available in USA (not approved by the FDA)(Brandstrom et al., 1998). The first author who studied ^{51}Cr-EDTA in humans is Garnett who was nuclearist in Southampton. These first data were published in The Lancet in 1967 (Garnett et al., 1967). This author injected one unique dose of ^{51}Cr-EDTA and described a mono-exponential decrease in ^{51}Cr-EDTA concentrations after 30 minutes. This author already evoked the plasma clearance (and the bolus injection) to measure GFR with ^{51}Cr-EDTA. Unhopefully, Garnett did not compare his results to inulin clearance but only to creatinine clearance. However, Garnett performed and compared 56 ^{51}Cr-EDTA urinary clearances with inulin urinary clearances. He found a correlation of 0.995 and asserted that ^{51}Cr-EDTA result were between ±5% of the inulin results which was really excellent. Thereafter, several studies were published on the same topic to compare performances of inulin clearance with urinary or plasma clearance of ^{51}Cr-EDTA. We resumed these studies in Table 2, restricting the data to studies in adults. However, once again, the following conclusions will be drawn from studies having used the most adequate statistical methods. Globally, the performance of ^{51}Cr-EDTA is good. Chantler, in 1969, showed that results of urinary clearance of ^{51}Cr-EDTA was within 5% of the results of inulin (Chantler et al., 1969). This excellent concordance between urinary clearances of ^{51}Cr-EDTA and inulin will be later confirmed by Froissart. This author showed a bias of +3 mL/min (^{51}Cr-EDTA thus slightly overestimating inulin) and a precision of ± 4 mL/min (95% of the ^{51}Cr-EDTA results will be + or - 8 mL/min around the bias)(Froissart et al., 2005b). The best study comparing ^{51}Cr-EDTA plasma clearance with inulin clearance is certainly published by Medeiros in 2009 (Medeiros et al., 2009). This author showed that bias between the two GFR was 3±6 mL/min. This is one of the rare studies where accuracy 30% results are given (defined as the percentage of patients having a ^{51}Cr-EDTA GFR within 30% of inulin GFR). Accuracy 30% for plasmatic clearance of ^{51}Cr-EDTA is 93%. The higher performance is obtained when late blood samples (at 6 or 8 h) are considered.

References	Sample	Population	GFR range (mL/min/ 1.73 m²)	GFR methods	Statistics	Results
(Garnett et al., 1967)	56	NA	± 0 to 180	Urinary clearance and constant infused rate	Regression Correlation	=1.075x-3.06 0.995
(Heath et al., 1968)	39	Healthy CKD Calcium troubles	10 to 150	Urinary clearance and constant infused rate	Correlation	0.995 ^{51}Cr-EDTA underestimates by de 14-16%
(Favre & Wing, 1968)	20	CKD	6 to 187	Urinary clearance and constant infused rate	Ratio Correlation BAr	1.02 0.992 1.5±8.7
(Lavender et al., 1969)	100 clearances in 28 subjects	CKD	± 0 to 150	Urinary clearance and constant infused rate	Ratio Regression Correlation	0.96 ± 0.0027 =0.96x+0.26 0.994
(Brochner-Mortensen et al., 1969)	17	2 healthy	± 10 to 130	Inulin: urinary clearance and constant infused rate ^{51}Cr-EDTA : plasmatic clearance: on 5 hours, samples every 15 min	Correlation Regression	0.974 =1.017x+1.6
(Chantler et al., 1969)	21	CKD	± 10 to 160	Urinary clearance and constant infused rate	Correlation Regression Ratio	0.977 =1.004x-0.032 1.004±0.013
(Stamp et al., 1970)	65 clearances in 56 subjects	15 healthy 41 calcium troubles	± 20 to 140	Urinary clearance and constant infused rate	Correlation Regression Ratio	0.91 =0.98x+6.5 0.96±0.02
(Ditzel et al., 1972)	20	NA	6 to 166	Inulin: urinary clearance and constant infused rate ^{51}Cr-EDTA : plasmatic clearance: samples at 5,10, 15, 20, 30, 60, 90, 120, 150, 180, 210, 240 min	Correlation Regression BAr	0.97 =0.85x+11.42 1.5±11.7
(Lingardh, 1972)	25	Healthy and CKD	±8 to 120	Inulin: urinary clearance and constant infused rate ^{51}Cr-EDTA : plasmatic clearance: samples timing not available	Correlation Regression Mean difference	0.984 =1.099x+4.96 6.2 mL/min

(Brochner-Mortensen, 1973)	89 clearances in 9 subjects	Healthy, before and after hyperglycemia	130 to 150	Urinary clearance and constant infused rate	Ratio	0.9±0.01
(Hagstam et al., 1974)	29	CKD	± 30 to 160	Urinary clearance and constant infused rate	Correlation Regression Ratio	0.97 =0.855x+7.555 0.96±0.07
(Hagstam et al., 1974)	31	CKD	± 30 to 160	Inulin: urinary clearance and constant infused rate ^{51}Cr-EDTA : plasmatic clearance: samples at 180, 200, 220 et 240 min + BM correction	Correlation Regression Ratio	0.97 =0.961x+2.908 1±0.11
(Winterborn et al., 1977)	16	Children and 4 healthy adults	± 5 to 120	Inulin: urinary clearance and constant infused rate ^{51}Cr-EDTA : urinary clearance:	Correlation Regression	0.99 =0.96x+3.5
(Jagenburg et al., 1978)	17	Severe CKD	2.6 to 11	Urinary clearance	Correlation Regression	0.97 =1.05x-0.3
(Rehling et al., 1986)	19	Nephrectomy	11 to 76	Inulin: urinary clearance and constant infused rate ^{51}Cr-EDTA : plasmatic clearance: 5 samples between 3 and 5 h+BM correction	Correlation Regression SD around the mean difference	0.96 =0.86x+2.4 4.3 mL/min
(Froissart et al., 2005b)	111	NA	NA	Urinary clearance and constant infused rate	BA	2.7±3.5
(Froissart et al., 2005a)	22	NA	NA	Urinary clearance and constant infused rate	BA	4±4.9
(Medeiros et al., 2009)	44	Renal grafted	±15 to 80	Inulin: urinary clearance and constant infused rate ^{51}Cr-EDTA : plasmatic clearance: samples at 2, 4, 6, 8 h + BM correction	t-test Correlation BA Exactitude 30%	NS 0.94 2.5±6.1 90.9%

Table 2. Studies comparing ^{51}Cr-EDTA with inulin. NA: not available, CKD: chronic kidney disease subjects, BA: Bland and Altman analysis, BAr: Bland and Altman analysis re-calculated by us, BM: Brochner-Mortensen.

5.3 Strengths and limitations

^{51}Cr-EDTA clearance was the first published alternative to inulin. Among the strengths of this marker, we have to underline the good performance of GFR measurement comparing to inulin (or to other markers). Physiological profile can also be considered as satisfying. This marker is yet easy to measure (especially according to its long half-life) and the precision of the measurement appears excellent. The costs, compared to other GFR markers, are acceptable. One important limitation is linked to the fact that ^{51}Cr-EDTA GFR must be done in a Nuclear Medicine department. The most important limitation of this marker is the non-use in USA, where ^{51}Cr-EDTA is not recognized by the FDA.

6. ^{99}Tc-DTPA (Diethylenetriaminepenta-acetic acid)

6.1 Physiological and analytical data

Like ^{51}Cr-EDTA, ^{99}Tc-DTPA is an isotopic marker with a low molecular weight (393 Da)(Durand et al., 2006). DTPA may be labeled with another isotopic marker (^{113m}Indium (Johansson & Falch, 1978; Reba et al., 1968; Piepsz et al., 1974), ^{169}Ytterbium (Perrone et al., 1990; Russell et al., 1985)) but technetium 99 is the most used up to now. The ^{99}Tc-DTPA is also used in Nuclear Imagery (isotopic nephrogram) for instance to measure separately the function or the right and left kidney (Biggi et al., 1995; Hilson et al., 1976; Kainer et al., 1979). However, we will only discuss GFR measurement based on plasma and/or urinary methods with ^{99}Tc-DTPA. GFR can also be estimated with external counting using gamma camera (namely the "Gates" method) (Gates, 1984; Russell, 1987) but this method is not precise enough to be considered as a reference method for measuring GFR. For some authors, the GFR estimation given by the Gates method is even less performing than the creatinine clearance (Owen et al., 1982; Goates et al., 1990; van de Wiele C. et al., 1999; Ma et al., 2007; Mulligan et al., 1990; Galli et al., 1994; Ginjaume et al., 1985; Rodby et al., 1992; Tepe et al., 1987; Aydin et al., 2008; De Santo et al., 1999; Fawdry et al., 1985; Durand et al., 2006).
Doses of injected ^{99}Tc-DTPA are totally safe (10 MBq)(Kempi & Persson, 1975; Durand et al., 2006). If the GFR measurement is coupled with nephrogram, the radioactive dose is however 40 to 200x higher than a simple GFR measurement with ^{51}Cr-EDTA (Kempi & Persson, 1975; Griffiths et al., 1988). The half-life of ^{99}Tc-DTPA is short (6.05 h) which imposes that the GFR measurement is realized quickly after the samplings, which is a practical inconvenient compared to ^{51}Cr-EDTA (Owen et al., 1982). The ^{99}Tc-DTPA measurement is as precise as other isotopic methods. The most relevant critic regarding ^{99}Tc-DTPA is its potential binding to protein. This aspect has been debated in the literature. Some authors described a binding to plasma proteins from 2 to 13%, which implies an underestimation of GFR, especially when GFR is measured by plasmatic clearance (Kempi & Persson, 1975; Agha & Persson, 1977; Klopper et al., 1972; Biggi et al., 1995; Houlihan et al., 1999; Rehling et al., 2001). These high percentages could however been explained by the lack of purity of the first available preparations of ^{99}Tc-DTPA (Rootwelt et al., 1980; Rehling et al., 2001; Fleming et al., 2004; Carlsen et al., 1980; Russell et al., 1983; Kempi & Persson, 1975). This hypothesis has been well illustrated in 1980 by Carlsen who studied and compared ^{51}Cr-EDTA clearances with 4 different commercial preparations of ^{99}Tc-DTPA. This author showed different results according to the preparation used (Carlsen et al., 1980). The binding to protein may also be studied by different methodologies (ultrafiltration, electrophoresis, precipitation, *in vitro* or *in vivo,* in humans or in animals etc)(Rehling et al.,

2001; Russell et al., 1983; Jeghers et al., 1990). For example, Rehling found a binding to protein of 10-13% but this author was also the only one who found a significant and comparable binding to protein for ^{51}Cr-EDTA and iothalamate (Rehling et al., 2001). The subject is finally still debated (Jeghers et al., 1990). Another potential critic about ^{99}Tc-DTPA is the very poor available data on its physiological handling. A study in a dog model argued for the absence of tubular secretion and reabsorption (Klopper et al., 1972).

6.2 Clinical data

There are hopefully much more clinical studies comparing ^{99}Tc-DTPA with other markers. After the preliminary study published by Hauser (Hauser et al., 1970), the performances of ^{99}Tc-DTPA clearance was studied from the seventies. Klopper may be considered as one of the pioneers with this markers (Klopper et al., 1972). The first studies were however comparing ^{99}Tc-DTPA with iothalamate and the samples were limited (Table 6)(Klopper et al., 1972; Rootwelt et al., 1980). The first study comparing ^{99}Tc-DTPA with inulin was published in 1984 (Rehling et al., 1984). In table 3, we resumed the results of studies comparing ^{99}Tc-DTPA with the gold standard method in adults. Two studies have compared with good statistical methods the urinary clearance of ^{99}Tc-DTPA and inulin. In the study published by Lewis in 1989, the bias was excellent bias (near to 0) but the precision was not satisfying (± 18 mL/min)(Lewis et al., 1989). One year later, Perrone showed excellent concordance between urinary clearances of ^{99}Tc-DTPA and inulin in 13 chronic kidney disease (CKD) patients. However, the results were less impressive in the 4 healthy subject where ^{99}Tc-DTPA clearances overestimate (+12 mL/min) inulin clearances. Definitive conclusion about the performance of ^{99}Tc-DTPA plasmatic clearance is difficult to draw and we clearly need additional studies on this topic.

6.3 Strengths and limitations

^{99}Tc-DTPA presents the advantages and inconvenient of other isotopic methods (see ^{51}Cr-EDTA paragraph). The dosage of the marker is relatively cheap and precise. His short half-time makes it a few less practicable than ^{51}Cr-EDTA. Among the most important advantages of ^{99}Tc-DTPA, we underline the fact that it is the only marker that can be coupled with nephrogram to give separated function between the two kidneys (Durand et al., 2006). Physiological data to confirm its role as a reference marker are however clearly lacking. We also think that global performance of ^{99}Tc-DTPA compared to inulin is probably a few less than the ^{51}Cr-EDTA, especially with plasma clearances (at least in part because ^{99}Tc-DTPA is binding to proteins).

7. Iothalamate

7.1 Physiological and analytical data

Iothalamate is an ionic contrast product which was particularly used for urography. Iothalamate is derived from the tri-iodobenzoic acid. Its molecular weight is 637 Da (Schwartz et al., 2006) and it is freely distributed into the extracellular volume (Visser et al., 2008). From a historical point of view, iothalamate was not the first contrast agent used to measure GFR. Other derivates from tri-iodobenzoic acid had been tested at the end of the fifties. Diatrizoate (Hypaque) was proposed by some authors as a potential GFR marker because it is fully excreted by the kidneys (Meschan et al., 1963; Burbank et al., 1963; Stokes et al., 1962; Mcchesney & Hoppe, 1957). However, other authors suggested that

References	Sample	Population	GFR range (mL/min/ 1.73 m²)	GFR methods	Statistics	Results
(Rehling et al., 1984)	20	Nephrectomy	11 to 76	Inulin: urinary and plasma clearance with bolus ^{99}Tc-DTPA: Urinary and plasma clearance: samples at 5, 10, 20, 40, 60, 90, 120, 150, 180, 210, 240, 270, 300 min	Wilcoxon Ratio urinary plasma ^{99}Tc-DTPA and urinary clearance of inulin Correlation Regression	urine : $p<0.05$ plasma : $p<0.05$ 0.97 0.97 =0.93x+6.8
(Shemesh et al., 1985)	45	NP	±10 to 140	Inulin: urinary clearance and constant infused rate ^{99}Tc-DTPA urinary clearance	Correlation Ratio	0,969 1,02±0,14
(Notghi et al., 1986)	37	Healthy and CKD	7 to 182	Inulin: urinary clearance and constant infused rate ^{99}Tc-DTPA plasma clearance: samples at: 60 and 150 min	Correlation Regression	0.77 =0.94x+33.7
(Petri et al., 1988)	NA	Lupus	23 to 123	Inulin: urinary clearance and constant infused rate ^{99}Tc-DTPA: urinary clearance with bolus	Correlation Regression r^2	0.96 =x+4.4 0.93
(Lewis et al., 1989)	29	10 heart grafted 11 renal grafted 10 donors	10 to 117	Inulin: urinary and plasma clearance with bolus ^{99}Tc-DTPA: urinary clearance with bolus	Correlation Regression BAr	0.85 =0.84x+8.4 0±18

(Perrone et al., 1990)	13	CKD	±5 to 130	Inulin: urinary clearance and constant infused rate ^{99}Tc-DTPA urinary clearance with bolus	Wilcoxon or t-test Correlation BA	P<0.001 from 0.93 to 0.98 Day 1 +0.5±3 Day 2 -2±3
	4	Healthy 2 successive days				Inulin (day 1 and 2): 108±14 96±8 ^{99}Tc-DTPA (day 1 and 2) 122±24 108±17
(Wharton, III et al., 1992)	18	Intensive care and CKD	2 to 69	Inulin: urinary clearance and constant infused rate ^{99}Tc-DTPA urinary clearance with bolus	Correlation Regression	0.85 =1.12x
(Gunasekera et al., 1996)	15	NA	±25 to 160	Bolus and plasma clearance for inulin and ^{99}Tc-DTPA: 6 samples within the first hours, 3 or 4 samples between 2 and 4 h	Correlation Regression	=0.98x-0.4 0.98

Table 3. Studies comparing ^{99}Tc-DTPA with inulin. NA: not available, CKD: chronic kidney disease subjects, BA: Bland and Altman analysis, BAr: Bland and Altman analysis re-calculated by us, BM: Brochner-Mortensen.

diatrizoate (as other derivates from tri-iodobenzoic acid) was secreted by renal tubules (Woodruff & Malvin, 1960; Harrow, 1956; Winter & Taplin, 1958). In 1961, Denneberg is the first to compare diatrizoate labeled with I^{131} and inulin in human (Denneberg et al., 1961). This author described a higher renal excretion and then confirmed that diatrizoate is secreted by renal tubules (Denneberg et al., 1961). Diatrizoate was still studied by some authors in the next years but the interest has definitively moved from diatrizoate to iothalamate (Burbank et al., 1963; Morris et al., 1965; Dalmeida & Suki, 1988; Owman & Olin, 1978; Donaldson, 1968).

As we will describe in the next paragraph, interest in iothalamate as a GFR marker has grown from the mid-sixties with the studies proposed by Sigman (Sigman et al., 1965a;

Sigman et al., 1965b). For this author, the binding of iothalamate to protein is less than 3% (Sigman et al., 1965b). Such result was confirmed by most of the authors thereafter (Anderson et al., 1968; Gagnon et al., 1971; Blaufox & Cohen, 1970; Prueksaritanont et al., 1986; Back et al., 1988b), except for Maher and Rehling (see ^{99}Tc-DTPA chapter)(Rehling et al., 2001; Maher & Tauxe, 1969). Rapidly, Sigman has proposed to move from labeling with I^{131} to labeling with I^{125}. I^{125} is actually more stable (Elwood & Sigman, 1967; Maher et al., 1971). I^{125}-Iothalamate is thus an isotopic method which is precise and safe. The half-life of ^{125}I is 60 days (Perrone et al., 1990). Physiological data on iothalamate have been published after the first clinical studies by Sigman. Iothalamate was then studied in aglomerular fishes and only 3% of injected iothalamate was found in urine. The absence of tubular secretion and reabsorption was confirmed in a dog model (Griep & Nelp, 1969). However, these reassuring results were not confirmed by Odlind in 1985. This author actually observed in rats a tubular secretion of iothalamate (comparing with ^{51}Cr-EDTA and using inhibitors of tubular secretion). In the same view, Odlind described, in 6 healthy subjects, that iothalamate clearance overestimates inulin clearance and that this overestimation is reversible after inhibition of tubular secretion by probenecid (Odlind et al., 1985). In anephric patients, Cangiano described an extra-renal excretion of iothalamate that reached 4 to 8 mL/min. This extra-renal excretion fall to 0 after thyroid saturation by iodine (Cangiano et al., 1971). A potential limited extra-renal clearance of iothalamate was thus suggested in the thyroid. Evans described a clearance of iothalamate of 3.1±1.8 mL/min in 7 dialysis patients (among these, 5 were anuric). In animal models, a limited biliary excretion is suggested by some authors (Owman & Olin, 1978; Prueksaritanont et al., 1986). Comparing the total (i.e. plasma) and the renal clearance of iothalamate in healthy subjects, Back calculated the extra-renal clearance at 6 mL/min (Back et al., 1988b). In the same experience, Dowling calculated extra-renal clearance at 10 ml/ml, which was constant for all the GFR levels (sample of 26 patients)(Dowling et al., 1999). In this last study, the plasma clearance was measured until 180 min, which may be considered as too short (Dowling et al., 1999). Visser has also calculated the urinary excretion of iothalamate on 24 h and estimated the extra-renal excretion at 14±12% (Visser et al., 2008). Such values of extra-renal clearances are thus not so negligible, especially when it is considered in patients with severe CKD. Actually, the relative importance of this extra-renal clearance will be higher when the GFR is yet low (Visser et al., 2008).

Iothalamate is a safe product but, of course, it will be not used in subjects presenting a known "true" allergy to contrast products (Heron et al., 1984). Regarding the isotopic method, the radioactive dose got by the patient is also very low (lower than the dose got for thorax radiography)(Hall & Rolin, 1995; Bajaj et al., 1996).

Because its relatively low molecular weight, iothalamate is a good marker (just like ^{51}Cr-EDTA) to be used in simplified protocols. Cohen was the first to use the bolus method instead of the constant rate infusing method in 1969 (Cohen et al., 1969). Several authors have showed that iothalamate could be used in plasma clearance (LaFrance et al., 1988; Welling et al., 1976; Back et al., 1988b; Gaspari et al., 1992) even if results are not fully comparable to urinary clearances (Agarwal et al., 2009). It must also be underlined that iothalamate is the only one marker which is frequently used with subcutaneous injection (Israelit et al., 1973). It had actually been shown that plasma iothalamate concentrations remain constant 60 to 90 min after a subcutaneous injection (so, equivalent to the constant infusion rate method but much easier) (Israelit et al., 1973; Adefuin et al., 1976; Tessitore et al., 1979; Sharma et al., 1997).

Iothalamate can yet be measured by "cold" non-isotopic methods. The first "cold" dosage of iothalamate was proposed in 1975 by Guesry (Guesry et al., 1975). This author used fluorescent excitation analysis or X ray fluorescence (XRF), which will be also used for iohexol measurement (see below). In this technique, iodine atoms are ionized by americanum. When the iodine atom comes back to neutral status, it will emit X ray that will be then quantified (Guesry et al., 1975). Guesry found an excellent correlation between isotopic and XRF iothalamate measurement. Iothalamate concentration can also be determined by electrophoresis but, to the best of our knowledge, this technique is only used in the Mayo Clinic (Wilson et al., 1997). The most used methods to measure iothalamate are HPLC methods (Boschi & Marchesini, 1981). The HPLC method seems specific, sensible and reproducible (CV intra-day lower than 2% and CV inter-day lower than 6%) (Boschi & Marchesini, 1981; Prueksaritanont et al., 1984; Weber et al., 1985; Reidenberg et al., 1988; Back et al., 1988b; Gaspari et al., 1991; Dowling et al., 1998; Agarwal, 1998; Kos et al., 2000; Agarwal et al., 2003; Farthing et al., 2005; Bi et al., 2007). A new technique based on mass spectrometry has recently been proposed to measure iothalamate (Seegmiller et al., 2010). These authors have compared 51 GFR results given by this new technique and by electrophoresis. The results are excellent in term of correlation and bias (0.8%). The SD around the bias, namely the precision, is however less negligible at 13.7%. That means that 95% of the results measures in the same patient may vary from ± 28% according the way iothalamate has been measured. Iothalamate measurement remain very stable (for two months at room temperature and at -4 and -20°C and for 1 year at -80°C) (Weber et al., 1985; Seegmiller et al., 2010).

7.2 Clinical data

Iothalamate (Conray°) was used as GFR marker for the first time by Sigman from the New York University in 1965 (Sigman et al., 1965a; Sigman et al., 1965b). In these articles, Sigman used iothalamate labeled with ^{131}I and compared its clearance with inulin clearance in 10 patients in the first publication (Sigman et al., 1965a) and in 16 in the second one (Sigman et al., 1965b). On this limited sample, Sigman described a ratio iothalamate/inulin near to 1, even though the ranges of this ratio are from 0.74 à 1 in the first study (Sigman et al., 1965a) and from 0.937 à 1.138 in the second one (Sigman et al., 1965b). These first interesting results were then confirmed by the same authors with ^{125}I-iothalamate (Elwood & Sigman, 1967). Other authors published thereafter their own data comparing performance of inulin and iothalamate clearances. We resumed the results obtained in adults in Table 4. It is probably right to write that iothalamate has been the most studied GFR marker and the marker for which several comparisons to inulin exist. Other authors have confirmed the good performance of iothalamate urinary clearances, especially in CKD patients (Maher et al., 1971; Perrone et al., 1990; Skov, 1970). In healthy subjects, the results are however more questionable and iothalamate seems to overestimate inulin (+20 mL/min)(Perrone et al., 1990) although precision is not optimal ±11 mL/min, as illustrated in the study by Botev (Botev et al., 2011). Data regarding the performance of the iothalamate plasma clearance are less numerous but is seems that bias is acceptable. However, precision is not optimal, especially in higher GFR levels. Additional studies could be of interest for the plasmatic method (Agarwal, 2003; Mirouze et al., 1972).

References	Sample	Population	GFR range (mL/min/1.73 m²)	GFR methods	Statistics	Results
(Sigman et al., 1965a)	10	NA	70 to 108	Inulin: urinary clearance and constant infused rate ^{131}iothalamate : urinary clearance and constant infused rate	Ratio It/inulin BAr	1.06 (0.74 to 1.23) 6±13
(Sigman et al., 1965b)	24 clearances in 16 subjects	NA	2 to 167	Inulin: urinary clearance and constant infused rate ^{131}iothalamate : urinary clearance and constant infused rate	t-test Ratio It/inulin BAr	NS 1.005 (from 0.937 to 1.138) 0.7±4
(Elwood & Sigman, 1967)	26 clearances in 21 subjects	NA	27 to 136	Inulin: urinary clearance and constant infused rate ^{125}iothalamate : urinary clearance and constant infused rate	Ratio It/inulin BAr	1 (from 0.93 to 1.09) 1±3
(Malamos et al., 1967)	19	Healthy and CKD	NA	Inulin: urinary clearance and constant infused rate ^{125}iothalamate : urinary clearance and constant infused rate	Ratio It/inulin Correlation (urinary) Regression	1.01±0.19 0.979 It=1.09inulin-0.65
(Anderson et al., 1968)	18	11 CKD and 8 healthy	3 to 139	Inulin: urinary clearance and constant infused rate ^{125}iothalamate : urinary clearance and constant infused rate	Regression BAr	=0.9x+6.7 -0.7±13

(Maher & Tauxe, 1969)	15	hypertensive	±55 to 120	Inulin: urinary clearance and constant infused rate ^{125}iothalamate : urinary clearance and constant infused rate	Ratio It/inulin Regression	0.92 (0.81 to 1.04) Inulin=1.08It
(Skov, 1970)	43 65 clearances in 22 subjects 38 clearances in 13 subjects 24 clearances in 8 subjects	CKD GFR<5 ml/ GFR between 5 et 15 mL/min GFR between 15 et 25 mL/min		Inulin: urinary clearance and constant infused rate ^{125}iothalamate : bolus and urinary clearance	Ratio It/inulin Correlation Regression BAr	Group 1 0.98±0.06 0.999 =0.972+0.01 0±0 Group 2 1 0±1 Group 3 0.92±0.071 0.968 =1.083+3.46 -2±1
(Gagnon et al., 1971)	78 clearances in 24 subjects	NA	±10 to 180	Inulin: urinary clearance and constant infused rate ^{125}iothalamate : urinary clearance and constant infused rate	Ratio It/inulin	1.01
(Cangiano et al., 1971)	49 clearances in 18 subjects	NA	±30 to 150	Inulin: urinary clearance and constant infused rate ^{125}iothalamate : urinary clearance and constant infused rate	Ratio It/inulin Correlation Regression	1.07 0.94 =1.06+1.17
(Maher et al., 1971)	198	NA	±5 to 150	Inulin: urinary clearance and constant infused rate ^{125}iothalamate : urinary clearance and constant infused rate	Bias Regression	-2.09 Inulin=1.022It+0.537

(Mirouze et al., 1972)	36 clearances in 23 subjects	hypertensive	±5 to 120	Inulin: urinary clearance and constant infused rate ^{125}iothalamate : urinary clearance and constant infused rate	Ratio It/inulin Correlation Regression	1.44±0.13 0.96 =1.18+8.43
(Mirouze et al., 1972)	15	hypertensive	±80 to 140	Inulin: urinary clearance and constant infused rate ^{125}iothalamate : plasma clearance: samples at 5, 10, 15, 20, 40, 60, 80, 100 et 120 min + correction	Ratio It/inulin Correlation Regression	1.23±0.16 0.77 =1.06+1.18
(Israelit et al., 1973)	22	20 CKD 2 healthy	6 to 125	Inulin: urinary clearance and constant infused rate ^{125}iothalamate : bolus SC and urinary clearance	Ratio It/inulin Correlation Regression	1.05±0.04 0.97 =1.054-3.069
(Rosenbaum et al., 1979)	7 healthy 9 renal grafted 8 donors after donation		96 to 147 35 to 87 42 to 98	Inulin: urinary clearance and constant infused rate ^{125}iothalamate : bolus and urinary clearance	Ratio It/inulin BAr	1.02±0.04 1.43±0.08 1.23±0.04 -1±13 -7±14 -4±13
(Ott, 1975)	84	CKD and donors	±10 to 150	Inulin: urinary clearance and constant infused rate ^{125}iothalamate : urinary clearance and constant infused rate	Correlation Regression	0.932 =1.04+2.11

(Ott, 1975)	100	CKD and donors	±5 to 150	Inulin: urinary clearance and constant infused rate ^{125}iothalamate: bolus SC and urinary clearance	Correlation Regression	0.982 =1.02-0.61
(Tessitore et al., 1979)	30	15 creatinine<1 mg/dL 15 creatinine<20 mg/dL	NA	Inulin: urinary clearance and constant infused rate ^{125}iothalamate: bolus SC and urinary clearance	Ratio It/inulin Correlation	1.07±0.05 0.96
(Notghi et al., 1986)	76 clearances in 40 subjects	Healthy and CKD	±10 to 180	Inulin: urinary clearance and constant infused rate ^{125}iothalamate: bolus SC and urinary clearance	Correlation Regression	0.86 =0.8x+19.5
(Petri et al., 1988)	NA	Lupus	23 to 123	Inulin: urinary clearance and constant infused rate Iothalamate (XRF): bolus and urinary clearance	Correlation Regression r^2	0.99 =0.9x-2.1 0.99
(Perrone et al., 1990)	13 4	CKD Healthy Two successive days	±5 to 130	Inulin: urinary clearance and constant infused rate ^{125}iothalamate: bolus SC and urinary clearance	Wilcoxon or t-test Correlation Means	P<0.001 from 0.93 to 0.98 Inulin : 108±14 day 1 96±8 day 2 ^{125}iothalamate 127±12 day 1 120±7 day 2
(al Uzri et al., 1992)	5	healthy	120 to 165	Inulin: urinary clearance and constant infused rate Iothalamate (HPLC): bolus and urinary clearance	ratio	1.00±0.06

(Isaka et al., 1992)	23	CKD	10 to 130	Inulin: urinary clearance and constant infused rate Iothalamate (HPLC): bolus and urinary clearance	Correlation Slope with 0 intercept	0.98 1.05±0.01
(Agarwal, 2003)	12 clearances in 3 subjects	CKD	± 20 to 110	Inulin: urinary clearance and constant infused rate Iothalamate (HPLC): plasma clearance on long time with insulin pomp	Bias (Inulin-It) CV	0.8 19.9%
(Botev et al., 2011) Data from 5 studies (Anderson et al., 1968; Elwood & Sigman, 1967; Perrone et al., 1990; Rosenbaum et al., 1979; Skov, 1970)	94	See above	± 5 to 140	See above	Correlation Regression BA (It-Inulin)	0.97 =1.04+2.334 +4.6±11

Table 4. Studies comparing iothalamate with inulin. NA: not available, CKD: chronic kidney disease subjects, BA: Bland and Altman analysis, BAr: Bland and Altman analysis re-calculated by us, BM: Brochner-Mortensen, HPLC: high pressure liquid chromatography, It: iothalamate, SC: subcutaneous, XRF: X ray fluorescence.

7.3 Strengths and limitations

Iothalamate can be measured either by HPLC or XRF methods or by isotopic methods. This is the only one marker where this choice is possible. However, there is no evidence that all the techniques of measurement are fully equivalent. Iothalamate is certainly the marker that has been the most deeply studied from a physiological point of view (with inulin). Unhopefully, there are strong reasons to believe that iothalamate is secreted by renal tubules. Moreover, extra-renal clearance of iothalamate is not so negligible. These limitations are confirmed by most of the clinical studies showing that iothalamate slightly overestimates inulin clearance, especially in the high levels of GFR. A clinical limitation concerns the patients who are allergic to contrast product. This marker remains however important because it is the most used marker in USA. For example, iothalamate has been used in trials having built the new creatinine-based equations (Levey et al., 1999).

8. Iohexol

8.1 Physiological and analytical data

Iohexol is a non-ionic contrast product, mainly used for myelography. Its molecular weight is 821 Da (Olsson et al., 1983; Schwartz et al., 2006). Iohexol is chronologically the last marker proposed for measuring GFR. Actually, the first human was receiving iohexol in 1980 (Aakhus et al., 1980). In this study, it was shown that the substance was safe and fully excreted by the kidneys (this assertion will be criticized thereafter, see below). However, these authors also describe (but data are not available) a higher urinary clearance of iohexol than ^{51}Cr-EDTA (Aakhus et al., 1980). The details of these comparison studies were published three years after (see clinical data)(Olsson et al., 1983). In the same study, the authors confirm that iohexol is distributed through the extracellular volume, which will be confirmed by other authors (including in CKD patients and in obese subjects) (Friedman et al., 2010; Nossen et al., 1995; Edelson et al., 1984; Back et al., 1988b; Olsson et al., 1983). Iohexol has not effect *per se* on GFR (Olofsson et al., 1996). Binding to protein seems very limited for iohexol. The first study described a binding to protein of only 1.5% (Mutzel et al., 1980). This will be thereafter confirmed (Back et al., 1988b; Krutzen et al., 1984). Physical properties of iohexol make it a good candidate to be used in simplified protocols like plasma clearance (Thomsen & Hvid-Jacobsen, 1991; Gaspari et al., 1995; Edelson et al., 1984). Contrary to the prior studies (Aakhus et al., 1980), several authors have shown that extra-renal clearance of iohexol is limited but not null (Arvidsson & Hedman, 1990; Krutzen et al., 1984). Back calculated at 6.2 mL/min the difference between total and urinary clearance of iohexol in healthy subjects (Back et al., 1988b). Frennby observed an extra-renal clearance lower than 2 mL/min in 6 anuric dialysis patients (Frennby et al., 1994; Frennby et al., 1995). These last very low results were also found by Nossen in 16 patients with severe CKD. Their mean measured GFR was 14 mL/min and the extra-renal clearance was estimated at 10% (Nossen et al., 1995). In 16 healthy subjects, Edelson estimated the extra-renal clearance of iohexol at 5% (Edelson et al., 1984). Contrary to iothalamate, there are very few physiological studies on the renal tubular handling of iohexol.

As for iothalamate, iohexol can be measured by several different techniques. Among these, HPLC and XRF are the most used ones. HPLC was historically the first method used (Aakhus et al., 1980) and described (Krutzen et al., 1984). As we have shown, iohexol measurements by HPLC are sensitive, specific and reproducible (Back et al., 1988c; Farthing et al., 2005; Cavalier et al., 2008). The high performance of such dosage notably enables the use of iohexol low doses and the measurement on finger-prick samples (Krutzen et al., 1990; Niculescu-Duvaz et al., 2006; Mafham et al., 2007; Cavalier et al., 2008; Aurell, 1994). Iohexol measurement is also pretty stable at room temperature and at -20°C(Krutzen et al., 1984; O'Reilly et al., 1988). Measurement of iohexol by XRF method is less validated and probably less performing, especially in low plasma concentrations (O'Reilly et al., 1986; Back & Nilsson-Ehle, 1993; Effersoe et al., 1990; Brandstrom et al., 1998; Aurell, 1994). We will not discuss into details the other methods for measuring iohexol: capillary electrophoresis (Shihabi & Constantinescu, 1992) and mass spectrometry (Lee et al., 2006; Annesley & Clayton, 2009; Denis et al., 2008; Stolz et al., 2010). The safety of iohexol is now confirmed (Heron et al., 1984; Aurell, 1994), notably by the largest series of iohexol measurements in Sweden (1500 GFR measurements/y)(Nilsson-Ehle & Grubb, 1994; Nilsson-Ehle, 2002). This safety profile is, at least in part, explained by the low dose of iohexol injected, and by the exclusion of patients with contrast products allergy.

8.2 Clinical data

The results of the first clinical study on iohexol as a reference GFR marker will be published in 1983 (Olsson et al., 1983). Actually, GFR was measured in 10 healthy subjects with urinary clearances of iohexol and ^{51}Cr-EDTA. In this study, the iohexol clearance was significantly higher than the ^{51}Cr-EDTA clearance (110 versus 96 mL/min). In this first study, large dose of iohexol was injected to the patient (from 375 to 500 mg I/kg)(Olsson et al., 1983). Thereafter, the doses of iohexol used will be drastically reduced but it has been well described that the physiologic handling of iohexol was identical if different dosages are used (Back et al., 1988a). In table 5, we resumed the study results having compared the performance of iohexol to inulin in adult subjects. To the best of our knowledge, only two studies have compared urinary clearances of iohexol and inulin. The results seem excellent but Bland and Altman analysis have not been realized (Brown & O'Reilly, 1991; Perrone et al., 1990). Contrary to other markers, iohexol plasmatic clearances have been the most studied. The relatively worst results obtained by Erley are explained by the patients included (Erley et al., 2001). Actually, the patients hospitalized in intensive care are prone to develop edema and, in this situation, plasmatic clearances are not accurate, whatever the marker (Skluzacek et al., 2003). The study published by Gaspari demonstrated a good performance of iohexol plasma clearance compared to inulin but the number of samples was high and these samples were drawn lately (after 10h)(Gaspari et al., 1995).

References	Sample	Population	GFR range (mL/min/1.73 m²)	GFR methods	Statistics	Results
(Lewis et al., 1989)	29	10 heart grafted 11 renal grafted 10 donors	9.6 to 116.8	Inulin: urinary clearance and constant infused rate Iohexol (XRF) Plasma clearance: bolus and samples after 3 and 4	Correlation Regression Ratio	0.86 =0.85x+8.79 1.09±0.06
(Brown & O'Reilly, 1991)	30	NA	±10 to 125	Inulin: urinary clearance and constant infused rate Iohexol (XRF) urinary clearance and plasma clearance: samples at 3 and 4 h +BM correction	Correlation Regression Ratio	Urinary 0.986 =0.998-2.309 Plasma 0.983 =0.947+4.92 =1.102±0.286

(Gaspari et al., 1995)	41	CKD	6 to 160	Inulin: urinary clearance and constant infused rate Iohexol (HPLC) Plasma clearance, samples at 5, 10, 20, 30, 45, 60, 90, 120, 180, 240, 300, 450, 600 min	Correlation Regression BA	0.97 =0.994x+2.339 1.02±7
(Erley et al., 2001)	31	intensive care	±10 to 130	Inulin: urinary clearance and constant infused rate Iohexol (XRF) Plasma clearance: samples at 150, 195, 240 + 360 min if estimated GFR under 30 mL/min	Correlation Regression BA	=0.971x+7.65 r^2=0.96 (Io-inulin) =8.67±7.21
(Sterner et al., 2008)	20	healthy	106 to 129	Inulin: urinary clearance and constant infused rate Iohexol (HPLC) Urinary clearance and constant infused rate	Wilcoxon	Not different

Table 5. Studies comparing iohexol with inulin. NA: not available, CKD: chronic kidney disease subjects, BA: Bland and Altman analysis, BAr: Bland and Altman analysis re-calculated by us, BM: Brochner-Mortensen, HPLC: high pressure liquid chromatography, Io: iohexol, SC: subcutaneous, XRF: X ray fluorescence.

8.3 Strengths and limitations

Iohexol is probably the easiest way to measure GFR. It can be used in all patients (except in patient with true allergy to contrast product). Its measurement by HPLC is probably one of the most precise compared to other cold method (inulin and iothalamate). Iohexol is the less expensive marker and the cost of HPLC is also low. More important, it must be underlined that an external quality control does exist for iohexol measurement (Equalis, Sweden). From unpublished data, it can be concluded that the inter-laboratory CV for iohexol measurement is very low (less than 5%). Such results don't exist for iothalamate and inulin, and, at least for inulin, we think that such good inter-laboratory results would not be reached (personal data). The limitations of iohexol are the lack of strong physiological data (notably regarding the tubular handling of the marker) and the relatively few studies having compared iohexol with inulin. More studies have actually compared iohexol with other GFR markers.

9. Studies comparing reference methods

In Table 6, we resumed the results of studies comparing reference markers (other than inulin). We selected studies in adults. We focused on studies having used the best statistical methods to analyze the results, i.e. the Bland and Altman analysis. It is difficult to interpret results from studies having compared different markers but also different methods (for example, plasmatic clearance of iothalamate with urinary clearance of ^{51}Cr-EDTA) because it is impossible to affirm that potential differences are due to difference in markers or to difference in methods. Another limitation of several studies is the relatively small sample of subjects included. If we take into account these two limitations, we can stress on some interesting results showing good concordance (bias±SD) between plasma clearances of ^{51}Cr-EDTA and ^{99}Tc-DTPA (1.91±6.1 mL/min), and between plasma clearances of ^{51}Cr-EDTA and iohexol (-0.16±6.17 mL/min in (Brandstrom et al., 1998), 4±7.9 mL/min in (Bird et al., 2009), 2±9.2 (Lundqvist et al., 1997), and -0.6±3.6 mL/min in (Pucci et al., 2001)).

References	Sample	Population	GFR range (mL/min/1.73 m²)	GFR methods	Statistics	Results
(Odlind et al., 1985)	11	Nephrectomy and CKD	37 to 137	Cp of Cr and ^{125}It: samples at 180, 210 and 240 min + BM correction	Wilcoxon Ratio It/Cr BAr It-Cr	It higher (p<0.001) 1.13 12±7.5
(Lewis et al., 1989)	29	10 heart grafted 11 renal grafted 10 donors	10 to 117	Cu of Dt and Io (XRF): samples at 3 and 4 h after bolus	Correlation Regression Ratio BAr Dt-Io	0.89 Io=0.89Dt+6.5 1.08±0.06 -0.7±14.8
(Goates et al., 1990)	16	NA	21 to 156	Cu ^{125}It: Cu after bolus IV and infusion Cp of Dt: samples at 60 and 180 min+ BM correction	Correlation BAr Io-Dt	0.99 3.2±6.1
(Effersoe et al., 1990)	15	urography	22 to 110	Cp of Io (XRF), Cr and Dt : samples at 0, 10, 20, 30, 120, 180, 240 and 300 min	Regression Correlation BA : Cr-Io Dt-Io Cr-Dt	Io=0.97Dt-11 0.96 Io=1.01Cr+8 0.95 -10.8±7.9 -9.4±6.9 -0.7±10.4

(Gaspari et al., 1992)	19	CKD	7 to 148	Cp of Cr and It (HPLC): bolus IV and samples at 5, 10, 20, 30, 40, 50, 60, 90, 120, 180, 240, 300, 450 and 600 min	Correlation Regression BAr It-Cr	0.995 It=1.007Cr-0.303 -0.1±4.7
(Lundqvist et al., 1994)	31	Para or tetraplegic	±70 to 130	Cp of Cr and Io (XRF): samples à 180, 210, 240 and 270 minutes+ BM correction day 1 and 2	BA Cr-Io	Day 1 : +2.1±10.2 Day 2 : +0.9±5.9
(Galli et al., 1994)	50	NA	±15 to 160	Cp of Cr and Dt: samples at 60 and 180 min	Regression BA Dt-Cr	Dt=0.982Cr+3.2 1.91±6.1
(Sambataro et al., 1996)	17	Diabetic	7 to 105	Cu of Cr and It (HPLC)	Regression BAr It-Cr	It=0.979Cr-3.04 1.3±5
(Lundqvist et al., 1997)	77	Urography	±25 to 125	Cp of Cr and Io (XRF): samples at 180, and 240 or 270 min+ BM correction	Correlation Regression BA (Io-Cr)	0.918 Io=0.892Cr+6.28 2±9.2
(Brandstrom et al., 1998)	49	GFR>40	±40 to 125	Cp of Cr and Io (HPLC and XRF): samples at 150, 195 and 240 min + BM correction	Regression Correlation BA Cr-Io	XRF Io=1.03Cr-1.79 0.97 0.58±4.95 HPLC Io=1.05Cr-4.43 0.96 -0.16±6.17
(Pucci et al., 1998)	32	Diabetic	13 to 151	Cp of Cr and Io (HPLC): samples at 5, 10, 15, 30, 60, 90, 120, 150, 180, 210, 240, 270, 300 + 360 and 420 if creatinine>2 mg/dL + 1440 min if>5mg/dL	Regression Correlation BA Cr-Io	0.995 Io=0.978Cr+2.45 -0.6±3.6

Houlihan (Houlihan et al., 1999)	21	Diabetic	50 to 145	Cp of Dt and Io (XRF): samples at 120, 165 and 210 for Dt samples at 120, 150, 180, 210 and 240 min for Io + BM correction	Regression Correlation BA Io-Dt	Io=0.9938Dt+4.916 0.97 4.3±7.7
(Pucci et al., 2001)	41	Diabetic	29 to 150	Cp of Cr and Io (HPLC): samples at 5, 10, 15, 30, 60, 90, 120, 150, 180, 210, 240, 270, 300 + 360 and 420 if creatinine>2 mg/dL + 1440 min if>5mg/dL	Regression Correlation BA Cr-Io	Type 1 Io=0.978Cr+0.132 0.999 Type 2 0.987 Io=0.078Cr+2.352 BA :-0.42±3.69
Bird (Bird et al., 2009)	56 19	CKD healthy	±15 to 140	Cp of Cr and Io (XRF): samples at 20, 40, 60, 120, 180 and 240 min	BA Cr-Io	4±7.9

Table 6. studies comparing different reference methods (other than inulin), NA = not available, BA: Bland and Altman, BAr: Bland and Altman recalculated by us, BM: Brochner Mortensen,Cr: ^{51}Cr-EDTA, Dt: ^{99}Tc-DTPA, Io: iohexol, It: iothalamate, Cp: plasma clearance, Cu: urinary clearance, IC: constant infusion rate, IB: bolus injection, IV: intravenous, SC: subcutaneous, AUC: area under the curve, NS: not significant, HPLC: high pressure liquid chromatography, XRF: X ray fluorescence.

10. Conclusions and perspectives

In this chapter, we reviewed all the reference methods available in 2011 to measure GFR. Among these methods, inulin clearance can certainly be considered as the gold-standard because it is historically the first method used and because this marker is certainly the best characterized from a physiological point of view. However, inulin is expensive and commercial sources are limited (Gaspari et al., 1997). Due to its high molecular weight, there are doubts to use inulin in simplified plasma clearance (urinary clearances with constant infusion rate remain necessary but are very cumbersome). Measurement of plasma inulin is neither easy nor standardized. For all these reasons, the use of inulin is and will always be relatively marginal. In 2011, it is maybe time to move from the perfect physiological marker (inulin) to markers, maybe less perfect in the renal physiologic handling, but less costly, easier to use everywhere in the world and with a standardized measurement. From our point of view, iohexol is probably the best marker with the best balance between physiological characteristics and practical advantages. Additional studies comparing references markers seem necessary in 2011. It seems also important to underline that GFR measurement is also subject to its own imprecision and to biological variation (Kwong et al., 2010). Therefore, it is illusionary to expect differences between different GFR methods of less than 10% (±2SD around the bias) and accuracy 10% over 85-90%. We must also keep these results in mind when we analyze the studies testing the performance of the creatinine-based equations (Kwong et al., 2010).

11. References

Aakhus, T., Sommerfelt, S.C., Stormorken, H. & Dahlstrom, K. (1980). Tolerance and excretion of iohexol after intravenous injection in healthy volunteers. Preliminary report, *Acta Radiol Suppl*, Vol.362, pp. 131-134

Adefuin, P.Y., Gur, A., Siegel, N.J., Spencer, R.P. & Hayslett, J.P. (1976). Single subcutaneous injection of iothalamate sodium I 125 to measure glomerular filtration rate, *JAMA*, Vol.235, No.14, pp. 1467-1469

Agarwal, R. (1998). Chromatographic estimation of iothalamate and p-aminohippuric acid to measure glomerular filtration rate and effective renal plasma flow in humans, *J Chromatogr B Biomed Sci Appl*, Vol.705, No.1, pp. 3-9

Agarwal, R. (2003). Ambulatory GFR measurement with cold iothalamate in adults with chronic kidney disease, *Am J Kidney Dis*, Vol.41, No.4, pp. 752-759

Agarwal, R., Bills, J.E., Yigazu, P.M., Abraham, T., Gizaw, A.B., Light, R.P., Bekele, D.M. & Tegegne, G.G. (2009). Assessment of iothalamate plasma clearance: duration of study affects quality of GFR, *Clin J Am Soc Nephrol*, Vol.4, No.1, pp. 77-85

Agarwal, R., Vasavada, N. & Chase, S.D. (2003). Liquid chromatography for iothalamate in biological samples, *J Chromatogr B Analyt Technol Biomed Life Sci*, Vol.785, No.2, pp. 345-352

Agha, N., Persson, R.B. (1977). Comparative labelling and biokinetic studies of 99mTc-EDTA(Sn) and 99mTc-DTPA(Sn), *Nuklearmedizin*, Vol.16, No.1, pp. 30-35

al Uzri, A., Holliday, M.A., Gambertoglio, J.G., Schambelan, M., Kogan, B.A. & Don, B.R. (1992). An accurate practical method for estimating GFR in clinical studies using a constant subcutaneous infusion, *Kidney Int*, Vol.41, No.6, pp. 1701-1706

Alving, A.S., Miller, B.F. & Rubin, J. (1939). A direct colorimetric method for the determination of inuline in blood and urine, *J Biol Chem*, Vol.127, No.3, pp. 609-616

Anderson, C.F., Sawyer, T.K. & Cutler, R.E. (1968). Iothalamate sodium I 125 vs cyanocobalamin Co 57 as a measure of glomerular filtration rate in man, *JAMA*, Vol.204, No.8, pp. 653-656

Annesley, T.M., Clayton, L.T. (2009). Ultraperformance liquid chromatography-tandem mass spectrometry assay for iohexol in human serum, *Clin Chem*, Vol.55, No.6, pp. 1196-1202

Arvidsson, A., Hedman, A. (1990). Plasma and renal clearance of iohexol--a study on the reproducibility of a method for the glomerular filtration rate, *Scand J Clin Lab Invest*, Vol.50, No.7, pp. 757-761

Aurell, M. (1994). Accurate and feasible measurements of GFR--is the iohexol clearance the answer?, *Nephrol Dial Transplant*, Vol.9, No.9, pp. 1222-1224

Aydin, F., Gungor, F., Cengiz, A.K., Tuncer, M., Mahsereci, E., Ozdem, S., Cenkci, M. & Karayalcin, B. (2008). Comparison of glomerular filtration rate measurements with the two plasma sample and single plasma sample, gamma camera Gates, creatinine clearance, and prediction equation methods in potential kidney donors with normal renal function, *Nucl Med Commun,* Vol.29, No.2, pp. 157-165

Baccard, N., Hoizey, G., Frances, C., Lamiable, D., Trenque, T. & Millart, H. (1999). Simultaneous determination of inulin and p-aminohippuric acid (PAH) in human plasma and urine by high-performance liquid chromatography, *Analyst,* Vol.124, No.6, pp. 833-836

Back, S.E., Krutzen, E. & Nilsson-Ehle, P. (1988a). Contrast media and glomerular filtration: dose dependence of clearance for three agents, *J Pharm Sci,* Vol.77, No.9, pp. 765-767

Back, S.E., Krutzen, E. & Nilsson-Ehle, P. (1988b). Contrast media as markers for glomerular filtration: a pharmacokinetic comparison of four agents, *Scand J Clin Lab Invest,* Vol.48, No.3, pp. 247-253

Back, S.E., Masson, P. & Nilsson-Ehle, P. (1988c). A simple chemical method for the quantification of the contrast agent iohexol, applicable to glomerular filtration rate measurements, *Scand J Clin Lab Invest,* Vol.48, No.8, pp. 825-829

Back, S.E., Nilsson-Ehle, P. (1993). Re: Iohexol clearance for the determination of glomerular filtration rate in clinical practice: evidence for a new gold standard, *J Urol,* Vol.149, No.2, pp. 378

Bailey, R.R., Rogers, T.G. & Tait, J.J. (1970). Measurement of glomerular filtration rate using a single injection of 51Cr-Edetic acid, *Australas Ann Med,* Vol.19, No.3, pp. 255-258

Bajaj, G., Alexander, S.R., Browne, R., Sakarcan, A. & Seikaly, M.G. (1996). 125Iodine-iothalamate clearance in children. A simple method to measure glomerular filtration, *Pediatr Nephrol,* Vol.10, No.1, pp. 25-28

Bi, D., Leary, K.J., Weitz, J.A., Cherstniakova, S.A., Reil, M.A., Roy, M.J. & Cantilena, L.R. (2007). High performance liquid chromatographic measurement of iothalamate in human serum and urine for evaluation of glomerular filtration rate, *J Chromatogr B Analyt Technol Biomed Life Sci,* Vol.856, No.1-2, pp. 95-99

Biggi, A., Viglietti, A., Farinelli, M.C., Bonada, C. & Camuzzini, G. (1995). Estimation of glomerular filtration rate using chromium-51 ethylene diamine tetra-acetic acid and technetium-99m diethylene triamine penta-acetic acid, *Eur J Nucl Med,* Vol.22, No.6, pp. 532-536

Bird, N.J., Peters, C., Michell, A.R. & Peters, A.M. (2009). Comparison of GFR measurements assessed from single versus multiple samples, *Am J Kidney Dis,* Vol.54, No.2, pp. 278-288

Bland, J.M., Altman, D.G. (1986). Statistical methods for assessing agreement between two methods of clinical measurement, *Lancet,* Vol.1, No.8476, pp. 307-310

Blaufox, M.D., Cohen, A. (1970). Single-injection clearances of iothalamate-131-I in the rat, *Am J Physiol,* Vol.218, No.2, pp. 542-544

Boschi, S., Marchesini, B. (1981). High-performance liquid chromatographic method for the simultaneous determination of iothalamate and o-iodohippurate, *J Chromatogr,* Vol.224, No.1, pp. 139-143

Botev, R., Mallie, J.P., Wetzels, J.F., Couchoud, C. & Schuck, O. (2011). The Clinician and Estimation of Glomerular Filtration Rate by Creatinine-based Formulas: Current Limitations and Quo Vadis, *Clin J Am Soc Nephrol,* Vol.6, No.4, pp. 937-950

Brandstrom, E., Grzegorczyk, A., Jacobsson, L., Friberg, P., Lindahl, A. & Aurell, M. (1998). GFR measurement with iohexol and 51Cr-EDTA. A comparison of the two favoured GFR markers in Europe, *Nephrol Dial Transplant,* Vol.13, No.5, pp. 1176-1182

Brochner-Mortensen, J. (1973). The glomerular filtration rate during moderate hyperglycemia in normal man, *Acta Med Scand,* Vol.1-2, No.1, pp. 31-37

Brochner-Mortensen, J. (1978). Routine methods and their reliability for assessment of glomerular filtration rate in adults, with special reference to total [51Cr]EDTA plasma clearance, *Dan Med Bull,* Vol.25, No.5, pp. 181-202

Brochner-Mortensen, J., Giese, J. & Rossing, N. (1969). Renal inulin clearance versus total plasma clearance of 51Cr-EDTA, *Scand J Clin Lab Invest,* Vol.23, No.4, pp. 301-305

Brochner-Mortensen, J., Rodbro, P. (1976). Comparison between total and renal plasma clearance of [51Cr] EDTA, *Scand J Clin Lab Invest,* Vol.36, No.3, pp. 247-249

Brown, S.C., O'Reilly, P.H. (1991). Iohexol clearance for the determination of glomerular filtration rate in clinical practice: evidence for a new gold standard, *J Urol,* Vol.146, No.3, pp. 675-679

Burbank, M.K., Tauxe, W.N., Maher, F.T. & Hunt, J.C. (1963). Utilisation des substances marquées dans les épreuves classiques de clearance rénale, *J Physiol (Paris),* Vol.55, pp. 433-444

Cangiano, J.L., Genuth, S.M., Renerts, L. & Berman, L.B. (1971). Simplified measurement of glomerular filtration rate, *Invest Urol,* Vol.9, No.1, pp. 34-38

Carlsen, J.E., Moller, M.L., Lund, J.O. & Trap-Jensen, J. (1980). Comparison of four commercial Tc-99m(Sn)DTPA preparations used for the measurement of glomerular filtration rate: concise communication, *J Nucl Med,* Vol.21, No.2, pp. 126-129

Cavalier, E., Rozet, E., Dubois, N., Charlier, C., Hubert, P., Chapelle, J.P., Krzesinski, J.M. & Delanaye, P. (2008). Performance of iohexol determination in serum and urine by HPLC: Validation, risk and uncertainty assessment, *Clin Chim Acta,*

Chantler, C., Garnett, E.S., Parsons, V. & Veall, N. (1969). Glomerular filtration rate measurement in man by the single injection methods using 51Cr-EDTA, *Clin Sci,* Vol.37, No.1, pp. 169-180

Cockcroft, D.W., Gault, M.H. (1976). Prediction of creatinine clearance from serum creatinine, *Nephron,* Vol.16, No.1, pp. 31-41

Cohen, M.L., Smith, F.G., Jr., Mindell, R.S. & Vernier, R.L. (1969). A simple, reliable method of measuring glomerular filtration rate using single, low dose sodium iothalamate I-131, *Pediatrics,* Vol.43, No.3, pp. 407-415

Corcoran, A.C. (1952). III. Determination of inulin clearance, *Methods Med Res,* Vol.5, pp. 246-248

Dall'Amico, R., Montini, G., Pisanello, L., Piovesan, G., Bottaro, S., Cracco, A.T., Zacchello, G. & Zacchello, F. (1995). Determination of inulin in plasma and urine by reversed-phase high-performance liquid chromatography, *J Chromatogr B Biomed Appl,* Vol.672, No.1, pp. 155-159

Dalmeida, W., Suki, W.N. (1988). Measurement of GFR with non-radioisotopic radio contrast agents, *Kidney Int,* Vol.34, No.5, pp. 725-728

Day, D.F., Workman, W.E. (1984). A simple inulin assay for renal clearance determination using an immobilized beta-fructofuranosidase, *Ann N Y Acad Sci*, Vol.434, pp. 504-507

De Santo, N.G., Anastasio, P., Cirillo, M., Santoro, D., Spitali, L., Mansi, L., Celentano, L., Capodicasa, D., Cirillo, E., Del, V.E., Pascale, C. & Capasso, G. (1999). Measurement of glomerular filtration rate by the 99mTc-DTPA renogram is less precise than measured and predicted creatinine clearance, *Nephron*, Vol.81, No.2, pp. 136-140

Delanaye, P., Cohen, E.P. (2008). Formula-based estimates of the GFR: equations variable and uncertain, *Nephron Clin Pract*, Vol.110, No.1, pp. c48-c53

Delanaye, P., Mariat, C., Maillard, N., Krzesinski, J.M. & Cavalier, E. (2011a). Are the creatinine-based equations accurate to estimate glomerular filtration rate in african american populations?, *Clin J Am Soc Nephrol*, Vol.6, No.4, pp. 906-912

Delanaye, P., Souvignet, M., Dubourg, L., Thibaudin, L., Maillard, N., Krzesinski, J.M., Cavalier, E. & Mariat, C. (2011b). Le dosage de l'inuline: mise au point, *Ann Biol Clin (Paris)*, Vol.69, No.3, pp. 273-284

Delanghe, J., Bellon, J., De Buyzere, M., Van Daele, G. & Leroux-Roels, G. (1991). Elimination of glucose interference in enzymatic determination of inulin, *Clin Chem*, Vol.37, No.11, pp. 2017-2018

Denis, M.C., Venne, K., Lesiege, D., Francoeur, M., Groleau, S., Guay, M., Cusson, J. & Furtos, A. (2008). Development and evaluation of a liquid chromatography-mass spectrometry assay and its application for the assessment of renal function, *J Chromatogr A*, Vol.1189, No.1-2, pp. 410-416

Denneberg, T., Ek, J. & Hedenskog, I. (1961). Comparison of the renal excretion of I-131-labelled hypaque and inulin, *Acta Med Scand*, Vol.170, pp. 169-181

Ditzel, J., Vestergaard, P. & Brinklov, M. (1972). Glomerular filtration rate determined by 51 Cr-EDTA-complex. A practical method based upon the plasma disappearance curve determined from four plasma samples, *Scand J Urol Nephrol*, Vol.6, No.2, pp. 166-170

Dodge, W.F., Travis, L.B. & Daeschner, C.W. (1967). Comparison of endogenous creatinine clearance with inulin clearance, *Am J Dis Child*, Vol.113, No.6, pp. 683-692

Donaldson, I.M. (1968). Comparison of the renal clearances of inulin and radioactive diatrizoate ("Hypaque") as measures of the glomerular filtration rate in man, *Clin Sci*, Vol.35, No.3, pp. 513-524

Dowling, T.C., Frye, R.F., Fraley, D.S. & Matzke, G.R. (1999). Comparison of iothalamate clearance methods for measuring GFR, *Pharmacotherapy*, Vol.19, No.8, pp. 943-950

Dowling, T.C., Frye, R.F. & Zemaitis, M.A. (1998). Simultaneous determination of p-aminohippuric acid, acetyl-p-aminohippuric acid and iothalamate in human plasma and urine by high-performance liquid chromatography, *J Chromatogr B Biomed Sci Appl*, Vol.716, No.1-2, pp. 305-313

Downes, A.M., McDonald, I.W. (1964). The chromium-51 Complex of ethylenediaminetetraacetic acid as a soluble rumen marker, *Br J Nutr*, Vol.18, pp. 153-162

Dubourg, L., Hadj-Aissa, A. & Ferrier, B. (2010). Adaptation of an enzymatic polyfructosan assay to clinical practice, *Anal Biochem*,

Durand, E., Chaumet-Riffaud, P., Archambaud, F., Moati, F. & Prigent, A. (2006). Mesure de la fonction rénale par les méthodes radio-isotopiques, *EMC,* Vol.Néphrologie, No.18-010-A-10, pp. 1-15

Edelson, J., Shaw, D. & Palace, G. (1984). Pharmacokinetics of iohexol, a new nonionic radiocontrast agent, in humans, *J Pharm Sci,* Vol.73, No.7, pp. 993-995

Effersoe, H., Rosenkilde, P., Groth, S., Jensen, L.I. & Golman, K. (1990). Measurement of renal function with iohexol. A comparison of iohexol, 99mTc-DTPA, and 51Cr-EDTA clearance, *Invest Radiol,* Vol.25, No.7, pp. 778-782

Eide, I. (1970). Renal excretion of 51Cr-EDTA studied with stop flow technique, *Scand J Clin Lab Invest,* Vol.26, No.4, pp. 373-380

Elwood, C.M., Sigman, E.M. (1967). The measurement of glomerular filtration rate and effective renal plasma flow in man by iothalamate 125-I and iodopyracet 131-I, *Circulation,* Vol.36, No.3, pp. 441-448

Erley, C.M., Bader, B.D., Berger, E.D., Vochazer, A., Jorzik, J.J., Dietz, K. & Risler, T. (2001). Plasma clearance of iodine contrast media as a measure of glomerular filtration rate in critically ill patients, *Crit Care Med,* Vol.29, No.8, pp. 1544-1550

Farthing, D., Sica, D.A., Fakhry, I., Larus, T., Ghosh, S., Farthing, C., Vranian, M. & Gehr, T. (2005). Simple HPLC-UV method for determination of iohexol, iothalamate, p-aminohippuric acid and n-acetyl-p-aminohippuric acid in human plasma and urine with ERPF, GFR and ERPF/GFR ratio determination using colorimetric analysis, *J Chromatogr B Analyt Technol Biomed Life Sci,* Vol.826, No.1-2, pp. 267-272

Favre, H.R., Wing, A.J. (1968). Simultaneous 51Cr edetic acid, inulin, and endogenous creatinine clearances in 20 patients with renal disease, *Br Med J,* Vol.1, No.5584, pp. 84-86

Fawdry, R.M., Gruenewald, S.M., Collins, L.T. & Roberts, A.J. (1985). Comparative assessment of techniques for estimation of glomerular filtration rate with 99mTc-DTPA, *Eur J Nucl Med,* Vol.11, No.1, pp. 7-12

Fleming, J.S., Zivanovic, M.A., Blake, G.M., Burniston, M. & Cosgriff, P.S. (2004). Guidelines for the measurement of glomerular filtration rate using plasma sampling, *Nucl Med Commun,* Vol.25, No.8, pp. 759-769

Foreman, H., Trujillo, T.T. (1954). The metabolism of C14-labeled ethylenediaminetetraacetic acid in human beings, *J Lab Clin Med,* Vol.43, pp. 566-574

Forland, M., Pullman, T.N., Lavender, A.R. & Aho, I. (1966). The renal excretion of ethylenediaminetetraacetate in the dog, *J Pharmacol Exp Ther,* Vol.153, No.1, pp. 142-147

Frennby, B., Sterner, G., Almen, T., Hagstam, K.E., Hultberg, B. & Jacobsson, L. (1995). The use of iohexol clearance to determine GFR in patients with severe chronic renal failure--a comparison between different clearance techniques, *Clin Nephrol,* Vol.43, No.1, pp. 35-46

Frennby, B., Sterner, G., Almen, T., Hagstam, K.E. & Jacobsson, L. (1994). Determination of low glomerular filtration rate using iohexol clearance, *Invest Radiol,* Vol.29 Suppl 2, pp. S234-S235

Friedman, A.N., Strother, M., Quinney, S.K., Hall, S., Perkins, S.M., Brizendine, E.J., Inman, M., Gomez, G., Shihabi, Z., Moe, S. & Li, L. (2010). Measuring the glomerular filtration rate in obese individuals without overt kidney disease, *Nephron Clin Pract,* Vol.116, No.3, pp. c224-c234

Froissart, M., Rossert, J., Jacquot, C., Paillard, M. & Houillier, P. (2005a). Predictive performance of the modification of diet in renal disease and Cockcroft-Gault equations for estimating renal function, *J Am Soc Nephrol,* Vol.16, No.3, pp. 763-773

Froissart, M.C., Rossert, J. & Houillier, P. (2005b). The new Mayo Clinic equation for estimating glomerular filtration rate, *Ann Intern Med,* Vol.142, No.8, pp. 679

Gagnon, J.A., Schrier, R.W., Weis, T.P., Kokotis, W. & Mailloux, L.U. (1971). Clearance of iothalamate-125 I as a measure of glomerular filtration rate in the dog, *J Appl Physiol,* Vol.30, No.5, pp. 774-778

Galli, G., Rufini, V., Meduri, G., Piraccini, R. & D'Andrea, G. (1994). Determination of glomerular filtration rate with 99mTc-DTPA in clinical practice, *J Nucl Biol Med,* Vol.38, No.4, pp. 556-565

Garnett, E.S., Parsons, V. & Veall, N. (1967). Measurement of glomerular filtration-rate in man using a 51Cr-edetic-acid complex, *Lancet,* Vol.1, No.7494, pp. 818-819

Gaspari, F., Mainardi, L., Ruggenenti, P. & Remuzzi, G. (1991). High-performance liquid chromatographic determination of iothalamic acid in human plasma and urine, *J Chromatogr,* Vol.570, No.2, pp. 435-440

Gaspari, F., Mosconi, L., Vigano, G., Perico, N., Torre, L., Virotta, G., Bertocchi, C., Remuzzi, G. & Ruggenenti, P. (1992). Measurement of GFR with a single intravenous injection of nonradioactive iothalamate, *Kidney Int,* Vol.41, No.4, pp. 1081-1084

Gaspari, F., Perico, N. & Remuzzi, G. (1997). Measurement of glomerular filtration rate, *Kidney Int Suppl,* Vol.63, pp. S151-S154

Gaspari, F., Perico, N., Ruggenenti, P., Mosconi, L., Amuchastegui, C.S., Guerini, E., Daina, E. & Remuzzi, G. (1995). Plasma clearance of nonradioactive iohexol as a measure of glomerular filtration rate, *J Am Soc Nephrol,* Vol.6, No.2, pp. 257-263

Gates, G.F. (1984). Computation of glomerular filtration rate with Tc-99m DTPA: an in-house computer program, *J Nucl Med,* Vol.25, No.5, pp. 613-618

Ginjaume, M., Casey, M., Barker, F. & Duffy, G. (1985). Measurement of glomerular filtration rate using technetium-99m DTPA, *J Nucl Med,* Vol.26, No.11, pp. 1347-1349

Goates, J.J., Morton, K.A., Whooten, W.W., Greenberg, H.E., Datz, F.L., Handy, J.E., Scuderi, A.J., Haakenstad, A.O. & Lynch, R.E. (1990). Comparison of methods for calculating glomerular filtration rate: technetium-99m-DTPA scintigraphic analysis, protein-free and whole-plasma clearance of technetium-99m-DTPA and iodine-125-iothalamate clearance, *J Nucl Med,* Vol.31, No.4, pp. 424-429

Griep, R.J., Nelp, W.B. (1969). Mechanism of excretion of radioiodinated sodium iothalamate, *Radiology,* Vol.93, No.4, pp. 807-811

Griffiths, P.D., Drolc, Z., Green, A., Taylor, C.M. & White, R.H. (1988). Comparison of 51Cr-EDTA and 99mTc-DTPA slope clearances in children with vesicoureteric reflux, *Child Nephrol Urol,* Vol.9, No.5, pp. 283-285

Guesry, P., Kaufman, L., Orloff, S., Nelson, J.A., Swann, S. & Holliday, M. (1975). Measurement of glomerular filtration rate by fluorescent excitation of non-radioactive meglumine iothalamate, *Clin Nephrol,* Vol.3, No.4, pp. 134-138

Gunasekera, R.D., Allison, D.J. & Peters, A.M. (1996). Glomerular filtration rate in relation to extracellular fluid volume: similarity between 99mTc-DTPA and inulin, *Eur J Nucl Med,* Vol.23, No.1, pp. 49-54

Gutman, Y., Gottschalk, C. & Lassiter, W.E. (1965). Micropuncture study of inulin absorption in the rat kidney, *Science*, Vol.147, pp. 753-754

Hagstam, K.E., Nordenfelt, I., Svensson, L. & Svensson, S.E. (1974). Comparison of different methods for determination of glomerular filtration rate in renal disease, *Scand J Clin Lab Invest*, Vol.34, No.1, pp. 31-36

Hall, P.M., Rolin, H. (1995). Iothalamate clearance and its use in large-scale clinical trials, *Curr Opin Nephrol Hypertens*, Vol.4, No.6, pp. 510-513

Handelsman, M.B., Sass, M. (1956). The use of capillary blood for estimating renal clearance of inulin and glucose excretion by means of an anthrone procedure, *J Lab Clin Med*, Vol.48, No.5, pp. 759-768

Harrow, B.R. (1956). Experiences in intravenous urography using hypaque, *Am J Roentgenol Radium Ther Nucl Med*, Vol.75, No.5, pp. 870-876

Hauser, W., Atkins, H.L., Nelson, K.G. & Richards, P. (1970). Technetium-99m DTPA: a new radiopharmaceutical for brain and kidney scanning, *Radiology*, Vol.94, No.3, pp. 679-684

Heath, D.A., Knapp, M.S. & Walker, W.H. (1968). Comparison between inulin and 51Cr-labelled edetic acid for the measurement of glomerular filtration-rate, *Lancet*, Vol.2, No.7578, pp. 1110-1112

Hendrix, J.P., Westfall, B.B. & Richards, A.N. (1937). Quantitative studies of the composition of glomerular urine. The glomerular excretion of inulin in frogs and Necturi, *J Biol Chem*, Vol.116, No.2, pp. 735-747

Heron, C.W., Underwood, S.R. & Dawson, P. (1984). Electrocardiographic changes during intravenous urography: a study with sodium iothalamate and iohexol, *Clin Radiol*, Vol.35, No.2, pp. 137-141

Heyrovsky, A. (1956). A new method for determination of inulin in plasma and urine, *Clin Chim Acta*, Vol.1, No.5, pp. 470-474

Hilson, A.J., Mistry, R.D. & Maisey, M.N. (1976). 99Tcm-DTPA for the measurement of glomerular filtration rate, *Br J Radiol*, Vol.49, No.585, pp. 794-796

Höber, R. (1930). Beweis selektiver Sekretion durch die Tubulusepithelien der Niere, *Arch f d ges Physiol*, Vol.224, pp. 72

Houlihan, C., Jenkins, M., Osicka, T., Scott, A., Parkin, D. & Jerums, G. (1999). A comparison of the plasma disappearance of iohexol and 99mTc-DTPA for the measurement of glomerular filtration rate (GFR) in diabetes, *Aust N Z J Med*, Vol.29, No.5, pp. 693-700

Hubbard, R.S., Loomis, T.A. (1942). The determination of inuline, *J Biol Chem*, Vol.145, pp. 641-645

Isaka, Y., Fujiwara, Y., Yamamoto, S., Ochi, S., Shin, S., Inoue, T., Tagawa, K., Kamada, T. & Ueda, N. (1992). Modified plasma clearance technique using nonradioactive iothalamate for measuring GFR, *Kidney Int*, Vol.42, No.4, pp. 1006-1011

Israelit, A.H., Long, D.L., White, M.G. & Hull, A.R. (1973). Measurement of glomerular filtration rate utilizing a single subcutaneous injection of 125I-iothalamate, *Kidney Int*, Vol.4, No.5, pp. 346-349

Jagenburg, R., Attman, P.O., Aurell, M. & Bucht, H. (1978). Determination of glomerular filtration rate in advanced renal insufficiency, *Scand J Urol Nephrol*, Vol.12, No.2, pp. 133-137

Jeghers, O., Piepsz, A. & Ham, H.R. (1990). What does protein binding of radiopharmaceuticals mean exactly?, *Eur J Nucl Med,* Vol.17, No.3-4, pp. 101-102

Johansson, R.S., Falch, D.K. (1978). 113mIn-DTPA, a useful compound for the determination of glomerular filtration rate (GFR). The binding of 113mIn to DTPA and a comparison between GFR estimated with 113mIn-DTPA and 125I-iothalamate, *Eur J Nucl Med,* Vol.3, No.3, pp. 179-181

Jung, K., Klotzek, S. & Schulze, B.D. (1990). Refinements of assays for low concentrations of inulin in serum, *Nephron,* Vol.54, No.4, pp. 360-361

Kainer, G., McIlveen, B., Hoschl, R. & Rosenberg, A.R. (1979). Assessment of individual renal function in children using 99mTc-DTPA, *Arch Dis Child,* Vol.54, No.12, pp. 931-936

Kempi, V., Persson, R.B. (1975). 99mTc-DTPA(Sn) dry-kit preparation. Quality control and clearance studies, *Nucl Med (Stuttg),* Vol.13, No.4, pp. 389-399

Klopper, J.F., Hauser, W., Atkins, H.L., Eckelman, W.C. & Richards, P. (1972). Evaluation of 99m Tc-DTPA for the measurement of glomerular filtration rate, *J Nucl Med,* Vol.13, No.1, pp. 107-110

Kos, T., Moser, P., Yilmatz, N., Mayer, G., Pacher, R. & Hallstrom, S. (2000). High-performance liquid chromatographic determination of p-aminohippuric acid and iothalamate in human serum and urine: comparison of two sample preparation methods, *J Chromatogr B Biomed Sci Appl,* Vol.740, No.1, pp. 81-85

Krutzen, E., Back, S.E., Nilsson-Ehle, I. & Nilsson-Ehle, P. (1984). Plasma clearance of a new contrast agent, iohexol: a method for the assessment of glomerular filtration rate, *J Lab Clin Med,* Vol.104, No.6, pp. 955-961

Krutzen, E., Back, S.E. & Nilsson-Ehle, P. (1990). Determination of glomerular filtration rate using iohexol clearance and capillary sampling, *Scand J Clin Lab Invest,* Vol.50, No.3, pp. 279-283

Kuehnle, H.F., von Dahl, K. & Schmidt, F.H. (1992). Fully enzymatic inulin determination in small volume samples without deproteinization, *Nephron,* Vol.62, No.1, pp. 104-107

Kwong, Y.T., Stevens, L.A., Selvin, E., Zhang, Y.L., Greene, T., Van, L.F., Levey, A.S. & Coresh, J. (2010). Imprecision of urinary iothalamate clearance as a gold-standard measure of GFR decreases the diagnostic accuracy of kidney function estimating equations, *Am J Kidney Dis,* Vol.56, No.1, pp. 39-49

Laake, H. (1954). Inulin clearance studies; concerning the cause of the reduced clearance figures in successive periods after one injection of inulin, *Acta Med Scand,* Vol.148, No.2, pp. 135-146

Ladegaard-Pedersen, H.J. (1972). Measurement of extracellular volume and renal clearance by a single injection of inulin, *Scand J Clin Lab Invest,* Vol.29, No.2, pp. 145-153

LaFrance, N.D., Drew, H.H. & Walser, M. (1988). Radioisotopic measurement of glomerular filtration rate in severe chronic renal failure, *J Nucl Med,* Vol.29, No.12, pp. 1927-1930

Lavender, S., Hilton, P.J. & Jones, N.F. (1969). The measurement of glomerular filtration-rate in renal disease, *Lancet,* Vol.2, No.7632, pp. 1216-1218

Lee, S.Y., Chun, M.R., Kim, D.J. & Kim, J.W. (2006). Determination of iohexol clearance by high-performance liquid chromatography-tandem mass spectrometry (HPLC-MS/MS), *J Chromatogr B Analyt Technol Biomed Life Sci,* Vol.839, No.1-2, pp. 124-129

Lentjes, E.G., Florijn, K.W., Chang, P.C. & van Dam, W. (1994). Inulin measurement in serum and urine with an autoanalyser, corrected for glucose interference, *Eur J Clin Chem Clin Biochem,* Vol.32, No.8, pp. 625-628

Levey, A.S., Bosch, J.P., Lewis, J.B., Greene, T., Rogers, N. & Roth, D. (1999). A more accurate method to estimate glomerular filtration rate from serum creatinine: a new prediction equation. Modification of Diet in Renal Disease Study Group, *Ann Intern Med,* Vol.130, No.6, pp. 461-470

Levey, A.S., Coresh, J., Greene, T., Stevens, L.A., Zhang, Y.L., Hendriksen, S., Kusek, J.W. & Van Lente, F. (2006). Using standardized serum creatinine values in the modification of diet in renal disease study equation for estimating glomerular filtration rate, *Ann Intern Med,* Vol.145, No.4, pp. 247-254

Levey AS, Madaio MP, Perrone RD 1991: Laboratory assessment of renal disease: clearance, urinalysis, and renal biopsy. In: Brenner BM, Rector FC (eds): The kidney. W.B. Saunders Company, Philadelphia, pp. 919-968

Levey, A.S., Stevens, L.A., Schmid, C.H., Zhang, Y.L., Castro, A.F., III, Feldman, H.I., Kusek, J.W., Eggers, P., Van Lente, F., Greene, T. & Coresh, J. (2009). A new equation to estimate glomerular filtration rate, *Ann Intern Med,* Vol.150, No.9, pp. 604-612

Lewis, R., Kerr, N., Van Buren, C., Lowry, P., Sandler, C., Frazier, O.H., Powers, P., Herson, J., Corriere, J., Jr., Kerman, R. & . (1989). Comparative evaluation of urographic contrast media, inulin, and 99mTc-DTPA clearance methods for determination of glomerular filtration rate in clinical transplantation, *Transplantation,* Vol.48, No.5, pp. 790-796

Lingardh, G. (1972). Renal clearance investigations with 51 Cr-EDTA and 125 I-hippuran, *Scand J Urol Nephrol,* Vol.6, No.1, pp. 63-71

Little, J.M. (1949). A modified diphenylamine procedure for the determination of inulin, *J Biol Chem,* Vol.180, No.2, pp. 747-754

Lundqvist, S., Hietala, S.O., Berglund, C. & Karp, K. (1994). Simultaneous urography and determination of glomerular filtration rate. A comparison of total plasma clearances of iohexol and 51Cr-EDTA in plegic patients, *Acta Radiol,* Vol.35, No.4, pp. 391-395

Lundqvist, S., Hietala, S.O., Groth, S. & Sjodin, J.G. (1997). Evaluation of single sample clearance calculations in 902 patients. A comparison of multiple and single sample techniques, *Acta Radiol,* Vol.38, No.1, pp. 68-72

Ma, Y.C., Zuo, L., Zhang, C.L., Wang, M., Wang, R.F. & Wang, H.Y. (2007). Comparison of 99mTc-DTPA renal dynamic imaging with modified MDRD equation for glomerular filtration rate estimation in Chinese patients in different stages of chronic kidney disease, *Nephrol Dial Transplant,* Vol.22, No.2, pp. 417-423

Mafham, M.M., Niculescu-Duvaz, I., Barron, J., Emberson, J.R., Dockrell, M.E., Landray, M.J. & Baigent, C. (2007). A practical method of measuring glomerular filtration rate by iohexol clearance using dried capillary blood spots, *Nephron Clin Pract,* Vol.106, No.3, pp. c104-c112

Maher, F.T., Nolan, N.G. & Elveback, L.R. (1971). Comparison of simultaneous clearances of 125-I-labeled sodium lothalamate (Glofil) and of inulin, *Mayo Clin Proc,* Vol.46, No.10, pp. 690-691

Maher, F.T., Tauxe, W.N. (1969). Renal clearance in man of pharmaceuticals containing radioactive iodine, *JAMA,* Vol.207, No.1, pp. 97-104

Malamos, B., Dontas, A.S., Koutras, D.A., Marketos, S., Sfontouris, J. & Papanicolaou, N. (1967). 125I-sodium iothalamate in the determination of the glomerular filtration rate, *Nucl Med (Stuttg)*, Vol.6, No.3, pp. 304-310

McChesney, E.W., Hoppe, J.O. (1957). Studies of the tissue distribution and excretion of sodium diatrizoate in laboratory animals, *Am J Roentgenol Radium Ther Nucl Med*, Vol.78, No.1, pp. 137-144

Medeiros, F.S., Sapienza, M.T., Prado, E.S., Agena, F., Shimizu, M.H., Lemos, F.B., Buchpiguel, C.A., Ianhez, L.E. & David-Neto, E. (2009). Validation of plasma clearance of 51Cr-EDTA in adult renal transplant recipients: comparison with inulin renal clearance, *Transpl Int*, Vol.22, No.3, pp. 323-331

Meschan, I., Deyton, W.E., Schmid, H.E. & Watts, F.C. (1963). The utilization of I 131-labeled renografin as an inulin substitute for renal clearance rate determination, *Radiology*, Vol.81, pp. 974-979

Mirouze, J., Barjon, P., Monnier, L. & Mimran, A. (1972). Détermination de la filtration glomérulaire par l'iothalamate radioactif: comparaison des méthodes par perfusion continue et injection unique rapide, *Vie Med Can Fr*, Vol.1, No.9, pp. 837-841

Möller, E., McIntosh, J.F. & Van Slycke, D.D. (1929). Studies of urea excretion. II. Relationship between urine volume and the rate of urea excretion by normal adults, *J Clin Invest*, Vol.6, No.3, pp. 427-465

Morgan, D.B., Dillon, S. & Payne, R.B. (1978). The assessment of glomerular function: creatinine clearance or plasma creatinine?, *Postgrad Med J*, Vol.54, No.631, pp. 302-310

Morris, A.M., Elwood, C., Sigman, E.M. & Catanzaro, A. (1965). The renal clearance of 131-I labeled meglumine diatrizoate (renografin) in man, *J Nucl Med*, Vol.6, pp. 183-191

Mulligan, J.S., Blue, P.W. & Hasbargen, J.A. (1990). Methods for measuring GFR with technetium-99m-DTPA: an analysis of several common methods, *J Nucl Med*, Vol.31, No.7, pp. 1211-1219

Mutzel, W., Siefert, H.M. & Speck, U. (1980). Biochemical-pharmacologic properties of iohexol, *Acta Radiol Suppl*, Vol.362, pp. 111-115

Niculescu-Duvaz, I., D'Mello, L., Maan, Z., Barron, J.L., Newman, D.J., Dockrell, M.E. & Kwan, J.T. (2006). Development of an outpatient finger-prick glomerular filtration rate procedure suitable for epidemiological studies, *Kidney Int*, Vol.69, No.7, pp. 1272-1275

Nilsson-Ehle, P. (2002). Iohexol clearance for the determination of glomerular filtration rate: 15 years' experience in clinical practice, *eJIFCC*, Vol.13, No.2,

Nilsson-Ehle, P., Grubb, A. (1994). New markers for the determination of GFR: iohexol clearance and cystatin C serum concentration, *Kidney Int Suppl*, Vol.47, pp. S17-S19

Nossen, J.O., Jakobsen, J.A., Kjaersgaard, P., Andrew, E., Jacobsen, P.B. & Berg, K.J. (1995). Elimination of the non-ionic X-ray contrast media iodixanol and iohexol in patients with severely impaired renal function, *Scand J Clin Lab Invest*, Vol.55, No.4, pp. 341-350

Nosslin, B. (1965). Determination of clearance and distribution volume with the single injection method, *Acta Med Scand Suppl*, Vol.442, pp. 97-101

Notghi, A., Merrick, M.V., Ferrington, C. & Anderton, J.L. (1986). A comparison of simplified and standard methods for the measurement of glomerular filtration rate and renal tubular function, *Br J Radiol*, Vol.59, No.697, pp. 35-39

O'Reilly, P.H., Brooman, P.J., Martin, P.J., Pollard, A.J., Farah, N.B. & Mason, G.C. (1986). Accuracy and reproducibility of a new contrast clearance method for the determination of glomerular filtration rate, *Br Med J (Clin Res Ed),* Vol.293, No.6541, pp. 234-236

O'Reilly, P.H., Jones, D.A. & Farah, N.B. (1988). Measurement of the plasma clearance of urographic contrast media for the determination of glomerular filtration rate, *J Urol,* Vol.139, No.1, pp. 9-11

Odlind, B., Hallgren, R., Sohtell, M. & Lindstrom, B. (1985). Is 125I iothalamate an ideal marker for glomerular filtration?, *Kidney Int,* Vol.27, No.1, pp. 9-16

Olofsson, P., Krutzen, E. & Nilsson-Ehle, P. (1996). Iohexol clearance for assessment of glomerular filtration rate in diabetic pregnancy, *Eur J Obstet Gynecol Reprod Biol,* Vol.64, No.1, pp. 63-67

Olsson, B., Aulie, A., Sveen, K. & Andrew, E. (1983). Human pharmacokinetics of iohexol. A new nonionic contrast medium, *Invest Radiol,* Vol.18, No.2, pp. 177-182

Ott, N.T. (1975). A simple technique for estimating glomerular filtration rate with subcutaneous injection of (125I)lothalamate, *Mayo Clin Proc,* Vol.50, No.11, pp. 664-668

Owen, J.E., Walker, R.G., Willems, D., Guignard, P.A. & d'Apice, A.J. (1982). Cadmium telluride detectors in the external measurement of glomerular filtration rate using 99mTc-DTPA (Sn): comparison with 51Cr-EDTA and 99mTc-DTPA (Sn) plasma sample methods, *Clin Nephrol,* Vol.18, No.4, pp. 200-203

Owman, T., Olin, T. (1978). Biliary excretion of urographic contrast media (iothalamate, diatrizoate, P 286 and metrizamide), *Ann Radiol (Paris),* Vol.21, No.4-5, pp. 309-314

Pastore, A., Bernardini, S., Dello, S.L., Rizzoni, G., Cortese, C. & Federici, G. (2001). Simultaneous determination of inulin and p-aminohippuric acid in plasma and urine by reversed-phase high-performance liquid chromatography, *J Chromatogr B Biomed Sci Appl,* Vol.751, No.1, pp. 187-191

Perrone, R.D., Steinman, T.I., Beck, G.J., Skibinski, C.I., Royal, H.D., Lawlor, M. & Hunsicker, L.G. (1990). Utility of radioisotopic filtration markers in chronic renal insufficiency: simultaneous comparison of 125I-iothalamate, 169Yb-DTPA, 99mTc-DTPA, and inulin. The Modification of Diet in Renal Disease Study, *Am J Kidney Dis,* Vol.16, No.3, pp. 224-235

Petri, M., Bockenstedt, L., Colman, J., Whiting-O'Keefe, Q., Fitz, G., Sebastian, A. & Hellmann, D. (1988). Serial assessment of glomerular filtration rate in lupus nephropathy, *Kidney Int,* Vol.34, No.6, pp. 832-839

Piepsz, A., Erbsmann, F., Vainsel, M. & Cantraine, F. (1974). Determination of glomerular filtration rate in children by external measurement of the disappearance of 113m-indium-DTPA in plasma, *Biomedicine,* Vol.20, No.3, pp. 192-197

Prueksaritanont, T., Chen, M.L. & Chiou, W.L. (1984). Simple and micro high-performance liquid chromatographic method for simultaneous determination of p-aminohippuric acid and iothalamate in biological fluids, *J Chromatogr,* Vol.306, pp. 89-97

Prueksaritanont, T., Lui, C.Y., Lee, M.G. & Chiou, W.L. (1986). Renal and non-renal clearances of iothalamate, *Biopharm Drug Dispos,* Vol.7, No.4, pp. 347-355

Pucci, L., Bandinelli, S., Penno, G., Nannipieri, M., Rizzo, L. & Navalesi, R. (1998). Iohexol plasma clearance in determining glomerular filtration rate in diabetic patients, *Ren Fail,* Vol.20, No.2, pp. 277-284

Pucci, L., Bandinelli, S., Pilo, M., Nannipieri, M., Navalesi, R. & Penno, G. (2001). Iohexol as a marker of glomerular filtration rate in patients with diabetes: comparison of multiple and simplified sampling protocols, *Diabet Med,* Vol.18, No.2, pp. 116-120

Reba, R.C., Hosain, F. & Wagner, H.N., Jr. (1968). Indium-113m diethylenetriaminepentaacetic acid (DTPA): a new radiopharmaceutical for study of the kidneys, *Radiology,* Vol.90, No.1, pp. 147-149

Rehberg, P.B. (1926a). Studies on Kidney Function: The Excretion of urea and chlorine analysed according to a modified filtration-reabsorption theory, *Biochem J,* Vol.20, No.3, pp. 461-482

Rehberg, P.B. (1926b). Studies on Kidney Function: The Rate of Filtration and Reabsorption in the Human Kidney, *Biochem J,* Vol.20, No.3, pp. 447-460

Rehling, M., Moller, M.L., Thamdrup, B., Lund, J.O. & Trap-Jensen, J. (1984). Simultaneous measurement of renal clearance and plasma clearance of 99mTc-labelled diethylenetriaminepenta-acetate, 51Cr-labelled ethylenediaminetetra-acetate and inulin in man, *Clin Sci (Lond),* Vol.66, No.5, pp. 613-619

Rehling, M., Moller, M.L., Thamdrup, B., Lund, J.O. & Trap-Jensen, J. (1986). Reliability of a 99mTc-DTPA gamma camera technique for determination of single kidney glomerular filtration rate. A comparison to plasma clearance of 51Cr-EDTA in one-kidney patients, using the renal clearance of inulin as a reference, *Scand J Urol Nephrol,* Vol.20, No.1, pp. 57-62

Rehling, M., Nielsen, B.V., Pedersen, E.B., Nielsen, L.E., Hansen, H.E. & Bacher, T. (1995). Renal and extrarenal clearance of 99mTc-MAG3: a comparison with 125I-OIH and 51Cr-EDTA in patients representing all levels of glomerular filtration rate, *Eur J Nucl Med,* Vol.22, No.12, pp. 1379-1384

Rehling, M., Nielsen, L.E. & Marqversen, J. (2001). Protein binding of 99Tcm-DTPA compared with other GFR tracers, *Nucl Med Commun,* Vol.22, No.6, pp. 617-623

Reidenberg, M.M., Lorenzo, B.J., Drayer, D.E., Kluger, J., Nestor, T., Regnier, J.C., Kowal, B.A. & Bekersky, I. (1988). A nonradioactive iothalamate method for measuring glomerular filtration rate and its use to study the renal handling of cibenzoline, *Ther Drug Monit,* Vol.10, No.4, pp. 434-437

Richards, A.N., Westfall, B.B. & Bott, P.A. (1934). Renal excretion of inulin, creatinine, and xylose in normal dogs., *Proc Soc Exp Biol Med,* Vol.32, pp. 73

Robson, J.S., Ferguson, M.H., Olbrich, O. & Stewart, C.P. (1949). The determination of the renal clearance of inulin in man, *Q J Exp Physiol,* Vol.35, No.2, pp. 111-134

Rodby, R.A., Ali, A., Rohde, R.D. & Lewis, E.J. (1992). Renal scanning 99mTc diethylene-triamine pentaacetic acid glomerular filtration rate (GFR) determination compared with iothalamate clearance GFR in diabetics. The Collaborative Study Group for The study of Angiotensin-Converting Enzyme Inhibition in Diabetic Nephropathy, *Am J Kidney Dis,* Vol.20, No.6, pp. 569-573

Roe, J.H. (1934). A colorimetric method for the determination of fructose in blood and urine, *J Biol Chem,* Vol.107, No.1, pp. 15-21

Rolf, D., Surtshin, A. & White, H.L. (1949). A modified diphenylamine procedure for fructose or inulin determination, *Proc Soc Exp Biol Med,* Vol.72, No.2, pp. 351-354

Rootwelt, K., Falch, D. & Sjokvist, R. (1980). Determination of glomerular filtration rate (GFR) by analysis of capillary blood after single shot injection of 99mTc-DTPA. A comparison with simultaneous 125I-iothalamate GFR estimation showing equal GFR but difference in distribution volume, *Eur J Nucl Med,* Vol.5, No.2, pp. 97-102

Rosenbaum, R.W., Hruska, K.A., Anderson, C., Robson, A.M., Slatopolsky, E. & Klahr, S. (1979). Inulin: an inadequate marker of glomerular filtration rate in kidney donors and transplant recipients?, *Kidney Int,* Vol.16, No.2, pp. 179-186

Ruo, T.I., Wang, Z., Dordal, M.S. & Atkinson, A.J., Jr. (1991). Assay of inulin in biological fluids by high-performance liquid chromatography with pulsed amperometric detection, *Clin Chim Acta,* Vol.204, No.1-3, pp. 217-222

Russell, C.D. (1987). Estimation of glomerular filtration rate using 99mTc-DTPA and the gamma camera, *Eur J Nucl Med,* Vol.12, No.11, pp. 548-552

Russell, C.D., Bischoff, P.G., Kontzen, F., Rowell, K.L., Yester, M.V., Lloyd, L.K., Tauxe, W.N. & Dubovsky, E.V. (1985). Measurement of glomerular filtration rate using 99mTc-DTPA and the gamma camera: a comparison of methods, *Eur J Nucl Med,* Vol.10, No.11-12, pp. 519-521

Russell, C.D., Bischoff, P.G., Rowell, K.L., Kontzen, F., Lloyd, L.K., Tauxe, W.N. & Dubovsky, E.V. (1983). Quality control of Tc-99m DTPA for measurement of glomerular filtration: concise communication, *J Nucl Med,* Vol.24, No.8, pp. 722-727

Sambataro, M., Thomaseth, K., Pacini, G., Robaudo, C., Carraro, A., Bruseghin, M., Brocco, E., Abaterusso, C., DeFerrari, G., Fioretto, P., Maioli, M., Tonolo, G.C., Crepaldi, G. & Nosadini, R. (1996). Plasma clearance rate of 51Cr-EDTA provides a precise and convenient technique for measurement of glomerular filtration rate in diabetic humans, *J Am Soc Nephrol,* Vol.7, No.1, pp. 118-127

Schanker, L.S., Hogben, C.A. (1961). Biliary excretion of inulin, sucrose, and mannitol: analysis of bile formation, *Am J Physiol,* Vol.200, pp. 1087-1090

Schwartz, G.J., Furth, S., Cole, S.R., Warady, B. & Munoz, A. (2006). Glomerular filtration rate via plasma iohexol disappearance: pilot study for chronic kidney disease in children, *Kidney Int,* Vol.69, No.11, pp. 2070-2077

Seegmiller, J.C., Burns, B.E., Fauq, A.H., Mukhtar, N., Lieske, J.C. & Larson, T.S. (2010). Iothalamate quantification by tandem mass spectrometry to measure glomerular filtration rate, *Clin Chem,* Vol.56, No.4, pp. 568-574

Shaffer, P.A., Somogoyi, M. (1933). Copper-iodometric reagents for sugar determination, *J Biol Chem,* Vol.100, pp. 695-713

Shannon, J.A. (1934). The excretion of inulin by the dogfish, *Squalus acanthias, J Cell and Comp Physiol,* Vol.5, No.3, pp. 301-310

Shannon, J.A., Smith, H.W. (1935). The excretion of inulin, xylose, and urea by normal and phorizinized man, *J Clin Invest,* Vol.14, No.4, pp. 393-401

Sharma, A.K., Mills, M.S., Grey, V.L. & Drummond, K.N. (1997). Infusion clearance of subcutaneous iothalamate versus standard renal clearance, *Pediatr Nephrol,* Vol.11, No.6, pp. 711-713

Shemesh, O., Golbetz, H., Kriss, J.P. & Myers, B.D. (1985). Limitations of creatinine as a filtration marker in glomerulopathic patients, *Kidney Int,* Vol.28, No.5, pp. 830-838

Shihabi, Z.K., Constantinescu, M.S. (1992). Iohexol in serum determined by capillary electrophoresis, *Clin Chem,* Vol.38, No.10, pp. 2117-2120

Sigman, E.M., Elwood, C., Reagan, M.E., MorrisS, A.M. & Catanzaro, A. (1965a). The renal clearance of of I-131 labelled iothalamate in man, *Invest Urol,* Vol.2, pp. 432-438

Sigman, E.M., Elwood, C.M. & Knox, F. (1965b). The measurement of glomerular filtration rate in man with sodium iothalamate 131-I (Conray), *J Nucl Med,* Vol.7, No.1, pp. 60-68

Skluzacek, P.A., Szewc, R.G., Nolan, C.R., III, Riley, D.J., Lee, S. & Pergola, P.E. (2003). Prediction of GFR in liver transplant candidates, *Am J Kidney Dis,* Vol.42, No.6, pp. 1169-1176

Skov, P.E. (1970). Glomerular filtration rate in patients with severe and very severe renal insufficiency. Determined by simultaneous inulin, creatinine and 125 iothalamate clearance, *Acta Med Scand,* Vol.187, No.5, pp. 419-428

Smith HW 1951a: Measurement of the filtration rate. The kidney: Structure and function in health and disease. Oxford University Press Inc, New York, pp. 39-62

Smith HW 1951b The kidney: Structure and function in health and disease. Oxford University Press Inc, New York

Smith HW 1951c: The reliability of inulin as a measure of glomerular filtration. The kidney: Structure and function in health and disease. Oxford University Press Inc, New York, pp. 231-238

Spencer, H., Samachson, J. & Laszlo, D. (1958). Effects of ethylenediaminetetraacetic acid on radiostrontium excretion in man, *Proc Soc Exp Biol Med,* Vol.97, pp. 565-567

Stacy, B.D., Thorburn, G.D. (1966). Chromium-51 ethylenediaminetetraacetate for estimation of globerular filtration rate, *Science,* Vol.152, No.725, pp. 1076-1077

Stamp, T.C., Stacey, T.E. & Rose, G.A. (1970). Comparison of glomerular filtration rate measurements using inulin, 51CrEDTA, and a phosphate infusion technique, *Clin Chim Acta,* Vol.30, No.2, pp. 351-358

Steinitz, K. (1938). A colorimetric method for the determination of inulin in blood plasma and urine, *J Biol Chem,* Vol.126, No.2, pp. 589-593

Sterner, G., Frennby, B., Mansson, S., Nyman, U., van Westen, D. & Almen, T. (2008). Determining 'true' glomerular filtration rate in healthy adults using infusion of inulin and comparing it with values obtained using other clearance techniques or prediction equations, *Scand J Urol Nephrol,* Vol.42, No.3, pp. 278-285

Stevens, L.A., Levey, A.S. (2009). Measured GFR as a confirmatory test for estimated GFR, *J Am Soc Nephrol,* Vol.20, No.11, pp. 2305-2313

Stokes, J.M., Conklin, J.W. & Huntley, H.C. (1962). Measurement of glomerular filtration rate by contrast media containing I-131 isotopes, *J Urol,* Vol.87, pp. 630-633

Stolz, A., Hoizey, G., Toupance, O., Lavaud, S., Vitry, F., Chanard, J. & Rieu, P. (2010). Evaluation of sample bias for measuring plasma iohexol clearance in kidney transplantation, *Transplantation,* Vol.89, No.4, pp. 440-445

Summerfield, A.L., Hortin, G.L., Smith, C.H., Wilhite, T.R. & Landt, M. (1993). Automated enzymatic analysis of inulin, *Clin Chem,* Vol.39, No.11 Pt 1, pp. 2333-2337

Tepe, P.G., Tauxe, W.N., Bagchi, A., Rezende, P. & Krishnaiah, P.R. (1987). Comparison of measurement of glomerular filtration rate by single sample, plasma disappearance slope/intercept and other methods, *Eur J Nucl Med,* Vol.13, No.1, pp. 28-31

Tessitore, N., Lo, S.C., Corgnati, A., Previato, G., Valvo, E., Lupo, A., Chiaramonte, S., Messa, P., D'Angelo, A., Zatti, M. & Maschio, G. (1979). 125I-iothalamate and creatinine clearances in patients with chronic renal diseases, *Nephron,* Vol.24, No.1, pp. 41-45

Thomsen, H.S., Hvid-Jacobsen, K. (1991). Estimation of glomerular filtration rate from low-dose injection of iohexol and a single blood sample, *Invest Radiol,* Vol.26, No.4, pp. 332-336

van de Wiele C., van den Eeckhaut A., Verweire, W., van Haelst, J.P., Versijpt, J. & Dierckx, R.A. (1999). Absolute 24 h quantification of 99Tcm-DMSA uptake in patients with severely reduced kidney function: a comparison with 51Cr-EDTA clearance, *Nucl Med Commun,* Vol.20, No.9, pp. 829-832

Visser, F.W., Muntinga, J.H., Dierckx, R.A. & Navis, G. (2008). Feasibility and impact of the measurement of extracellular fluid volume simultaneous with GFR by 125I-iothalamate, *Clin J Am Soc Nephrol,* Vol.3, No.5, pp. 1308-1315

Weber, A.F., Lee, D.W., Opheim, K. & Smith, A.L. (1985). Quantitation of iothalamate in serum and urine by high-performance liquid chromatography, *J Chromatogr,* Vol.337, No.2, pp. 434-440

Welling, P.G., Mosegaard, A., Dobrinska, M.R. & Madsen, P.O. (1976). Pharmacokinetics of 125I-iothalamate and 131I-o-iodohippurate in man, *J Clin Pharmacol,* Vol.16, No.2-3, pp. 142-148

Wharton, W.W., III, Sondeen, J.L., McBiles, M., Gradwohl, S.E., Wade, C.E., Ciceri, D.P., Lehmann, H.G., Stotler, R.E., Henderson, T.R., Whitaker, W.R. & . (1992). Measurement of glomerular filtration rate in ICU patients using 99mTc-DTPA and inulin, *Kidney Int,* Vol.42, No.1, pp. 174-178

Wilson, D.M., Bergert, J.H., Larson, T.S. & Liedtke, R.R. (1997). GFR determined by nonradiolabeled iothalamate using capillary electrophoresis, *Am J Kidney Dis,* Vol.30, No.5, pp. 646-652

Winter, C.C., Taplin, G.V. (1958). A clinical comparison and analysis of radioactive diodarast, hypaque, miokon and urokon renograms as tests of kidney function, *J Urol,* Vol.79, No.3, pp. 573-579

Winterborn, M.H., Beetham, R. & White, R.H. (1977). Comparison of plasma disappearance and standard clearance techniques for measuring glomerular filtration rate in children with and without vesico-ureteric reflux, *Clin Nephrol,* Vol.7, No.6, pp. 262-270

Woodruff, M.W., Malvin, R.L. (1960). Localization of renal contrast media excretion by stop flow analysis, *J Urol,* Vol.84, pp. 677-684

3

Effects of Preterm Birth on the Kidney

Mary Jane Black, Megan R. Sutherland and Lina Gubhaju
Department of Anatomy and Developmental Biology, Monash University
Australia

1. Introduction

Preterm birth is the leading cause of morbidity and mortality in the neonatal period (Ward and Beachy 2003) and in childhood overall (McCormick, 1985). Over recent decades both the incidence of preterm birth and survival rates of preterm infants has increased, with babies born as early as 25 weeks gestation now having about an 80% chance of survival (Kutz et al., 2009). Preterm birth is defined as birth prior to 37 weeks of gestation; it can be further sub-classified as moderately preterm (birth between 32 and 37 weeks gestation) very preterm (birth < 32 weeks gestation) and extremely preterm (birth at < 28 weeks gestation) (Tucker and McGuire, 2004).

Due to the immaturity of the organs at the time of birth, preterm infants exhibit an increased risk of developing a number of postnatal complications including renal insufficiency and in severe cases renal failure (Drukker and Guignard, 2002; Choker and Gouyon, 2004); the mortality rate in these infants is very high (Drukker and Guignard, 2002; Andreoli, 2004). There is also evidence that preterm birth adversely affects nephrogenesis (the formation of nephrons) in the developing kidney; if this is the case, this has the potential to not only adversely affect renal function in the early postnatal period but to also increase the risk of renal disease later in life. Certainly, there are many studies linking a reduced nephron endowment early in life with hypertension (Keller et al., 2003; Luyckx and Brenner, 2005) and vulnerability to secondary renal insults in adulthood (Nenov et al., 2000; Zimanyi et al., 2006; Hoppe et al., 2007). In this regard, there is substantial recent epidemiological evidence linking preterm birth with an increase in blood pressure in adulthood (Siewert-Delle and Ljungman, 1998; Kistner et al., 2000; Kistner et al., 2002; Doyle et al., 2003; Bonamy et al., 2005; Hack et al., 2005; Johansson et al., 2005; Dalziel et al., 2007; Cooper et al., 2008; Keijzer-Veen et al., 2010b); these observations may be due to a reduced nephron endowment in preterm individuals.

In this chapter, we review the current knowledge of the effects of preterm birth on nephrogenesis in the developing kidney and on renal function postnatally.

2. The effects of preterm birth on nephrogenesis

The human kidney develops from a ridge of mesodermal tissue (known as the nephrogenic cord) which is found along the posterior wall of the abdominal cavity on either side of the primitive aorta (Blackburn, 2003). Development of the permanent kidney involves the formation of the pronephros and mesonephros (transitory organs) and the metanephros (the permanent kidney) (Saxen, 1987; Clark and Bertram, 1999; Sweeney and Avner, 2004; Moritz et al., 2008). Development of the metanephros, begins at approximately week 5 of gestation with the outgrowth of the ureteric bud from the Wolffian duct (Saxen, 1987). Subsequent events include invasion of the mass of metanephric mesenchyme by the ureteric bud, followed by reciprocal inductive interactions between the ureteric bud and metanephric mesenchyme that lead to both dichotomous branching of the ureteric bud and the formation of nephrons at the ureteric bud tips (Moritz et al., 2008). Formation of the functional units of the kidney, the nephron, commences at approximately week 9 of gestation (Figure 1)(Blackburn, 2003).

As shown in the timeline in Figure 1, nephrogenesis in the human kidney is not complete until ~34-36 weeks of gestation with the majority of nephrons formed during the third trimester (from ~20 weeks of gestation onwards) (Hinchliffe et al., 1991). In very preterm and extremely preterm neonates, nephrogenesis is still on-going at the time of birth and continues in the *ex-utero* environment. Hence it is imperative to get a good understanding of how preterm birth affects the developing kidney and in particular the effects on nephrogenesis.

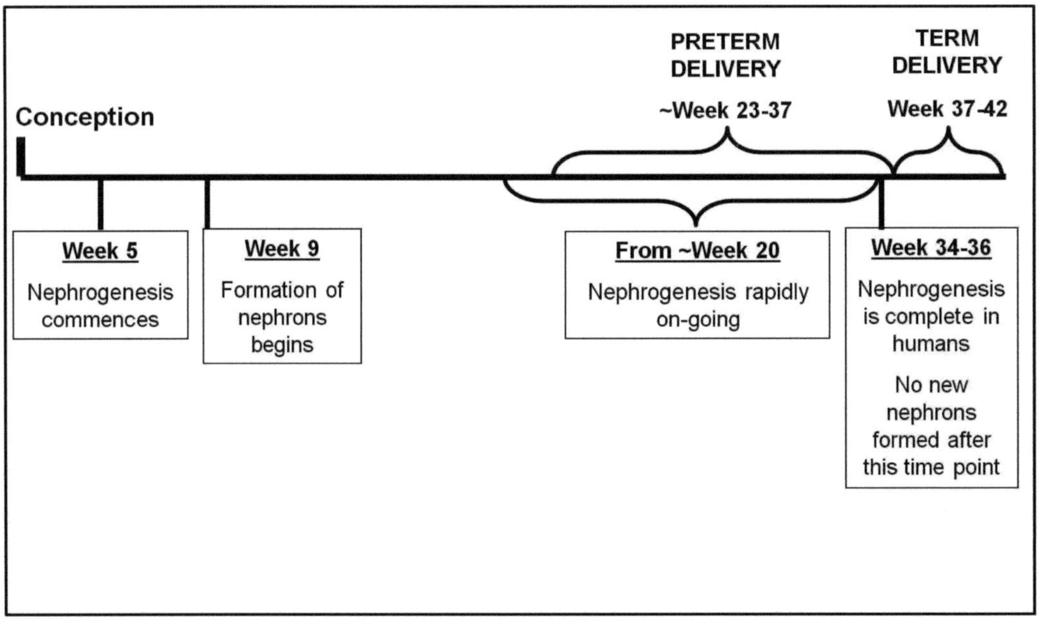

Fig. 1. A timeline of human nephrogenesis during gestation. Nephrogenesis is rapidly on-going at the time when most preterm neonates are delivered.

To date, there have been few studies examining the effects of preterm birth on nephrogenesis. *In vivo,* clinical studies have utilised renal ultrasound and magnetic resonance imaging (MRI) to estimate kidney size as a proxy measure of nephron endowment. However, such extrapolations should be treated with caution. Although kidney size is generally a good predictor of nephron number, this may not be the case in the preterm infant, with kidney size likely to be influenced by glomerular and tubular hypertrophy and increased interstitial mass due to the increased postnatal functional demands. Hence, it is often difficult to make predictions based on parameters such as kidney size (Lodrup et al., 2008). In this regard, autopsy studies in deceased preterm neonates have provided insight into how preterm birth affects the structure of the kidney and the number of glomerular generations formed within the kidney. As well, carefully controlled experimental studies in the nonhuman primate provide valuable insight into the effects of preterm birth on nephrogenesis and on the total number of nephrons formed.

2.1 Clinical *in vivo* studies

Table 1 summarizes the main *in vivo* clinical studies that have investigated the effects of preterm birth on kidney length and volume. Overall, the findings in relation to the effects of preterm birth on kidney size are conflicting; however, it is difficult to compare between studies due to the varying time points of assessment and the differences in the control groups used in each study.

In order to establish the normal expected renal growth in preterm neonates, in a recent study van Venrooji *et al* (2010) examined kidney lengths and volumes of 30 very preterm neonates (gestational age ranging from 23.6 weeks to 30.6 weeks) at 1, 4 and 8 weeks after birth through ultrasound measurements. Significant correlations were found between average renal size (volume and length) with both body weight and age. The study also found no significant difference in growth rates between the extremely low birth weight group (<1.0 kg; GA 23.6 - 27.1 weeks) and the very low birth weight group (1.0 - 1.5 kg; GA 26.1 - 30.6 weeks). In another study, Huang and colleagues (2007) compared postnatal kidney growth in preterm neonates (<34 weeks gestation) to kidney growth *in utero* in a control group (28-40 weeks of gestation). Kidney volumes were measured in 56 preterm neonates at postnatal time points ranging from 14 to 96 days after birth. In the control group, kidney volumes were measured within 48 hours of birth. Kidney volumes of preterm neonates with a postconceptional age (defined as the sum of gestational age and postnatal age) equivalent to less than 31 weeks of gestation were significantly larger compared to controls, whereas the preterm neonates with a postconceptional age greater than 31 weeks of gestation had a significantly smaller kidney volume compared to controls. In the preterm infants where kidney volume increased, it is likely that the increase in kidney size is indicative of the response of the neonatal kidney to increased functional demands. However, if this is the case, it is unclear why the renal response was different in the preterm neonates greater than 31 weeks of postconceptional age where kidney volume was significantly less than controls. Another study by Kent *et al* (2009) compared MRI measurements of kidney volume and kidney volume relative to body weight in extremely preterm neonates (25-28 weeks gestation) to term-born controls. Kidney volumes in the preterm neonates were measured once they reached term-corrected age (37-40 weeks gestation) and within the first 4 weeks of life in the term controls. Interestingly in that study, no differences were found between groups.

Findings from older preterm infants, children and adults have been more consistent across studies and generally demonstrate a decrease in kidney size (relative to body size) compared to term controls. Firstly, Schmidt *et al* (2005) reported significantly smaller relative kidney volumes in preterm infants (born at less than 37 weeks of gestation) at 3 months of term-corrected age compared to 3-month-old term infants. Furthermore, preterm children at 18 months of term-equivalent age had slimmer shaped kidneys compared to term-born infants perhaps suggestive of decreased glomerular generations. In the most comprehensive study of renal growth in preterm infants to date, (involving 466 infants from 3 months through to two years of age), Drougia *et al* (2009) showed that kidney length was

Author & Year	Gestational age at birth (weeks), range	Age at assessment	Study Groups and sample size	Outcomes on renal size
Huang (2007)	24-36	14-96 days	Preterm (n=56) Gestational controls (n=44)	Larger relative volume in preterm <31 weeks PCA Smaller relative volume in preterm >31 weeks PCA
Van Venrooij (2010)	23-30	1, 4, 8 weeks	ELBW (n=14) VLBW (n=16)	No differences in volume or length
Kent (2009)	25-28	37-40 weeks (term equivalent)	Preterm (n=17) Term (n=13)	No differences in volume
Drougia (2008)	28-41	36 and 40 weeks (term equivalent) 3, 6, 12 and 24 months	Preterm 28-34 weeks (SGA: n=100 AGA: n=54) Preterm 34-36 weeks (SGA: n=80 AGA: n=61) Term (AGA: n=90 SGA: n=81)	Smaller right kidney length in preterm SGA 28-34 week group compared to AGA group at all postnatal time points
Schmidt (2005)	<37	40 weeks 3 and 18 months	Preterm (n=59) Term (n=801)	Smaller relative volumes at 3 and 18 months
Zaffanello (2010)	26-31	5-6 years	ELBW (n=36) VLBW (n=43)	ELBW have smaller volumes (Right, Left, Total) ELBW have smaller length (Right and Left)
Kwinta (2011)	26-29	6-7 years	ELBW (n=78) Term (n=38)	ELBW have smaller volume
Rakow (2008)	<32 (mean=27)	9-12 years	Preterm (n=33) Term (n=37)	Smaller absolute volume; not significant when adjusted for body surface area
Rodriguez-Soriano (2005)	23-35	6-12 years	Preterm (n=27)	Length and volume appeared to be in normal range; no comparison group
Keijzer-Veen (2010)	<32 (mean=31)	20 years	Preterm SGA (n=22) Preterm AGA (n=29) Term AGA (n=30)	Smaller length and volume in preterm (SGA and AGA) female group compared to term

Table 1. The main studies that have examined renal size (volume and length) in preterm neonates, children and adults (PCA=post-conceptional age, ELBW=extremely low birth weight, VLBW=very low birth weight, SGA=small for gestational age, AGA=appropriately grown for gestational age)

significantly decreased in small-for-gestational age preterm infants (born 28-34 weeks of gestation) compared to those born at term. In addition, Kwinta *et al* (2011) recently reported in 6 to 7 year old children, reduced absolute and relative kidney volumes in those born extremely low birth weight (26 – 29 weeks of gestation) compared to children born full-term. Furthermore, extremely low birth weight (birth weight <1.0kg; 26.3 - 27.7 weeks of gestation) children in a similar age group (5-6 year olds), had significantly reduced right and left kidney volumes and lengths compared to very low birth weight children (birth weight 1.0-1.5 kg; 29.9 - 31.3 weeks of gestation) (Zaffanello et al., 2010). This is the only study to date demonstrating significant differences in kidney size due to severity of prematurity.

To our knowledge, there has only been one study to date examining kidney size in preterm individuals in adulthood. In that study, 20-year-old adults born preterm (less than 32 weeks of gestation) had significantly smaller absolute and relative left kidney lengths and volumes compared to 20 year-old term controls; the difference was only significant in females (Keijzer-Veen et al., 2010a).

2.2 Human autopsy studies

There have been three published human autopsy studies (apart from case studies) that have examined the effect of preterm birth on postnatal nephrogenesis (Rodriguez et al., 2004; Faa et al., 2010; Sutherland et al., 2011b). Since non-uniform portions of the kidney are usually collected at autopsy, stereological methods cannot be accurately employed. Under these circumstances, the medullary ray glomerular generation counting method (Hinchliffe et al., 1992b) (also referred to as radial glomerular count or glomerular generation count) is a useful technique to provide insight into renal maturity and potentially nephron endowment. The method involves counting all developed glomeruli along one side of clearly distinguishable medullary rays in histological renal sections. Glomeruli are counted from the inner to outer renal cortex. Importantly, in our studies we have found a strong correlation between glomerular generation number and nephron number, which supports the validity of the technique (Sutherland et al., 2011a).

In one of the first autopsy studies conducted, the number of radial glomerular counts in kidneys from extremely preterm neonates (56 neonates) was compared to 10 full-term infants (Rodriguez et al., 2004). Radial glomerular counts were found to be significantly reduced in preterm infants; however, since many of the preterm infants were also intrauterine growth restricted (IUGR) it is difficult to determine the effects of preterm birth *per se* from this study. In a smaller study, Faa *et al* (2010) have reported significantly reduced radial glomerular counts and marked inter-individual variability in the number of glomerular generations among the kidneys from preterm neonates compared to term newborns. In that study, 8 human fetuses, 12 preterm neonates and 3 full-term neonates were examined; it is unknown whether any of the neonates were also IUGR.

As follow on to these studies, we have recently undertaken a study examining kidneys obtained at autopsy from 28 preterm infants and 32 still-born gestational controls (Sutherland et al., 2011b); the preterm group included 6 infants that were also IUGR. Importantly, analyses comparing growth restricted and non-growth restricted kidneys demonstrated no significant differences, although the findings are limited by the small sample of growth restricted neonates. In contrast to the studies described above, we found accelerated nephrogenesis in the preterm group demonstrated by an increase in the number of glomerular generations, a decreased nephrogenic zone width (suggesting earlier cessation of nephrogenesis postnatally) and a decreased proportion of glomeruli in the immature V (vesicle) -stage of maturation compared to still-born gestational controls. Furthermore, mean renal corpuscle cross sectional area was significantly larger in the preterm kidneys. Of particular concern, kidneys from preterm infants had a higher percentage of structurally abnormal glomeruli compared to the gestational controls with up to 13.7% of glomeruli affected. These abnormal glomeruli exhibited a dilated Bowman's space and shrunken glomerular tuft. The factors associated with the development of abnormal glomeruli are yet unknown and this is an important area of future research.

2.3 Nonhuman primate animal studies

We have shown that the baboon is an ideal model to study human kidney development, as the ontogeny of the kidney very closely matches that of the human (Gubhaju and Black, 2005). Similar to the human, nephrogenesis in the baboon commences at approximately 30 days of gestation (Hendrickx et al., 1971) and ceases prior to term by 175 days gestation (Term = 185 days gestation) (Gubhaju and Black, 2005). Similar to the wide range in nephron number found in human kidneys, in the kidneys we examined total nephron number ranged from 193,983 to 334,316 in baboons delivered at term.

In collaboration with researchers at the Southwest Foundation for Biomedical Research (San Antonio, Texas, U.S.A) we have examined the kidneys from fetal baboons that have been prematurely delivered and ventilated after birth in a neonatal intensive care unit (NICU) in a similar manner to human preterm babies (Gubhaju et al., 2009). These appropriate weight-for-gestational age baboons were delivered extremely preterm (125 days of gestation); equivalent to approximately 27 weeks gestation in humans. After birth, all preterm neonates were intubated, administered 100 mg/kg surfactant (Survanta; donated by Ross Products, Columbus, OH), and ventilated with pressure limited infant ventilators (InfantStar; donated by Infrasonics, San Diego, CA). All preterm neonates were also treated with ampicillin and gentamicin for the first 7–10 days of life (Thomson et al., 2004). Further doses of antibiotics were only administered in cases of clinically suspected infection. Following birth, the baboon neonates were ventilated in the NICU for a maximum period of 21 days.

In this model, kidney volume, nephron number and size of the renal corpuscle were estimated using unbiased stereology, the gold standard method for the determination of nephron number (Bertram, 2001; Sutherland et al., 2011a). One of the most significant findings from the nonhuman primate studies was the clear evidence that nephrogenesis was on-going in the extrauterine environment following preterm birth. There was structural evidence of on-going nephrogenesis in the outer renal cortex (branching of the ureteric bud, metanephric mesenchyme and Comma and S-shaped bodies) and this was accompanied by a significant increase in the number of glomerular generations and nephron number in the postnatal environment by postnatal day 21 (Gubhaju et al., 2009). Furthermore, kidney weight and volume relative to body weight were significantly higher in the preterm baboon neonates compared to gestational age-matched controls; a finding that has been previously reported in human studies (Huang et al., 2007). There was a significant decrease in glomerular density (glomeruli/gram of kidney) in the kidney from preterm baboon neonates compared to gestational controls suggestive of altered renal growth and potentially an increase in tubular mass.

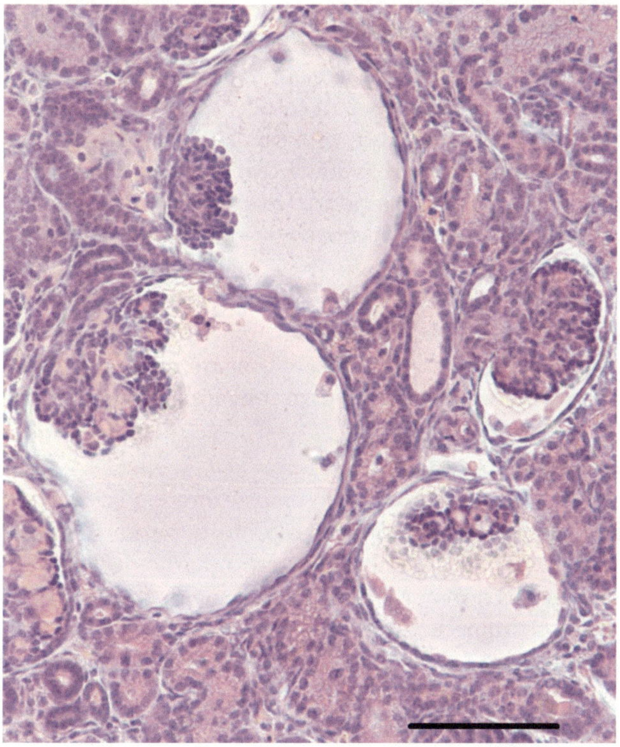

Fig. 2. A representative photomicrograph of a histological renal section from a preterm baboon showing abnormal glomeruli in the outer renal cortex; these morphologically immature glomeruli exhibited a shrunken glomerular tuft and enlarged Bowman's space. Scale bar = 100 μm

Similar to the findings from the human autopsy studies, morphologically abnormal glomeruli were also found in kidneys from preterm baboon neonates; with up to 18% of glomeruli affected (Figure 2). High proportions of abnormal glomeruli were only found in those kidneys from preterm baboons, whereas in gestational controls the proportion of abnormal glomeruli was negligible. The observed abnormal glomeruli were only present in the superficial outer cortex of the preterm kidney suggesting that it is the glomeruli that are recently formed (possibly those formed in the extrauterine environment) that are 'at risk.' Further immunohistochemical analyses demonstrated that the abnormal glomeruli were poorly vascularised (lack of endothelial cell marker, CD31 immunostaining). In addition, immunostaining with the podocyte marker, WT-1, revealed that the abnormal glomeruli were in a relatively immature stage of development since the glomerular tuft contained WT-1 positive cells surrounding a mass of relatively undifferentiated cells. Importantly, there were a large number of parietal epithelial cells surrounding the Bowman's capsule; previous human studies have reported a similar morphology in atubular glomeruli (Gibson et al., 1996; Bariety et al., 2006). If the abnormal glomeruli in the preterm kidneys are atubular, then they will never be functional. Further studies are required to determine whether this is the case. Certainly, a large proportion of non-functional glomeruli in the preterm kidney is likely to have adverse consequences on renal function both in the neonatal period and in the long-term (by reducing the functional reserve of nephrons).

3. Renal function in the preterm neonate

There have been a number of studies that have examined the effects of preterm birth on renal function. However, it must be kept in mind when interpreting the data from these studies that the function of the immature preterm kidney is likely to be quite different to that of the term infant, which in turn is likely to be quite different to the adult. Hence, although the 'normal' levels of the standard markers of renal function (such as serum creatinine and urinary albumin) have been well-established for the adult population, the standard levels in the neonate, especially those of the preterm neonate, are not clearly defined. This often makes the clinical assessment of renal function in the preterm neonate difficult. In future research, it is necessary to establish the 'normal' levels of renal function in the preterm infant and to identify robust biomarkers for the early diagnosis of renal injury in the neonatal period, which may in turn prevent long-term renal dysfunction.

3.1 Fluid and electrolyte homeostasis

An imbalance of fluid and electrolyte intake versus excretion is very common in premature neonates, and can lead to significant morbidity and mortality (Bhatia, 2006); hypernatraemia, for example, can result in severe neurological injury (Moritz and Ayus, 2005). Insensible fluid loss is a major factor (Bhatia, 2006), and is primarily transcutaneous due to the developmental immaturity of the skin and a high body surface area to body water mass ratio (Baumgart and Costarino, 2000). Equally, the delayed loss of extracellular fluid volume following preterm birth is also associated with an increased risk of morbidity, in particular bronchopulmonary dysplasia (Oh et al., 2005) and patent ductus arteriosus (Bell and Acarregui, 2008).

Three phases of fluid and electrolyte homeostasis have been observed in the immediate period following preterm birth; these phases occurred similarly in extremely low birth weight infants and those at older gestational ages (Lorenz et al., 1982; Lorenz et al., 1995). As described by Lorenz *et al.*, (1982; 1995) in the first 24 hours following birth, a period known as the pre-diuretic stage, urine output is minimal and sodium excretion is low. On postnatal days 2-3, termed the diuretic phase, sodium excretion and urine output significantly increase, which occurs independently of fluid intake. From approximately days 4-5 of life, the post-diuretic phase, urine output changes in response to fluid intake (Lorenz et al., 1982; Lorenz et al., 1995). Importantly, however, the postnatal time-point that these phases occur, and their duration, differ between individual neonates (Lorenz et al., 1995), as does the amount of insensible fluid loss; together, this highlights the need for an individualised approach to fluid therapy in preterm neonates.

Urine output is the most commonly and easily measured indicator of renal function in the preterm neonate. Urine output less than 0.5 ml/kg/h, known as oliguria, can be indicative of acute kidney injury (AKI). AKI, however, can also be non-oliguric, therefore urine output is not a very specific indicator of renal function. Furthermore, from the post-diuretic phase of fluid homeostasis urine output is highly dependent upon fluid intake; high intakes may artificially increase urine output, while not accurately reflecting renal functional capacity.

The most common measure of electrolyte balance in the neonate is the calculation of the fractional excretion of sodium (FENa), which is the percentage of sodium that is excreted and not taken up through tubular reabsorption. The calculation of FENa takes into account the levels of both serum and urine sodium, and it is corrected for serum and urine creatinine levels. Therefore, high urine sodium levels may be indicative of structural immaturity of the renal tubule (short length of the tubules, and changes in the density and structure of transporter proteins) (Jones and Chesney, 1992), or due to renal injury (Ueda and Shah, 2000; Bonventre, 2007).

Studies that have assessed FENa during the neonatal period have determined that sodium excretion is significantly higher in preterm neonates compared to term controls (Siegel and Oh, 1976; Aperia et al., 1981), and significantly decreases with increasing gestational (Gallini et al., 2000) and postnatal age (Ross et al., 1977; Sulyok et al., 1979; Aperia et al., 1981; Gallini et al., 2000; Giapros et al., 2007). Therefore, with increasing renal maturity a positive sodium balance (low FENa) is achieved, which is essential for the growth and development of the neonate and the maintenance of fluid homeostasis (Engle, 1986).

3.2 Glomerular filtration rate

Endogenous creatinine is the most practical and commonly used marker of renal function, with calculated creatinine clearance widely used as an estimate of glomerular filtration rate (GFR). In the clinical setting, repeated serum creatinine levels are used to gauge renal function in neonates; this is an easily obtainable measure via routine blood collection and does not rely on timed urine samples or additional invasive procedures. This method does, however, have significant limitations. Immediately following birth, serum creatinine levels are equivalent to the fetal levels, which during the third trimester of gestation rise from 42 μmol/L at 23 weeks to 47 μmol/L at term; the increase likely reflecting an increase in muscle mass (Moniz et al., 1985). In the first forty-eight hours following birth, however, serum creatinine levels significantly increase (Bueva and Guignard, 1994; Miall et al., 1999). This is considered to be due, in part, to tubular creatinine reabsorption, as has been evidenced in a neonatal animal model (Matos et al., 1998), and also due to the inadequacy of glomerular filtration during the early postnatal period (Miall et al., 1999). Peak serum creatinine levels are reached at postnatal day 2-4 of life, with the highest levels and most delayed timing of the peak creatinine level seen in neonates at the lowest gestational ages (Miall et al., 1999).

During the first week of life following preterm birth, GFR is significantly lower in preterm neonates than in term-born controls (Siegel and Oh, 1976; Finney et al., 2000; Schreuder et al., 2009), and is significantly positively correlated with both gestational age at birth, and postnatal age (Clark et al., 1989; Gordjani et al., 1998; Iacobelli et al., 2009). Compared to term neonates, the rate of increase in GFR after birth is slower in neonates born preterm (Gordjani et al., 1998). Up until two months of age there are similar findings, with a number of studies observing an increase in GFR concurrent to increasing gestational and postnatal ages (Ross et al., 1977; Fawer et al., 1979; Sulyok et al., 1979; Aperia et al., 1981; Wilkins, 1992; Bueva and Guignard, 1994; Gallini et al., 2000; Cuzzolin et al., 2006; Thayyil et al., 2008). Although a number of studies have now been performed in this area, there is still a lack of clear definition regarding expected GFR values in the preterm neonate. Recently published standard curves of GFRs in neonates born at 27-31 weeks gestational age, from 7 to 28 days of life, will go some way in aiding in the clinical interpretation of renal function in this particular group of neonates (Vieux et al., 2010).

Given that age has been found to be a strong determinant of GFR, the low GFR observed in the preterm neonate after birth is likely the result of renal immaturity (a low number of filtering glomeruli), and it is also likely to be influenced by differences in renal blood flow and vascular resistance. It is essential that GFR is monitored in the postnatal period following preterm birth, as a very low GFR is likely to impair renal drug clearance, leading to nephrotoxicity.

3.3 Acute kidney injury

Acute kidney injury (AKI; previously referred to as acute renal failure) is reported to occur in 8% to 24% of preterm neonates admitted to neonatal intensive care units (Stapleton et al., 1987; Hentschel et al., 1996). The current diagnosis of AKI is primarily based on the RIFLE system, which categorises the stages of increasing AKI severity: Risk, Injury, Failure, Loss and End-stage kidney disease (ESKD) (Bellomo et al., 2004). This system was further modified following recommendations from the acute kidney injury network (AKIN) (Mehta et al., 2007). The initial clinical indication of AKI risk includes a 50% increase in serum creatinine (or ≥ 0.3 mg/dl within a 48 hour period), and/or a urine output less than 0.5 mg/kg/hr for a period of six hours (Bellomo et al., 2004; Mehta et al., 2007), which are changes indicative of a significantly reduced GFR. Classifications for the definition of AKI in a neonatal specific population, however, have not been developed.

The causes of AKI in the preterm neonate are primarily pre-renal in origin, arising from conditions which affect renal perfusion such as hypotension, hypoxia and sepsis (Stapleton et al., 1987; Cataldi et al., 2005). These in turn lead to apoptotic, necrotic and inflammatory processes within the kidney (Ueda and Shah, 2000; Bonventre, 2007). Importantly, AKI in the preterm neonate may subsequently lead to long-term chronic renal disease (Abitbol et al., 2003).

In a study involving 172 preterm neonates by Cataldi *et al.* 2005, the risk factors for AKI were found to be maternal and neonatal drug administration (non-steroidal anti-inflammatory drugs (NSAIDs) and antibiotics, especially ceftazidime), a low Apgar score, and a patent ductus arteriosus. Interestingly, gestational age did not affect risk of AKI, however, the majority of AKI cases (79%) weighed < 1.5 kg at birth (Cataldi et al., 2005). In a larger study by Cuzzolin *et al.* (2006), involving 281 preterm neonates, a number of risk factors for AKI were also identified. These included maternal NSAID administration, low Apgar score, respiratory distress syndrome, neonatal drug administration (antibiotics and NSAIDs), and a number of clinical interventions (intubation at birth, catheterization, phototherapy, and mechanical ventilation).

Given the importance of the early diagnosis and treatment of AKI, there has been much recent focus on the discovery of novel urinary biomarkers. The expectation of a new biomarker is to enable the diagnosis of cellular injury before a decline in renal function occurs. For example, serum creatinine is not elevated until 48-72 hours after an acute injury has occurred (Moran and Myers, 1985); such a prolonged delay before diagnosis and treatment likely results in further renal injury. As Rosner (2009) describes, it would be optimal if a biomarker could be developed to: 1) assess the response to, and any adverse effects of therapeutic interventions 2) indicate the severity of renal injury 3) inform on the etiology of the injury and 4) identify the location of injured cells. In a systematic review of the current literature, Parikh *et al.* (2010) determined that the molecules with the most promise for the diagnosis of established AKI include interleukin-18 (IL-18), kidney injury molecule-1 (KIM-1), N-acetyl-beta-D-glucosaminidase (NAG) and neutrophil gelatinase-associated lipocalin (NGAL). NGAL, IL-18, fatty acid binding protein (FABP), and cystatin-C are the most encouraging biomarkers for the early diagnosis of AKI, given that the upregulation of these molecules following injury onset precedes the rise in serum creatinine by many hours (Parikh et al., 2010).

In the preterm neonate, a small number of studies have been conducted for the assessment of urinary NGAL levels, with mixed results. These studies have shown that the highest NGAL levels are evident in the neonates that are critically ill, with and without evidence of renal dysfunction (Lavery et al., 2008; Parravicini, 2010); in particular, NGAL shows potential as a promising biomarker of late-onset sepsis (Lavery et al., 2008; Parravicini et al., 2010). Urinary NGAL levels also strongly correlated with gestational and postnatal age (Lavery et al., 2008; Huynh et al., 2009), perhaps reflecting the renal production of NGAL during nephrogenesis (Gwira et al., 2005) which is often still ongoing during the early postnatal period. Normative values for urinary NGAL in preterm neonates with uncomplicated clinical courses have also been published, with the results indicating a greater variation in females than males (Huynh et al., 2009).

3.4 Proteinuria

Proteinuria, the presence of high levels of protein in the urine, may be of glomerular and/or tubular origin. The number of different proteins that have been identified in the adult urinary proteome is 1,543, and these are primarily of membrane, extracellular and lysosomal origin (Adachi et al., 2006). Despite this large number, unless renal function is impaired, proteins are normally only present at very low levels in urine, due to the function of the glomerular filtration barrier and tubular reabsorption capabilities.

Presence of high molecular weight (HMW) proteins in the urine, such as albumin traditionally indicates a disruption in the integrity of the glomerular filtration barrier. Recent debate, however, has suggested that the contribution of tubular reabsorption of albumin from the filtrate may be greater than previously considered (Comper et al., 2008). In general, albuminuria is a strong marker for renal and cardiovascular disease, and a risk factor for mortality (Matsushita et al., 2010; Methven et al., 2011). Normally, adults excrete less than 30 mg of albumin per 24 hours (Mathieson, 2004). Urinary albumin levels between 30 - 300 mg in 24 hours is considered microalbuminuria, with levels greater than 300 mg classified as macroalbuminuria (Mathieson, 2004). Traditionally, 24 hour urine samples were required for reliable estimates of urinary protein. However, single random spot samples with protein levels corrected for urine creatinine, have been shown to be significantly correlated with results from 24 hour collections, and are equally effective in the prediction of outcomes (Ralston et al., 1988; Methven et al., 2011). In neonates, 24 hour urine collection is difficult, therefore analysis of urinary protein levels are undertaken using spot urine samples obtained using urine collection bags.

Low molecular weight (LMW) proteins, such as α1-microglobulin, β2-microglobulin and retinol binding protein pass freely through the glomerular filter and undergo reuptake via proximal tubule cells (Tomlinson, 1992). Megalin and cubulin have been identified as important receptors involved in tubular protein uptake, with mutations in the receptors resulting in proteinuria (Christensen and Birn, 2001). To date, LMW protein levels in the urine are not routinely measured in the clinical setting. Importantly, however, amongst the LMW proteins there may be potential novel biomarkers of tubular cell injury and this requires further research (Rosner, 2009; Parikh et al., 2010).

In the preterm neonate, few studies have been conducted to examine urine protein excretion. In general, there is a high variability in urine albumin levels between individual neonates (Clark et al., 1989; Fell et al., 1997), with the highest levels exhibited by those with a low gestational age at birth and those that are clinically unstable (Galaske, 1986; Clark et al., 1989; Tsukahara et al., 1994; Fell et al., 1997; Awad et al., 2002b). The majority of studies have only been conducted during the first week of life following preterm birth. However, in a study by Tsukahara *et al.* (1994) urine albumin levels were assessed in preterm and term neonates over the first 28 days of life. Urine albumin levels were found to remain relatively stable postnatally over the one month period in the term neonates, whereas in the preterm neonates, urine albumin was seen to decrease with increasing postnatal age. These findings suggest that the glomerular filtration barrier following preterm birth is structurally immature, until beyond one month of age.

Urinary β2-microglobulin levels have also been shown to be significantly greater in the preterm infant compared to term-born infants throughout the first month of life (Aperia et al., 1981; Tsukahara et al., 1990; Tsukahara et al., 1994), and are decreased with increasing gestational and postnatal age (Takieddine et al., 1983). Similarly, levels of α1-microglobulin and RBP are higher in preterm neonates than neonates born at term (Clark et al., 1989; Fell et al., 1997; Awad et al., 2002a). To date, however, it remains unclear whether the increased urinary high- and low- molecular weight protein levels reported in preterm neonates are associated with renal immaturity and/or injury. The high variability in urinary protein levels may also reflect differences in the postnatal clinical course in preterm neonates; further studies are necessary to verify whether this is the case.

3.5 Long-term effects of preterm birth on renal function

Renal function in preterm-born children and adults, has to date only been investigated in a small number of studies, with inconclusive results. In school-aged children, Rakow *et al.* (2008) found no difference in GFR or urinary levels of both HMW and LMW proteins between children born less than 32 weeks gestational age, and those that were born at term. Similarly, Vanpee *et al.* (1992) determined no difference in renal function in preterm and term-born children at 8 years of age, despite lower GFR and higher urine albumin levels being evident in the preterm group at 9 months of age. In contrast, however, a study by Rodriguez-Soriano and colleagues (2005) reported that GFR was significantly reduced in preterm-born children compared to term controls, with impairments in electrolyte excretion also evident. Furthermore, in children examined at 6-8 years of age, Iacobelli et al. (2007) demonstrated microalbuminuria in 8.3% of the preterm neonates, which was associated with postnatal factors such as neonatal hypotension and increased catch-up growth. Increased risk of renal demise was also evident in individuals born preterm who were obese during childhood (Abitbol et al., 2009).

Two studies have also been conducted to examine renal function in young adults (20-30 years of age), with both Keijzer-Veen *et al.* (2007) and Kistner *et al.* (Kistner et al., 2000) finding no effect of preterm birth on GFR or albuminuria. To the contrary, in a cohort of 19 year old young adults, those who were born preterm as well as IUGR, there was a significant reduction in GFR (Keijzer-Veen et al., 2005). Given these results in preterm-born children and adults, there is some suggestion that preterm birth adversely affects the growth and functional capacity of the kidney and may result in progressive renal failure later in life. Importantly, adverse consequences appear to be more likely to occur in combination with other insults. Therefore, future research must be directed towards identifying these insults and their effects on the structure and function of the kidney.

4. Preterm birth leads to glomerular abnormalities – Areas of future research

One of the most important findings we have shown thus far, is the presence of abnormal glomeruli in both the human and nonhuman primate (baboon) preterm kidney. These abnormal glomeruli are located in the outer renal cortex and are in the most immature stage of development (stage 1); they are composed of an undifferentiated glomerular anlage of cells (foundation group of cells) surrounded by a layer of podocytes with scant, if any, capillarisation. Our findings thus strongly suggest that it is the very immature glomeruli (possibly those formed in the extrauterine environment) that are particularly vulnerable to preterm birth. Given the gross abnormalities observed in these glomeruli, it is unlikely that these glomeruli will ever be functional and thus, it is expected that they will be subsequently resorbed into the surrounding tissue. In the short-term, such abnormalities will likely lead to marked impairment of renal function in the neonate if a high proportion of the nephrons are affected, or to minor impairment if only a small proportion are abnormal. When the kidney is severely affected this will adversely impact on the number of functional nephrons at the beginning of life and thus reduce the long-term functional reserve of the kidney, rendering it vulnerable to hypertension and secondary life style insults.

The cause(s) of the glomerular abnormalities in the preterm infant is currently unknown. Importantly in this regard, we have shown that there is a wide variation in the proportion of abnormal glomeruli within the kidneys of preterm infants, with the kidneys of some preterm infants appearing morphologically normal whereas in others a large proportion of the glomeruli appear abnormal (Sutherland et al., 2011b). Given the wide variation in the proportion of abnormal glomeruli within the kidneys of preterm infants, this suggests that it is not preterm birth *per se* that leads to the glomerular abnormalities; instead they are likely due to factors often associated with preterm birth as shown in Figure 3. It is likely that these deleterious effects may relate to: 1) adverse factors in the *in utero* environment that have led to premature delivery, 2) factors in the neonatal care of the preterm infant and 3) pharmacological interventions/therapies administered to mothers prior to birth and/or the infant after birth. There are many factors which apply to each of these categories; below we have selected some that we consider are important for future research.

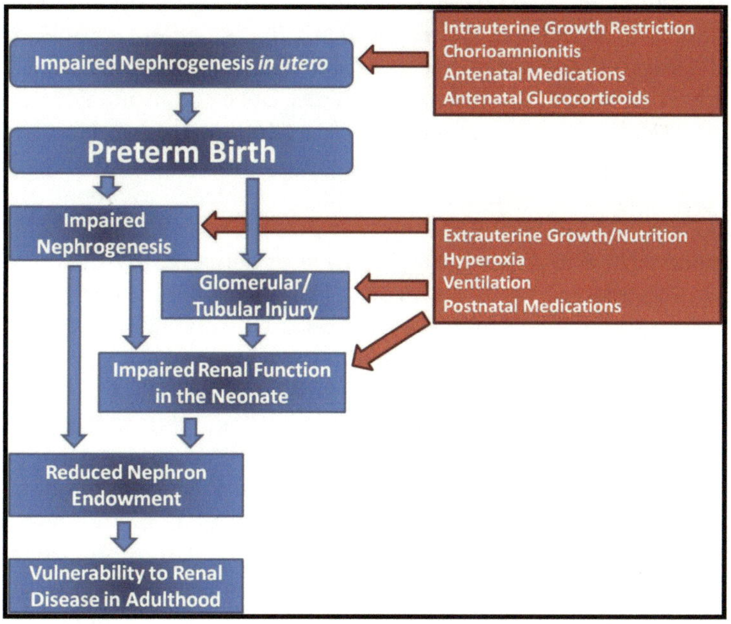

Fig. 3. Depiction of the potential factors that may contribute to impaired nephrogenesis in the preterm kidney and consequently lead to a reduced nephron endowment and vulnerability to renal disease in adulthood

4.1 Adverse factors in the *in utero* environment

Two potential factors in the *in utero* environment that may render the preterm kidney vulnerable are IUGR and/or exposure to chorioamnionitis.

4.1.1 Intrauterine growth restriction

IUGR (growth below the 10th percentile for gestational age) is often a co-morbidity of preterm birth. Certainly, it is well described in both human and experimental models that IUGR leads to a reduced nephron endowment at birth (Hinchliffe et al., 1992a; Merlet-Benichou et al., 1994; Manalich et al., 2000; Zimanyi et al., 2004; Zohdi et al., 2007). This is likely due to the reduced growth of the fetal kidney (with the number of nephrons directly proportional to kidney size). In this regard, there is often redistribution of blood flow in the growth-restricted fetus, leading to preferential blood flow to the brain (termed brain sparing) and reduced blood flow to organs such as the kidneys (Behrman et al., 1970; Gunnarsson et al., 1998). To our knowledge the impact of reduced blood flow to the formation of nephrons in the IUGR fetal kidney has not been investigated. Given the dramatic change in hemodynamics at the time of birth (elevation in blood pressure and increased renal blood flow) it is conceivable that the recently formed glomeruli in the IUGR kidney (with a reduced renal blood flow prenatally) may be particularly vulnerable to the haemodynamic transition at birth. This is an important area of research that needs to be thoroughly investigated.

4.1.2 Chorioamnionitis

Chorioamnionitis (a bacterial infection of the chorion and amnion) is a common antecedent of preterm birth (Romero et al., 2006; Goldenberg et al., 2008), especially in births prior to 30 weeks of gestation (Lahra and Jeffery, 2004); it is often complicated by IUGR. Chorioamnionitis may manifest as either a clinical or subclinical condition. When severe, it can ultimately give rise to the fetal inflammatory response syndrome which is characterised by funisitis, fetal vasculitis and an increase in of pro-inflammatory cytokines in fetal blood and amniotic fluid (Romero et al., 1998; Romero et al., 2003; Gotsch et al., 2007). It is likely that the fetal systemic inflammatory response will lead to renal inflammation in chorioamnionitis-exposed infants; conceivably if present *in utero* this will have deleterious effects on nephrogenesis, and if present at the time of delivery, it will adversely impact on renal function. In this regard, we have recent evidence in fetal sheep to demonstrate that exposure to chorioamnionitis late in gestation does adversely affect nephrogenesis, leading to a 23% and 18% reduction in nephron endowment in singleton and twin-exposed fetuses, respectively (Galinsky et al., 2011). It is important to note that we did not observe any morphological abnormalities in the glomeruli of these fetal kidneys. However, it is conceivable, that if renal inflammation is present at the time of birth, that this will further compromise postnatal nephrogenesis and renal function in the neonate. Following the hemodynamic transition at birth, it may be then that glomerular morphological abnormalities develop in these already compromised kidneys. Importantly in this regard, a multiple logistic regression analysis of 2508 preterm neonates, treated with indomethacin, showed a significant correlation between intrauterine inflammation and prevalence of renal and electrolyte abnormalities (Itabashi et al., 2003), thus suggesting that intrauterine inflammation in concert with postnatal indomethacin treatment can lead to renal dysfunction. Certainly our results support the idea that prematurity, when complicated with chorioamnionitis, is likely to exacerbate postnatal renal dysfunction and further studies are required to determine whether renal inflammation at the time of birth is associated with the formation of abnormal glomeruli in the neonatal period.

4.2 Factors in the neonatal care of the infant

4.2.1 Hyperoxia

The administration of supplemental oxygen to preterm infants experiencing respiratory distress is standard therapy, however, the effects of high levels of oxygen in the bloodstream on the development of organs is not well understood. Although the levels of supplemental oxygen administered to the preterm infant have been substantially reduced in recent years, the levels of oxygen in the bloodstream remain elevated above normal; hence it is important that research is conducted into the effects of hyperoxia on nephrogenesis in the preterm infant. Certainly, experimental studies in the lung have shown that hyperoxia can lead to the generation of oxygen free radicals, infiltration of inflammatory cells, collagen deposition, cellular apoptosis and subsequent tissue injury (McGrath-Morrow and Stahl, 2001; Dieperink et al., 2006; Alejandre-Alcazar et al., 2007; Chen et al., 2007; Chetty et al., 2008). Whether this is also the case in other tissues has not been examined.

4.2.2 Ventilation

The mode of ventilation of the preterm infant also has the potential to impact on the developing kidney, since alterations in airway pressure are reported to lead to significant cardiopulmonary haemodynamic changes (Polglase et al., 2009) which may subsequently affect renal perfusion. For instance, mechanical ventilation has been shown to alter renal hemodynamics by leading to an increase in intrathoracic pressure, therefore decreasing cardiac output, leading to renal vasoconstriction and decreased GFR (Arant, 1987). It is likely that changes in renal blood flow will directly influence the growth of the kidney. Hence, it is important in future research to determine the effects of altered renal hemodynamics on growth of the developing kidney and how this is influenced by different modes of ventilation.

4.2.3 Extrauterine growth / nutrition

In general, postnatal growth of the preterm infant is markedly attenuated when compared to the term infant and when compared to the normal rate of growth *in utero* for the same post-conceptional age (Ehrenkranz, 2000; Clark et al., 2003). Extrauterine growth restriction in premature neonates (defined as growth below the 10th percentile of intrauterine growth expectation) is likely to directly influence nephrogenesis. In support of this concept, Bacchetta et al (2009) reported lower GFRs (albeit in the normal range) in 7 year old children who had been born very preterm (< 30 weeks gestation) and who were either IUGR or extrauterine growth restricted. However, it is important to note that in some preterm infants there can be a disproportional increase in kidney size (relative to body weight) after birth (Huang et al., 2007; Sutherland et al., 2011b) most probably due to the increased functional demands on the kidney. Importantly we have shown in our preterm baboon studies that under these circumstances, there remains a significant correlation between kidney size and nephron number (Gubhaju et al., 2009).

Taken together, these studies highlight the importance that neonatal nutrition can potentially have on kidney development in the preterm infant. Since nephrogenesis is ongoing after birth in the preterm infant, this provides a window of opportunity whereby early postnatal nutrition in the intensive care unit may be able to directly influence the number of nephrons formed within the kidney. Hence optimising nutrition in the neonatal period, with an aim to maximising nephron endowment in the preterm newborn, is an important area for future research. At this stage, there is no known maternal nutrient supplementation that can improve renal outcomes in the fetus; it is critical to investigate this.

4.3 Pharmacological treatments to the mother prior to birth and / or the infant after birth

There are a number of medications routinely administered to women during pregnancy and to preterm infants. Some of the most commonly used are: 1) antenatal glucocorticoids which are routinely administered either to the mother 'at risk' of preterm delivery (Vidaeff et al., 2003) or to the preterm infant immediately after delivery to accelerate lung maturation in the infant, 2) antibiotics, often administered to the mother with chorioamnionitis and to the infant with postnatal conditions such as necrotising enterocolitis (Gortner et al., 1991) 3) non steroidal anti-inflammatory drugs (such as ibuprofen and indomethacin) which are often administered to close a patent ductus arteriosus (Ellison et al., 1983) and 4) inotropes (such as dopamine and dobutamine) which are administered in cases of hypotension and poor blood flow (Osborn et al., 2002). Importantly, and of concern, all these medications have the potential to adversely impact on nephrogenesis.

4.3.1 Glucocorticoids

In addition to leading to lung maturation in the preterm infant, administration of glucocorticoids has been favourably reported to accelerate renal maturation thus establishing an adequate GFR and efficient tubular reabsorption (Ervin et al., 1996; Ervin et al., 1998; Petershack et al., 1999). However, the question remains: 'Does this acceleration in renal maturation lead to an abnormal and rapid cessation of nephrogenesis which would ultimately affect nephron endowment? In support of this, a number of experimental studies (conducted in animal models) have shown that exposure of the fetus to maternal glucocorticoids can lead to reduced nephron endowment in the offspring (Celsi et al., 1998; Ortiz et al., 2001; Moritz et al., 2002). As follow up to these studies, in a carefully controlled study in our baboon model we have examined the effect of administration of antenatal betamethasone (intramuscular injection of 6mg at 48 hours and 24 hours prior to preterm delivery) on nephrogenesis in the neonatal baboon kidney (Gubhaju et al., 2009). We found that although there was acceleration of glomerular maturation in the betamethasone-treated baboons, the total number of nephrons was within the normal range and importantly we demonstrated that fetal exposure to maternal glucocorticoids was not the cause of the glomerular abnormalities associated with preterm birth.

4.3.2 Antibiotics

The use of antibiotics is often essential in the treatment of the mother during pregnancy and of the preterm infant after birth. Alarmingly, it has been shown that antibiotics, such as the aminoglycosides, can be nephrotoxic in the newborn with the preterm infant most vulnerable (Giapros et al., 2003). This is of concern, given that aminoglycosides are not metabolised in the body and thus accumulate in the kidney where they are eventually eliminated (Nagai and Takano, 2004). In experimental studies antibiotics are also linked with impairment of nephrogenesis (Gilbert et al., 1990; Gilbert et al., 1994; Cullen et al., 2000; Nathanson et al., 2000). For instance, it has been shown that incubation of metanephroi in culture with gentamicin leads to decreased branching morphogenesis of the ureteric tree; this is a likely mediator of the reduction in the number of nephrons formed (Cullen et al., 2000). Given that antibiotics can readily cross the placenta, plus their wide use in the neonatal care of the preterm infant, it is imperative in future studies to gain a more precise understanding of the dose, duration and class of antibiotic treatment that leads to adverse effects in the neonatal kidney; such information would likely influence the care in the neonatal intensive care unit.

4.3.3 Non steroidal anti-inflammatory drugs

NSAIDs, such as ibuprofen and indomethacin are usually administered to preterm neonates to stimulate closure of a patent ductus arteriosus; this can occur in up to 80% of extremely preterm infants (Ellison et al., 1983). Importantly, there have been a number of studies that have reported adverse effects on both the structure and function of the preterm kidney following treatment with NSAIDs. For example, renal insufficiency, demonstrated by a significant increase in serum creatinine has been reported in infants following either antenatal or postnatal exposure to NSAIDs (Kang et al., 1999; Butler-O'Hara and D'Angio, 2002). Of concern, in a case-controlled study where renal impairment was reported in preterm neonates that had received indomethacin treatment for a patent ductus arteriosus, 24% of the babies suffered acute renal failure (Akima et al., 2004). In addition, in the rat model where, similar to the preterm infant, nephrogenesis is ongoing after birth, exposure to indomethacin, ibuprofen and gentamicin have all been shown to lead to renal injury in the immature kidneys. There was evidence of vacuolization of epithelium and loss of microvilli in proximal tubules, effacement of podocyte foot processes and irregularities of the basement membrane in the glomeruli and edema within the interstitium (Kent et al., 2007).

4.3.4 Inotropes

At birth, there is a marked change in hemodynamics, with a subsequent rise in blood pressure and heart rate (Teitel et al., 1987; Louey et al., 2000). Preterm birth causes an abrupt and premature shift in the circulation from the fetal to postnatal configuration at a time when the cardiovascular system is still relatively immature; as a result, it is often necessary for inotropes to be administered to preterm neonates when blood pressure remains abnormally low after birth (Kluckow and Evans, 2001; Osborn et al., 2002). Given the importance of renal blood flow to growth of the kidney it is important that future research examines how the hemodyamic transition at birth affects the development of the immature renal vasculature and/or nephrogenesis and what effect the administration of inotropes have on the developing kidney.

5. Conclusion

Over the past decade, considerable advances have been made in our understanding of the effects of preterm birth on the developing kidney. Encouragingly, it has clearly been demonstrated that nephrogenesis continues after birth in the preterm neonate, however, glomerular abnormalities are commonly observed. Future research should be directed into the causes of these abnormalities, so that strategies can be implemented to maximise the number of functional nephrons at the beginning of life in the preterm infant in order to ensure long-term renal health. It is important that renal clinicians are made aware of the potential deleterious effects of preterm birth on developing glomerui, so they are aware of the renal vulnerability in subjects that are born preterm.

6. References

Abitbol, CL, Bauer, CR, Montane, B, Chandar, J, Duara, S & Zilleruelo, G. (2003). Long-term follow-up of extremely low birth weight infants with neonatal renal failure. *Pediatr Nephrol*, Vol. 18, No. 9, (Sep 2003), pp. 887-893, 0931-041X (Print)

Abitbol, CL, Chandar, J, Rodriguez, MM, Berho, M, Seeherunvong, W, Freundlich, M & Zilleruelo, G. (2009). Obesity and preterm birth: additive risks in the progression of kidney disease in children. *Pediatr Nephrol*, Vol. 24, No. 7, (Jul 2009), pp. 1363-1370, 1432-198X (Electronic)

Adachi, J, Kumar, C, Zhang, Y, Olsen, JV & Mann, M. (2006). The human urinary proteome contains more than 1500 proteins, including a large proportion of membrane proteins. *Genome Biol*, Vol. 7, No. 9, 2006), pp. R80, 1465-6914 (Electronic)

Akima, S, Kent, A, Reynolds, G, Gallagher, M & Falk, M. (2004). Indomethacin and renal impairment in neonates. *Pediatr Nephrol*, Vol. 19, No. 5, (May 2004), pp. 490-493, 0931-041X (Print)

Alejandre-Alcazar, MA, Kwapiszewska, G, Reiss, I, Amarie, OV, Marsh, LM, Sevilla-Perez, J, Wygrecka, M, Eul, B, Kobrich, S, Hesse, M, Schermuly, RT, Seeger, W, Eickelberg, O & Morty, RE. (2007). Hyperoxia modulates TGF-beta/BMP signaling in a mouse model of bronchopulmonary dysplasia. *Am J Physiol Lung Cell Mol Physiol*, Vol. 292, No. 2, (Feb 2007), pp. L537-549, 1040-0605 (Print)

Andreoli, SP. (2004). Acute renal failure in the newborn. *Semin Perinatol*, Vol. 28, No. 2, (Apr 2004), pp. 112-123, 0146-0005 (Print)

Aperia, A, Broberger, O, Elinder, G, Herin, P & Zetterstrom, R. (1981). Postnatal development of renal function in pre-term and full-term infants. *Acta Paediatr Scand*, Vol. 70, No. 2, (Mar 1981), pp. 183-187, 0001-656X (Print)

Arant, BS, Jr. (1987). Postnatal development of renal function during the first year of life. *Pediatr Nephrol*, Vol. 1, No. 3, (Jul 1987), pp. 308-313, 0931-041X (Print)

Awad, H, el-Safty, I, el-Barbary, M & Imam, S. (2002a). Evaluation of renal glomerular and tubular functional and structural integrity in neonates. *American Journal of the Medical Sciences*, Vol. 324, No. 5, (Nov 2002a), pp. 261-266,

Awad, H, el-Safty, I, el-Barbary, M & Imam, S. (2002b). Evaluation of renal glomerular and tubular functional and structural integrity in neonates. *Am J Med Sci*, Vol. 324, No. 5, (Nov 2002b), pp. 261-266, 0002-9629 (Print)

Bacchetta, J, Harambat, J, Dubourg, L, Guy, B, Liutkus, A, Canterino, I, Kassai, B, Putet, G & Cochat, P. (2009). Both extrauterine and intrauterine growth restriction impair renal function in children born very preterm. *Kidney Int*, Vol. 76, No. 4, (Aug 2009), pp. 445-452, 1523-1755 (Electronic)

Bariety, J, Mandet, C, Hill, G & Bruneval, P. (2006). Parietal podocytes in normal human glomeruli. *J Am Soc Nephrol*, Vol. 17, No. (Oct 2006), pp. 2770-2780, 1046-6673 (Print)

Baumgart, S & Costarino, AT. (2000). Water and electrolyte metabolism of the micropremie. *Clin Perinatol*, Vol. 27, No. 1, (Mar 2000), pp. 131-146, vi-vii, 0095-5108 (Print)

Behrman, RE, Lees, MH, Peterson, EN, De Lannoy, CW & Seeds, AE. (1970). Distribution of the circulation in the normal and asphyxiated fetal primate. *Am J Obstet Gynecol*, Vol. 108, No. 6, (Nov 15 1970), pp. 956-969, 0002-9378 (Print)

Bell, EF & Acarregui, MJ. (2008). Restricted versus liberal water intake for preventing morbidity and mortality in preterm infants. *Cochrane Database Syst Rev*, Vol. No. 1, 2008), pp. CD000503, 1469-493X (Electronic)

Bellomo, R, Ronco, C, Kellum, JA, Mehta, RL & Palevsky, P. (2004). Acute renal failure - definition, outcome measures, animal models, fluid therapy and information technology needs: the Second International Consensus Conference of the Acute Dialysis Quality Initiative (ADQI) Group. *Crit Care*, Vol. 8, No. 4, (Aug 2004), pp. R204-212, 1466-609X (Electronic)

Bertram, JF. (2001). Counting in the kidney. *Kidney Int*, Vol. 59, No. 2, (Feb 2001), pp. 792-796, 0085-2538 (Print)

Bhatia, J. (2006). Fluid and electrolyte management in the very low birth weight neonate. *J Perinatol*, Vol. 26 Suppl 1, No. (May 2006), pp. S19-21, 0743-8346 (Print)

Blackburn, S. 2003. Renal system and fluid and electrolyte homeostasis. In: Maternal, fetal and neonatal physiology, 2 ed: Saunders.

Bonamy, A, Bendito, A, Martin, H, Andolf, E, Sedin, G & Norman, M. (2005). Preterm Birth Contributes to Increased Vascular Resistance and Higher Blood Pressure in Adolescent Girls. *Pediatr Res*, Vol. 58, No. 5, 2005), pp. 845–849, 0031-3998 (Print)

Bonventre, JV. (2007). Pathophysiology of acute kidney injury: roles of potential inhibitors of inflammation. *Contrib Nephrol*, Vol. 156, No. 2007), pp. 39-46, 0302-5144 (Print)

Bueva, A & Guignard, J. (1994). Renal Function in the Preterm Neonates. *Pediatr Res*, Vol. 36, No. 5, 1994), pp. 572-577, 0031-3998 (Print)

Butler-O'Hara, M & D'Angio, CT. (2002). Risk of persistent renal insufficiency in premature infants following the prenatal use of indomethacin for suppression of preterm labor. *J Perinatol*, Vol. 22, No. 7, (Oct-Nov 2002), pp. 541-546, 0743-8346 (Print)

Cataldi, L, Leone, R, Moretti, U, De Mitri, B, Fanos, V, Ruggeri, L, Sabatino, G, Torcasio, F, Zanardo, V, Attardo, G, Riccobene, F, Martano, C, Benini, D & Cuzzolin, L. (2005). Potential risk factors for the development of acute renal failure in preterm newborn infants: a case-control study. *Arch Dis Child Fetal Neonatal Ed*, Vol. 90, No. 2005), pp. F514-519, 1359-2998 (Print)

Celsi, G, Kistner, A, Aizman, R, Eklof, AC, Ceccatelli, S, de Santiago, A & Jacobson, SH. (1998). Prenatal dexamethasone causes oligonephronia, sodium retention, and higher blood pressure in the offspring. *Pediatr Res*, Vol. 44, No. 3, (Sep 1998), pp. 317-322, 0031-3998 (Print)

Chen, CM, Wang, LF, Chou, HC, Lang, YD & Lai, YP. (2007). Up-regulation of connective tissue growth factor in hyperoxia-induced lung fibrosis. *Pediatr Res*, Vol. 62, No. 2, (Aug 2007), pp. 128-133, 0031-3998 (Print)

Chetty, A, Cao, GJ, Severgnini, M, Simon, A, Warburton, R & Nielsen, HC. (2008). Role of matrix metalloprotease-9 in hyperoxic injury in developing lung. *Am J Physiol Lung Cell Mol Physiol*, Vol. 295, No. 4, (Oct 2008), pp. L584-592, 1040-0605 (Print)

Choker, G & Gouyon, JB. (2004). Diagnosis of acute renal failure in very preterm infants. *Biol Neonate*, Vol. 86, No. 3, 2004), pp. 212-216, 0006-3126 (Print)

Christensen, EI & Birn, H. (2001). Megalin and cubilin: synergistic endocytic receptors in renal proximal tubule. *Am J Physiol Renal Physiol*, Vol. 280, No. 4, (Apr 2001), pp. F562-573, 1931-857X (Print)

Clark, AT & Bertram, JF. (1999). Molecular regulation of nephron endowment. *Am J Physiol*, Vol. 276, No. 4 Pt 2, (Apr 1999), pp. F485-497, 0002-9513 (Print)

Clark, PM, Bryant, TN, Hall, MA, Lowes, JA & Rowe, DJ. (1989). Neonatal renal function assessment. *Arch Dis Child*, Vol. 64, No. 9, (Sep 1989), pp. 1264-1269, 1468-2044 (Electronic)

Clark, R, Thomas, P & Peabody, J. (2003). Extrauterine growth restriction remains a serious problem in prematurely born neonates. *Pediatrics*, Vol. 111, No. 2003), pp. 986-990, 1098-4275 (Electronic)

Comper, WD, Haraldsson, B & Deen, WM. (2008). Resolved: normal glomeruli filter nephrotic levels of albumin. *J Am Soc Nephrol*, Vol. 19, No. 3, (Mar 2008), pp. 427-432, 1533-3450 (Electronic)

Cooper, R, Atherton, K & Power, C. (2008). Gestational age and risk factors for cardiovascular disease: evidence from the 1958 British birth cohort followed to mid-life. *Int J Epidemiol*, Vol. No. (Jul 25 2008), pp. 1464-3685 (Electronic)

Cullen, L, Young, R & Bertram, J. (2000). Studies on the effects of gentamicin on rat metanephric development *in vitro*. *Nephrology*, Vol. 5, No. 2000), pp. 115-123, 1440-1797

Cuzzolin, L, Fanos, V, Pinna, B, di Marzio, M, Perin, M, Tramontozzi, P, Tonetto, P & Cataldi, L. (2006). Postnatal renal function in preterm newborns: a role of diseases, drugs and therapeutic interventions. *Pediatr Nephrol*, Vol. 21, No. 7, 2006), pp. 931-938, 0931-041X (Print)

Dalziel, S, Parag, V, Rodgers, A & Harding, J. (2007). Cardiovascular risk factors at age 30 following pre-term birth. *Int J Epidemiol*, Vol. 36, No. 4, 2007), pp. 907-915, 0300-5771 (Print)

Dieperink, HI, Blackwell, TS & Prince, LS. (2006). Hyperoxia and apoptosis in developing mouse lung mesenchyme. *Pediatr Res*, Vol. 59, No. 2, (Feb 2006), pp. 185-190, 0031-3998 (Print)

Doyle, LW, Faber, B, Callanan, C & Morley, R. (2003). Blood pressure in late adolescence and very low birth weight. *Pediatrics*, Vol. 111, No. 2, (Feb 2003), pp. 252-257, 1098-4275 (Electronic)

Drougia, A, Giapros, V, Hotoura, E, Papadopoulou, F, Argyropoulou, M & Andronikou, S. (2009). The effects of gestational age and growth restriction on compensatory kidney growth. *Nephrol Dial Transplant*, Vol. 24, No. 1, (Jan 2009), pp. 142-148, 1460-2385 (Electronic)

Drukker, A & Guignard, JP. (2002). Renal aspects of the term and preterm infant: a selective update. *Curr Opin Pediatr*, Vol. 14, No. 2, (Apr 2002), pp. 175-182, 1040-8703 (Print)

Ehrenkranz, RA. (2000). Growth outcomes of very low-birth weight infants in the newborn intensive care unit. *Clin Perinatol*, Vol. 27, No. 2, (Jun 2000), pp. 325-345, 0095-5108 (Print)

Ellison, RC, Peckham, GJ, Lang, P, Talner, NS, Lerer, TJ, Lin, L, Dooley, KJ & Nadas, AS. (1983). Evaluation of the preterm infant for patent ductus arteriosus. *Pediatrics*, Vol. 71, No. 3, (Mar 1983), pp. 364-372, 0031-4005 (Print)

Engle, W. (1986). Development of fetal and neonatal renal function. *Semin Perinatol*, Vol. 10, No. 1986), pp. 113-124, 0146-0005 (Print)

Ervin, MG, Berry, LM, Ikegami, M, Jobe, AH, Padbury, JF & Polk, DH. (1996). Single dose fetal betamethasone administration stabilizes postnatal glomerular filtration rate and alters endocrine function in premature lambs. *Pediatr Res*, Vol. 40, No. 5, (Nov 1996), pp. 645-651, 0031-3998 (Print)

Ervin, MG, Seidner, SR, Leland, MM, Ikegami, M & Jobe, AH. (1998). Direct fetal glucocorticoid treatment alters postnatal adaptation in premature newborn baboons. *Am J Physiol*, Vol. 274, No. 4 Pt 2, (Apr 1998), pp. R1169-1176, 0002-9513 (Print)

Faa, G, Gerosa, C, Fanni, D, Nemolato, S, Locci, A, Cabras, T, Marinelli, V, Puddu, M, Zaffanello, M, Monga, G & Fanos, V. (2010). Marked interindividual variability in renal maturation of preterm infants: lessons from autopsy. *J Matern Fetal Neonatal Med*, Vol. No. (Sep 14 2010), pp. 1476-4954 (Electronic)

Fawer, CL, Torrado, A & Guignard, JP. (1979). Maturation of renal function in full-term and premature neonates. *Helv Paediatr Acta*, Vol. 34, No. 1, (Feb 1979), pp. 11-21, 0018-022X (Print)

Fell, JM, Thakkar, H, Newman, DJ & Price, CP. (1997). Measurement of albumin and low molecular weight proteins in the urine of newborn infants using a cotton wool ball collection method. *Acta Paediatr*, Vol. 86, No. 5, (May 1997), pp. 518-522, 0803-5253 (Print)

Finney, H, Newman, DJ, Thakkar, H, Fell, JM & Price, CP. (2000). Reference ranges for plasma cystatin C and creatinine measurements in premature infants, neonates, and older children. *Arch Dis Child*, Vol. 82, No. 1, (Jan 2000), pp. 71-75, 1468-2044 (Electronic)

Galaske, RG. (1986). Renal functional maturation: renal handling of proteins by mature and immature newborns. *Eur J Pediatr*, Vol. 145, No. 5, (Oct 1986), pp. 368-371, 0340-6199 (Print)

Galinsky, R, Moss, TJ, Gubhaju, L, Hooper, SB, Black, MJ & Polglase, GR. (2011). Effect of intra-amniotic lipopolysaccharide on nephron number in preterm fetal sheep. *Am J Physiol Renal Physiol*, Vol. No. (May 18 2011), pp. 1522-1466 (Electronic)

Gallini, F, Maggio, L, Romagnoli, C, Marrocco, G & Tortorolo, G. (2000). Progression of renal function in preterm neonates with gestational age < or = 32 weeks. *Pediatr Nephrol*, Vol. 15, No. 1-2, (Nov 2000), pp. 119-124, 0931-041X (Print)

Giapros, V, Papadimitriou, P, Challa, A & Andronikou, S. (2007). The effect of intrauterine growth retardation on renal function in the first two months of life. *Nephrol Dial Transplant*, Vol. 22, No. 1, (Jan 2007), pp. 96-103, 0931-0509 (Print)

Giapros, VI, Andronikou, SK, Cholevas, VI & Papadopoulou, ZL. (2003). Renal function and effect of aminoglycoside therapy during the first ten days of life. *Pediatr Nephrol*, Vol. 18, No. 1, (Jan 2003), pp. 46-52, 0931-041X (Print)

Gibson, I, Downie, T, More, I & Lindop, G. (1996). Atubular glomeruli and glomerular cysts - a possible pathway for nephron loss in the human kidney? *J Pathol*, Vol. 179, No. (Aug 1996), pp. 421-426, 0022-3417 (Print)

Gilbert, T, Gaonach, S, Moreau, E & Merlet-Benichou, C. (1994). Defect of nephrogenesis induced by gentamicin in rat metanephric organ culture. *Lab Invest*, Vol. 70, No. 5, (May 1994), pp. 656-666, 0023-6837 (Print)

Gilbert, T, Lelievre-Pegorier, M & Merlet-Benichou, C. (1990). Immediate and long-term renal effects of fetal exposure to gentamicin. *Pediatr Nephrol*, Vol. 4, No. 4, (Jul 1990), pp. 445-450, 0931-041X (Print)

Goldenberg, RL, Culhane, JF, Iams, JD & Romero, R. (2008). Epidemiology and causes of preterm birth. *Lancet*, Vol. 371, No. 9606, (Jan 5 2008), pp. 75-84, 1474-547X (Electronic)

Gordjani, N, Burghard, R, Leititis, J & Brandis, M. (1998). Serum creatinine and creatinine clearance in healthy neonates and prematures during the first 10 days of life. *Eur J Pediatr*, Vol. 148, No. 1998), pp. 143-145, 0340-6199 (Print)

Gortner, L, Bernsau, U, Brand, M, Hellwege, HH, Hieronimi, G, Jorch, G, Reiter, HL & Versmold, H. (1991). Drug utilization in very premature infants in neonatal intensive care units. *Dev Pharmacol Ther*, Vol. 17, No. 3-4, 1991), pp. 167-171, 0379-8305 (Print)

Gotsch, F, Romero, R, Kusanovic, J, Mazaki-Tovi, S, Pineles, B, Erez, O, Espinoza, J & Hassan, S. (2007). The fetal inflammatory response syndrome. *Clin Obstet Gynecol*, Vol. 50, No. 2007), pp. 652-683, 0009-9201 (Print)

Gubhaju, L & Black, MJ. (2005). The baboon as a good model for studies of human kidney development. *Pediatr Res*, Vol. 58, No. 2005), pp. 505-509, 0031-3998 (Print)

Gubhaju, L, Sutherland, MR, Yoder, BA, Zulli, A, Bertram, JF & Black, MJ. (2009). Is nephrogenesis affected by preterm birth? Studies in a non-human primate model. *Am J Physiol Renal Physiol*, Vol. 297, No. 6, (Dec 2009), pp. F1668-1677, 1522-1466 (Electronic)

Gunnarsson, GO, Gudmundsson, S, Hokegard, K, Stale, H, Kjellmer, I, Hafstrom, O & Marsal, K. (1998). Cerebral Doppler blood flow velocimetry and central hemodynamics in the ovine fetus during hypoxemia-acidemia. *J Perinat Med*, Vol. 26, No. 2, 1998), pp. 107-114, 0300-5577 (Print)

Gwira, JA, Wei, F, Ishibe, S, Ueland, JM, Barasch, J & Cantley, LG. (2005). Expression of neutrophil gelatinase-associated lipocalin regulates epithelial morphogenesis in vitro. *J Biol Chem*, Vol. 280, No. 9, (Mar 4 2005), pp. 7875-7882, 0021-9258 (Print)

Hack, M, Schluchter, M, Cartar, L & Rahman, M. (2005). Blood pressure among very low birth weight (<1.5 kg) young adults. *Pediatr Res*, Vol. 58, No. 4, (Oct 2005), pp. 677-684, 0031-3998 (Print)

Hendrickx, A, Bollert, J & Houston, M. (1971). *Embryology of the Baboon* The University of Chicago Press, 0226327124/0-226-32712-4, London.

Hentschel, R, Lodige, B & Bulla, M. (1996). Renal insufficiency in the neonatal period. *Clin Nephrol*, Vol. 46, No. 1, (Jul 1996), pp. 54-58, 0301-0430 (Print)

Hinchliffe, SA, Lynch, MR, Sargent, PH, Howard, CV & Van Velzen, D. (1992a). The effect of intrauterine growth retardation on the development of renal nephrons. *Br J Obstet Gynaecol*, Vol. 99, No. 4, (Apr 1992a), pp. 296-301, 0306-5456 (Print)

Hinchliffe, SA, Sargent, PH, Chan, YF, van Velzen, D, Howard, CV, Hutton, JL & Rushton, DI. (1992b). "Medullary ray glomerular counting" as a method of assessment of human nephrogenesis. *Pathol Res Pract*, Vol. 188, No. 6, (Aug 1992b), pp. 775-782, 0344-0338 (Print)

Hinchliffe, SA, Sargent, PH, Howard, CV, Chan, YF & van Velzen, D. (1991). Human intrauterine renal growth expressed in absolute number of glomeruli assessed by the disector method and Cavalieri principle. *Laboratory Investigation*, Vol. 64, No. 6, (Jun 1991), pp. 777-784, 0023-6837 (Print)

Hoppe, CC, Evans, RG, Moritz, KM, Cullen-McEwen, LA, Fitzgerald, SM, Dowling, J & Bertram, JF. (2007). Combined prenatal and postnatal protein restriction influences adult kidney structure, function, and arterial pressure. *Am J Physiol Regul Integr Comp Physiol*, Vol. 292, No. 1, (Jan 2007), pp. R462-469, 0363-6119 (Print)

Huang, HP, Tsai, IJ, Lai, YC, Cheng, CH & Tsau, YK. (2007). Early postnatal renal growth in premature infants. *Nephrology*, Vol. 12, No. 6, (Dec 2007), pp. 572-575, 1320-5358 (Print)

Huynh, TK, Bateman, DA, Parravicini, E, Lorenz, JM, Nemerofsky, SL, Sise, ME, Bowman, TM, Polesana, E & Barasch, JM. (2009). Reference values of urinary neutrophil gelatinase-associated lipocalin in very low birth weight infants. *Pediatr Res*, Vol. 66, No. 5, (Nov 2009), pp. 528-532, 1530-0447 (Electronic)

Iacobelli, S, Bonsante, F, Ferdinus, C, Labenne, M & Gouyon, JB. (2009). Factors affecting postnatal changes in serum creatinine in preterm infants with gestational age <32 weeks. *J Perinatol*, Vol. 29, No. 3, (Mar 2009), pp. 232-236, 1476-5543 (Electronic)

Iacobelli, S, Loprieno, S, Bonsante, F, Latorre, G, Esposito, L & Gouyon, JB. (2007). Renal function in early childhood in very low birthweight infants. *Am J Perinatol*, Vol. 24, No. 10, (Nov 2007), pp. 587-592, 0735-1631 (Print)

Itabashi, K, Ohno, T & Nishida, H. (2003). Indomethacin responsiveness of patent ductus arteriosus and renal abnormalities in preterm infants treated with indomethacin. *J Pediatr*, Vol. 143, No. 2, (Aug 2003), pp. 203-207, 0022-3476 (Print)

Johansson, S, Iliadou, A, Bergvall, N, Tuvemo, T, Norman, M & Cnattingius, S. (2005). Risk of high blood pressure among young men increases with the degree of immaturity at birth. *Circulation*, Vol. 112, No. 2005), pp. 3430-3436, 1524-4539 (Electronic)

Jones, DP & Chesney, RW. (1992). Development of tubular function. *Clin Perinatol*, Vol. 19, No. 1, (Mar 1992), pp. 33-57, 0095-5108 (Print)

Kang, NS, Yoo, KH, Cheon, H, Choi, BM, Hong, YS, Lee, JW & Kim, SK. (1999). Indomethacin treatment decreases renal blood flow velocity in human neonates. *Biol Neonate*, Vol. 76, No. 5, (Nov 1999), pp. 261-265, 0006-3126 (Print)

Keijzer-Veen, M, Schrevel, M, Finken, M, Dekker, F, Nauta, J, Hille, E, Frolich, M & van der Heijden, B. (2005). Microalbuminuria and lower glomerular filtration rate at young adult age in subjects born very premature and after intrauterine growth retardation. *J Am Soc Nephrol*, Vol. 16, No. 9, 2005), pp. 2762-2768, 1046-6673 (Print)

Keijzer-Veen, MG, Devos, AS, Meradji, M, Dekker, FW, Nauta, J & van der Heijden, BJ. (2010a). Reduced renal length and volume 20 years after very preterm birth. *Pediatr Nephrol*, Vol. 25, No. (Mar 2010a), pp. 499-507, 1432-198X (Electronic)

Keijzer-Veen, MG, Dulger, A, Dekker, FW, Nauta, J & van der Heijden, BJ. (2010b). Very preterm birth is a risk factor for increased systolic blood pressure at a young adult age. *Pediatr Nephrol*, Vol. 25, No. 3, 2010b), pp. 509-516, 1432-198X (Electronic)

Keijzer-Veen, MG, Kleinveld, HA, Lequin, MH, Dekker, FW, Nauta, J, de Rijke, YB & van der Heijden, BJ. (2007). Renal function and size at young adult age after intrauterine growth restriction and very premature birth. *Am J Kidney Dis*, Vol. 50, No. 4, (Oct 2007), pp. 542-551, 1523-6838 (Electronic)

Keller, G, Zimmer, G, Mall, G, Ritz, E & Amann, K. (2003). Nephron number in patients with primary hypertension. *N Engl J Med*, Vol. 348, No. 2, (Jan 9 2003), pp. 101-108, 1533-4406 (Electronic)

Kent, AL, Jyoti, R, Robertson, C, Gonsalves, L, Meskell, S, Shadbolt, B & Falk, MC. (2009). Does extreme prematurity affect kidney volume at term corrected age? *J Matern Fetal Neonatal Med*, Vol. 22, No. 5, (May 2009), pp. 435-438, 1476-4954 (Electronic)

Kent, AL, Maxwell, LE, Koina, ME, Falk, MC, Willenborg, D & Dahlstrom, JE. (2007). Renal glomeruli and tubular injury following indomethacin, ibuprofen, and gentamicin exposure in a neonatal rat model. *Pediatr Res*, Vol. 62, No. 3, (Sep 2007), pp. 307-312, 0031-3998 (Print)

Kistner, A, Celsi, G, Vanpee, M & Jacobson, SH. (2000). Increased blood pressure but normal renal function in adult women born preterm. *Pediatr Nephrol*, Vol. 15, No. 3-4, (Dec 2000), pp. 215-220, 0931-041X (Print)

Kistner, A, Jacobson, L, Jacobson, S, Svensson, E & Hellstrom, A. (2002). Low gestational age associated with abnormal retinal vascularization and increased blood pressure in adult women. *Pediatr Res*, Vol. 51, No. 6, 2002), pp. 675–680, 0031-3998 (Print)

Kluckow, M & Evans, N. (2001). Low systemic blood flow in the preterm infant. *Semin Neonatol*, Vol. 6, No. 1, (Feb 2001), pp. 75-84, 1084-2756 (Print)

Kutz, P, Horsch, S, Kuhn, L & Roll, C. (2009). Single-centre vs. population-based outcome data of extremely preterm infants at the limits of viability. *Acta Paediatr*, Vol. 98, No. 9, (Sep 2009), pp. 1451-1455, 1651-2227 (Electronic)

Kwinta, P, Klimek, M, Drozdz, D, Grudzien, A, Jagla, M, Zasada, M & Pietrzyk, JJ. (2011). Assessment of long-term renal complications in extremely low birth weight children. *Pediatr Nephrol*, Vol. 26, No. 7, (Jul 2011), pp. 1095-1103, 1432-198X (Electronic)

Lahra, MM & Jeffery, HE. (2004). A fetal response to chorioamnionitis is associated with early survival after preterm birth. *Am J Obstet Gynecol*, Vol. 190, No. 1, (Jan 2004), pp. 147-151, 0002-9378 (Print)

Lavery, AP, Meinzen-Derr, JK, Anderson, E, Ma, Q, Bennett, MR, Devarajan, P & Schibler, KR. (2008). Urinary NGAL in premature infants. *Pediatr Res*, Vol. 64, No. 4, (Oct 2008), pp. 423-428, 1530-0447 (Electronic)

Lodrup, AB, Karstoft, K, Dissing, TH, Nyengaard, JR & Pedersen, M. (2008). The association between renal function and structural parameters: a pig study. *BMC Nephrol*, Vol. 9, No. 2008), pp. 18, 1471-2369 (Electronic)

Lorenz, JM, Kleinman, LI, Ahmed, G & Markarian, K. (1995). Phases of fluid and electrolyte homeostasis in the extremely low birth weight infant. *Pediatrics*, Vol. 96, No. 3 Pt 1, (Sep 1995), pp. 484-489, 0031-4005 (Print)

Lorenz, JM, Kleinman, LI, Kotagal, UR & Reller, MD. (1982). Water balance in very low-birth-weight infants: relationship to water and sodium intake and effect on outcome. *J Pediatr*, Vol. 101, No. 3, (Sep 1982), pp. 423-432, 0022-3476 (Print)

Louey, S, Cock, ML, Stevenson, KM & Harding, R. (2000). Placental insufficiency and fetal growth restriction lead to postnatal hypotension and altered postnatal growth in sheep. *Pediatr Res*, Vol. 48, No. 6, (Dec 2000), pp. 808-814, 0031-3998 (Print)

Luyckx, VA & Brenner, BM. (2005). Low birth weight, nephron number, and kidney disease. *Kidney Int Suppl*, Vol. No. 97, (Aug 2005), pp. S68-77, 0098-6577 (Print)

Manalich, R, Reyes, L, Herrera, M, Melendi, C & Fundora, I. (2000). Relationship between weight at birth and the number and size of renal glomeruli in humans: a histomorphometric study. *Kidney Int*, Vol. 58, No. 2, (Aug 2000), pp. 770-773, 0085-2538 (Print)

Mathieson, P. (2004). The cellular basis of albuminuria. *Clin Sci*, Vol. 107, No. 2004), pp. 533 - 538,

Matos, P, Duarte-Silva, M, Drukker, A & Guignard, JP. (1998). Creatinine reabsorption by the newborn rabbit kidney. *Pediatr Res*, Vol. 44, No. 5, (Nov 1998), pp. 639-641, 0031-3998 (Print)

Matsushita, K, van der Velde, M, Astor, BC, Woodward, M, Levey, AS, de Jong, PE, Coresh, J & Gansevoort, RT. (2010). Association of estimated glomerular filtration rate and albuminuria with all-cause and cardiovascular mortality in general population cohorts: a collaborative meta-analysis. *Lancet*, Vol. 375, No. 9731, (Jun 12 2010), pp. 2073-2081, 1474-547X (Electronic)

McCormick, MC. (1985). The contribution of low birth weight to infant mortality and childhood morbidity. *N Engl J Med*, Vol. 312, No. 2, (Jan 10 1985), pp. 82-90, 0028-4793 (Print)

McGrath-Morrow, SA & Stahl, J. (2001). Apoptosis in neonatal murine lung exposed to hyperoxia. *Am J Respir Cell Mol Biol*, Vol. 25, No. 2, (Aug 2001), pp. 150-155, 1044-1549 (Print)

Mehta, RL, Kellum, JA, Shah, SV, Molitoris, BA, Ronco, C, Warnock, DG & Levin, A. (2007). Acute Kidney Injury Network: report of an initiative to improve outcomes in acute kidney injury. *Crit Care*, Vol. 11, No. 2, 2007), pp. R31, 1466-609X (Electronic)

Merlet-Benichou, C, Gilbert, T, Muffat-Joly, M, Lelievre-Pegorier, M & Leroy, B. (1994). Intrauterine growth retardation leads to a permanent nephron deficit in the rat. *Pediatr Nephrol*, Vol. 8, No. 2, (Apr 1994), pp. 175-180, 0931-041X (Print)

Methven, S, MacGregor, MS, Traynor, JP, Hair, M, O'Reilly, DS & Deighan, CJ. (2011). Comparison of urinary albumin and urinary total protein as predictors of patient outcomes in CKD. *Am J Kidney Dis*, Vol. 57, No. 1, (Jan 2011), pp. 21-28, 1523-6838 (Electronic)

Miall, LS, Henderson, MJ, Turner, AJ, Brownlee, KG, Brocklebank, JT, Newell, SJ & Allgar, VL. (1999). Plasma creatinine rises dramatically in the first 48 hours of life in preterm infants. *Pediatrics*, Vol. 104, No. 6, (Dec 1999), pp. e76, 1098-4275 (Electronic)

Moniz, CF, Nicolaides, KH, Bamforth, FJ & Rodeck, CH. (1985). Normal reference ranges for biochemical substances relating to renal, hepatic, and bone function in fetal and maternal plasma throughout pregnancy. *J Clin Pathol*, Vol. 38, No. 4, (Apr 1985), pp. 468-472, 0021-9746 (Print)

Moran, SM & Myers, BD. (1985). Course of acute renal failure studied by a model of creatinine kinetics. *Kidney Int*, Vol. 27, No. 6, (Jun 1985), pp. 928-937, 0085-2538 (Print)

Moritz, KM, Johnson, K, Douglas-Denton, R, Wintour, EM & Dodic, M. (2002). Maternal glucocorticoid treatment programs alterations in the renin-angiotensin system of the ovine fetal kidney. *Endocrinology*, Vol. 143, No. 11, (Nov 2002), pp. 4455-4463, 0013-7227 (Print)

Moritz, KM, Wintour, EM, Black, MJ, Bertram, JF & Caruana, G. (2008). Factors influencing mammalian kidney development: implications for health in adult life. *Adv Anat Embryol Cell Biol*, Vol. 196, No. 2008), pp. 1-78, 0301-5556 (Print)

Moritz, ML & Ayus, JC. (2005). Preventing neurological complications from dysnatremias in children. *Pediatr Nephrol*, Vol. 20, No. 12, (Dec 2005), pp. 1687-1700, 0931-041X (Print)

Nagai, J & Takano, M. (2004). Molecular aspects of renal handling of aminoglycosides and strategies for preventing the nephrotoxicity. *Drug Metab Pharmacokinet*, Vol. 19, No. 3, (Jun 2004), pp. 159-170, 1347-4367 (Print)

Nathanson, S, Moreau, E, Merlet-Benichou, C & Gilbert, T. (2000). In utero and in vitro exposure to beta-lactams impair kidney development in the rat. *J Am Soc Nephrol*, Vol. 11, No. 5, (May 2000), pp. 874-884, 1046-6673 (Print)

Nenov, VD, Taal, MW, Sakharova, OV & Brenner, BM. (2000). Multi-hit nature of chronic renal disease. *Curr Opin Nephrol Hypertens*, Vol. 9, No. 2, (Mar 2000), pp. 85-97, 1062-4821 (Print)

Oh, W, Poindexter, BB, Perritt, R, Lemons, JA, Bauer, CR, Ehrenkranz, RA, Stoll, BJ, Poole, K & Wright, LL. (2005). Association between fluid intake and weight loss during the first ten days of life and risk of bronchopulmonary dysplasia in extremely low birth weight infants. *J Pediatr*, Vol. 147, No. 6, (Dec 2005), pp. 786-790, 0022-3476 (Print)

Ortiz, LA, Quan, A, Weinberg, A & Baum, M. (2001). Effect of prenatal dexamethasone on rat renal development. *Kidney Int*, Vol. 59, No. 5, (May 2001), pp. 1663-1669, 0085-2538 (Print)

Osborn, D, Evans, N & Kluckow, M. (2002). Randomized trial of dobutamine versus dopamine in preterm infants with low systemic blood flow. *J Pediatr*, Vol. 140, No. 2, (Feb 2002), pp. 183-191, 0022-3476 (Print)

Parikh, CR, Lu, JC, Coca, SG & Devarajan, P. (2010). Tubular proteinuria in acute kidney injury: a critical evaluation of current status and future promise. *Ann Clin Biochem*, Vol. 47, No. Pt 4, (Jul 2010), pp. 301-312, 1758-1001 (Electronic)

Parravicini, E. (2010). The clinical utility of urinary neutrophil gelatinase-associated lipocalin in the neonatal ICU. *Curr Opin Pediatr*, Vol. 22, No. 2, (Apr 2010), pp. 146-150, 1531-698X (Electronic)

Parravicini, E, Nemerofsky, SL, Michelson, KA, Huynh, TK, Sise, ME, Bateman, DA, Lorenz, JM & Barasch, JM. (2010). Urinary neutrophil gelatinase-associated lipocalin is a promising biomarker for late onset culture-positive sepsis in very low birth weight infants. *Pediatr Res*, Vol. 67, No. 6, (Jun 2010), pp. 636-640, 1530-0447 (Electronic)

Petershack, JA, Nagaraja, SC & Guillery, EN. (1999). Role of glucocorticoids in the maturation of renal cortical Na+-K+-ATPase during fetal life in sheep. *Am J Physiol*, Vol. 276, No. 6 Pt 2, (Jun 1999), pp. R1825-1832, 0002-9513 (Print)

Polglase, GR, Hooper, SB, Gill, AW, Allison, BJ, McLean, CJ, Nitsos, I, Pillow, JJ & Kluckow, M. (2009). Cardiovascular and pulmonary consequences of airway recruitment in preterm lambs. *J Appl Physiol*, Vol. 106, No. 4, (Apr 2009), pp. 1347-1355, 8750-7587 (Print)

Rakow, A, Johansson, S, Legnevall, L, Sevastik, R, Celsi, G, Norman, M & Vanpee, M. (2008). Renal volume and function in school-age children born preterm or small for gestational age. *Pediatr Nephrol*, Vol. 23, No. 8, (Aug 2008), pp. 1309-1315, 0931-041X (Print)

Ralston, SH, Caine, N, Richards, I, O'Reilly, D, Sturrock, RD & Capell, HA. (1988). Screening for proteinuria in a rheumatology clinic: comparison of dipstick testing, 24 hour urine quantitative protein, and protein/creatinine ratio in random urine samples. *Ann Rheum Dis*, Vol. 47, No. 9, (Sep 1988), pp. 759-763, 0003-4967 (Print)

Rodriguez-Soriano, J, Aguirre, M, Oliveros, R & Vallo, A. (2005). Long-term renal follow-up of extremely low birth weight infants. *Pediatr Nephrol*, Vol. 20, No. 2005), pp. 579-584, 0931-041X (Print)

Rodriguez, MM, Gomez, AH, Abitbol, CL, Chandar, JJ, Duara, S & Zilleruelo, GE. (2004). Histomorphometric Analysis of Postnatal Glomerulogenesis in Extremely Preterm Infants. *Pediatr Dev Pathol*, Vol. 7, No. 2004), pp. 17-25, 1093-5266 (Print)

Romero, R, Chaiworapongsa, T & Espinoza, J. (2003). Micronutrients and intrauterine infection, preterm birth and the fetal inflammatory response syndrome. *J Nutr*, Vol. 133, No. 5 Suppl 2, (May 2003), pp. 1668S-1673S, 0022-3166 (Print)

Romero, R, Espinoza, J, Goncalves, LF, Kusanovic, JP, Friel, LA & Nien, JK. (2006). Inflammation in preterm and term labour and delivery. *Semin Fetal Neonatal Med*, Vol. 11, No. 5, (Oct 2006), pp. 317-326, 1744-165X (Print)

Romero, R, Gomez, R, Ghezzi, F, Yoon, BH, Mazor, M, Edwin, SS & Berry, SM. (1998). A fetal systemic inflammatory response is followed by the spontaneous onset of preterm parturition. *Am J Obstet Gynecol*, Vol. 179, No. 1, (Jul 1998), pp. 186-193, 0002-9378 (Print)

Rosner, MH. (2009). Urinary biomarkers for the detection of renal injury. *Adv Clin Chem*, Vol. 49, No. 2009), pp. 73-97, 0065-2423 (Print)

Ross, B, Cowett, R & Oh, W. (1977). Renal functions of low birth weight infants during the first two months of life. *Pediatr Res*, Vol. 11, No. 1977), pp. 1162-1164, 0031-3998 (Print)

Saxen, L. (1987). *Organogenesis of the Kidney* Cambridge University Press, Cambridge.

Schmidt, I, Chellakooty, M, Boisen, K, Damgaard, I, Kai, C, Olgaard, K & Main, K. (2005). Impaired kidney growth in low-birth-weight children: Distinct effects of maturity and weight for gestational age. *Kidney Int*, Vol. 68, No. 2005), pp. 731-740, 0085-2538 (Print)

Schreuder, MF, Wilhelm, AJ, Bokenkamp, A, Timmermans, SM, Delemarre-van de Waal, HA & van Wijk, JA. (2009). Impact of gestational age and birth weight on amikacin clearance on day 1 of life. *Clin J Am Soc Nephrol*, Vol. 4, No. 11, (Nov 2009), pp. 1774-1778, 1555-905X (Electronic)

Siegel, SR & Oh, W. (1976). Renal function as a marker of human fetal maturation. *Acta Paediatr Scand*, Vol. 65, No. 4, (Jul 1976), pp. 481-485, 0001-656X (Print)

Siewert-Delle, A & Ljungman, S. (1998). The impact of birth weight and gestational age on blood pressure in adult life. A population-based study of 49-year-old men. *Am J Hypertens*, Vol. 11, No. 1998), pp. 946-953, 0895-7061 (Print)

Stapleton, F, Jones, D & Green, R. (1987). Acute renal failure in neonates: Incidence, etiology and outcome. *Pediatr Nephrol*, Vol. 1, No. 1987), pp. 314-320, 0931-041X (Print)

Sulyok, E, Varg, F, Gyory, E, Jobst, K & Czaba, I. (1979). Postnatal development of renal sodium handling in premature infants. *J Pediatr*, Vol. 95, No. 1979), pp. 787-792, 0022-3476 (Print)

Sutherland, MR, Gubhaju, L & Black, MJ. (2011a). Stereological assessment of renal development in a baboon model of preterm birth. *Am J Nephrol*, Vol. 33 Suppl 1, No. 2011a), pp. 25-33, 1421-9670 (Electronic)

Sutherland, MR, Gubhaju, L, Moore, L, Kent, AL, Dahlstrom, JE, Horne, RS, Hoy, WE, Bertram, JF & Black, MJ. (2011b). Accelerated Maturation and Abnormal Morphology in the Preterm Neonatal Kidney. *J Am Soc Nephrol*, Vol. No. (Jun 2 2011b), pp. 1533-3450 (Electronic)

Sweeney, W & Avner, E. 2004. The kidney - Embryogenesis and anatomic development of the kidney. In: Polin R, Fox W, Abman S, editors. Fetal and Nenatal Physiology, 3 ed: Saunders (Elsevier).

Takieddine, F, Tabbara, M, Hall, P, Sokol, RJ & King, KC. (1983). Fetal renal maturation. Studies on urinary beta 2 microglobulin the neonate. *Acta Obstet Gynecol Scand*, Vol. 62, No. 4, 1983), pp. 311-314, 0001-6349 (Print)

Teitel, DF, Iwamoto, HS & Rudolph, AM. (1987). Effects of birth-related events on central blood flow patterns. *Pediatr Res*, Vol. 22, No. 5, (Nov 1987), pp. 557-566, 0031-3998 (Print)

Thayyil, S, Sheik, S, Kempley, ST & Sinha, A. (2008). A gestation- and postnatal age-based reference chart for assessing renal function in extremely premature infants. *J Perinatol*, Vol. 28, No. 3, (Mar 2008), pp. 226-229, 0743-8346 (Print)

Thomson, MA, Yoder, BA, Winter, VT, Martin, H, Catland, D, Siler-Khodr, TM & Coalson, JJ. (2004). Treatment of immature baboons for 28 days with early nasal continuous positive airway pressure. *Am J Respir Crit Care Med*, Vol. 169, No. 9, (May 1 2004), pp. 1054-1062, 1073-449X (Print)

Tomlinson, PA. (1992). Low molecular weight proteins in children with renal disease. *Pediatr Nephrol*, Vol. 6, No. 6, (Nov 1992), pp. 565-571, 0931-041X (Print)

Tsukahara, H, Fujii, Y, Tsuchida, S, Hiraoka, M, Morikawa, K, Haruki, S & Sudo, M. (1994). Renal handling of albumin and beta-2-microglobulin in neonates. *Nephron*, Vol. 68, No. 2, 1994), pp. 212-216, 0028-2766 (Print)

Tsukahara, H, Yoshimoto, M, Saito, M, Sakaguchi, T, Mitsuyoshi, I, Hayashi, S, Nakamura, K, Kikuchi, K & Sudo, M. (1990). Assessment of tubular function in neonates using urinary beta 2-microglobulin. *Pediatr Nephrol*, Vol. 4, No. 5, (Sep 1990), pp. 512-514, 0931-041X (Print)

Tucker, J & McGuire, W. (2004). Epidemiology of preterm birth. *BMJ*, Vol. 329, No. 7467, (Sep 18 2004), pp. 675-678, 1468-5833 (Electronic)

Ueda, N & Shah, SV. (2000). Tubular cell damage in acute renal failure-apoptosis, necrosis, or both. *Nephrol Dial Transplant*, Vol. 15, No. 3, (Mar 2000), pp. 318-323, 0931-0509 (Print)

van Venrooij, NA, Junewick, JJ, Gelfand, SL, Davis, AT, Crumb, TL & Bunchman, TE. (2010). Sonographic assessment of renal size and growth in premature infants. *Pediatr Radiol*, Vol. 40, No. 9, (Sep 2010), pp. 1505-1508, 1432-1998 (Electronic)

Vanpee, M, Blennow, M, Linne, T, Herin, P & Aperia, A. (1992). Renal function in very low birth weight infants: normal maturity reached during early childhood. *J Pediatr*, Vol. 121, No. 5 Pt 1, (Nov 1992), pp. 784-788, 0022-3476 (Print)

Vidaeff, AC, Doyle, NM & Gilstrap, LC, 3rd. (2003). Antenatal corticosteroids for fetal maturation in women at risk for preterm delivery. *Clin Perinatol*, Vol. 30, No. 4, (Dec 2003), pp. 825-840, vii, 0095-5108 (Print)

Vieux, R, Hascoet, JM, Merdariu, D, Fresson, J & Guillemin, F. (2010). Glomerular filtration rate reference values in very preterm infants. *Pediatrics*, Vol. 125, No. 5, (May 2010), pp. e1186-1192, 1098-4275 (Electronic)

Wilkins, BH. (1992). Renal function in sick very low birthweight infants: 1. Glomerular filtration rate. *Arch Dis Child*, Vol. 67, No. 10 Spec No, (Oct 1992), pp. 1140-1145, 1468-2044 (Electronic)

Zaffanello, M, Brugnara, M, Bruno, C, Franchi, B, Talamini, G, Guidi, G, Cataldi, L, Biban, P, Mella, R & Fanos, V. (2010). Renal function and volume of infants born with a very low birth-weight: a preliminary cross-sectional study. *Acta Paediatr*, Vol. 99, No. 8, (Aug 2010), pp. 1192-1198, 1651-2227 (Electronic)

Zimanyi, MA, Bertram, JF & Black, MJ. (2004). Does a nephron deficit in rats predispose to salt-sensitive hypertension? *Kidney Blood Press Res*, Vol. 27, No. 4, 2004), pp. 239-247, 1420-4096 (Print)

Zimanyi, MA, Denton, KM, Forbes, JM, Thallas-Bonke, V, Thomas, MC, Poon, F & Black, MJ. (2006). A developmental nephron deficit in rats is associated with increased susceptibility to a secondary renal injury due to advanced glycation end-products. *Diabetologia*, Vol. 49, No. 4, (Apr 2006), pp. 801-810, 0012-186X (Print)

Zohdi, V, Moritz, KM, Bubb, KJ, Cock, ML, Wreford, N, Harding, R & Black, MJ. (2007). Nephrogenesis and the renal renin-angiotensin system in fetal sheep: effects of intrauterine growth restriction during late gestation. *Am J Physiol Regul Integr Comp Physiol*, Vol. 293, No. 3, (Sep 2007), pp. R1267-1273, 0363-6119 (Print)

4

Renal Potassium Handling and Associated Inherited Tubulopathies Leading to Hypokalemia

Jelena Stojanovic and John Sayer
Institute of Genetic Medicine
Newcastle University
Newcastle upon Tyne
United Kingdom

1. Introduction

Regulation of intracellular and extracellular potassium concentration is a fundamental process vital for cellular metabolism. Potassium intake, from the diet, is carefully balanced with excretion of potassium via the renal tract and gastrointestinal losses. Following a potassium load, extra-renal buffering of potassium occurs in peripheral tissues prior to its excretion. Thus potassium regulation is achieved by both short term and long term mechanisms. It has become clear that a series of potassium ion channels and transporter proteins have physiologically important roles throughout the length of the nephron. Our knowledge of normal physiological mechanisms has been increased by studying molecular defects responsible for variety of disorders associated with potassium transport. Studying renal tubular epithelial cell proteins and their regulation has improved the understanding of inherited tubular disorders which may cause hypokalemia.

Here, we review the normal renal tubular handling of potassium and discuss the molecular basis of clinical syndromes associated with hypokalemic alkalosis and hypokalemic forms of hypertension.

2. Renal tubular handling of potassium

2.1 Glomerular filtration and proximal tubule

Glomerular filtration produces >160 L of filtrate per day in a healthy adult, and 99% of this volume and majority of filtered solutes are reabsorbed along the nephron. The filtrate is identical to that of plasma with respect to water and solutes of low molecular weight, such as glucose, chloride, sodium, phosphate, urea, uric acid, creatinine and potassium.

The proximal convoluted tubule is responsible for reabsorption of glucose, amino acids, phosphate, sodium and low-molecular weight proteins. Around 65% of filtered sodium is reabsorbed in the proximal tubule. Potassium reabsorption is closely coupled to sodium transport (driven passively by the electrical gradient) and around 75% of filtered potassium is reabsorbed by the proximal convoluted tubule. The proximal straight tubule may secrete some potassium into the urine, and this secretion can be upregulated significantly in patients with chronic kidney disease. Generalized defects in proximal tubule handling of solutes result in Fanconi syndrome syndrome. Specific proximal tubular handling defects leading to hypokalemia include proximal renal tubular acidosis, and have been recently reviewed elsewhere (Fry &Karet, 2007).

2.2 Potassium movement in the thin loop of Henle

Potassium may be secreted in the thin descending loops of Henle that penetrate the inner medulla, whilst the thin ascending loop is permeable to sodium and potassium and allows some uptake.

The thin ascending limbs of the loops of Henle (among other nephron segments) express the CLC-KA chloride channel, with its subunit Barttin. Polymorphisms in *CLCNKA* have recently been associated with a hyperreninemic hyperaldosteronism, implicating a key role for this channel in regulating renal salt handling and determining a set point for renin and angiotensin levels (Cappola, et al., 2011).

2.3 Potassium movement in thick ascending loop of Henle

In this part of nephron, ~25% of filtered sodium is reabsorbed together with ~15% of the filtered potassium. Transcellular sodium and potassium transport is achieved by the $Na^+K^+2Cl^-$ cotransporter (NKCC2) in the apical membrane, driven by the basolateral Na^+K^+ATPase pump. Alternative names for NKCC2 include the bumetanide sensitive co-transporter, (BSC). NKCC2 is exclusively expressed in kidney tissue and is encoded by *SLC12A1* gene (Simon, et al., 1996a). The NKCC2 transporter may also transport ammonium ions, which compete with potassium ions.

Potassium entering the cell via NKCC2 is recycled back into tubule lumen via the apical membrane channel, ROMK1 (Simon, et al., 1996b), generating a lumen positive potential driving paracellular resorption of calcium and magnesium. Tight junction proteins, such as paracellin 1, mediate this divalent cation transport. ROMK1, also known as a KCNJ, is an ATPase sensitive potassium channel. Functional coupling of ROMK1 with NKCC2 is essential for NaCl reabsorption. Chloride exits the basolateral membrane of the TAL via the CLC chloride channel, CLC-KB, which is co-expressed with the subunit Barttin.

2.4 The distal convoluted tubule

The distal convoluted tubule is responsible for ~8% of filtered sodium reabsorption. This is achieved via an apical Na^+Cl^- cotransporter (NCCT, alias the thiazide sensitive sodium chloride transporter). This transporter is regulated by a group of serine-threonine protein kinases, incluidng WNK4. In healthy individuals, WNK4 inhibits NCCT function by reducing its expression on the membrane.

Recent data has suggested that potassium channels control DCT function. An apically expressed potassium channel Kv1.1 is postulated to stabilise the luminal membrane potential in this nephron segment (Glaudemans, et al., 2009). and facilitates effective magnesium transport via the apical TRPM6 magnesium channel. At the basolateral membrane of the DCT a potassium channel Kir4.1 is thought to allow potassium recycling, allowing maintenance of the basolateral Na^+K^+ATPase activity, the driving force for NaCl reabsorption via NCCT in this nephron segment (Bockenhauer, et al., 2009, Scholl, et al., 2009).

2.5 The collecting ducts

The connecting tubules, initial collecting tubule and the cortical collecting duct, are major sites of regulated potassium secretion. Indeed, potassium secretion in these nephron segments may be upregulated to exceed the filtered load of potassium. In addition, if potassium reabsorption is required, this part of the nephron and regions of the medullary collecting duct may reabsorb potassium. In the cortical collecting duct two important cell types mediate potassium transport: principal cells and intercalated cells.

In principal cells, sodium entry occurs via selective sodium channels (ENaCs), located on apical membrane. Potassium secretion in these cells occurs by a transcellular movement of potassium, mediated by a basolateral Na^+K^+ATPase pump and apical ROMK potassium channels. Potassium secretion is directly linked to sodium entry via ENaC.

The distribution of ENaC channels within the apical membrane is regulated by effects of aldosterone on the mineralocorticoid receptor. The ENaC channel has three subunits: alpha, beta and gamma encoded by genes *SCNN1A, SCNN1B* and *SCNN1C.* Alpha-intercalated cells in the cortical collecting duct mediate potassium reabsorption. An apical H^+K^+ATPase pump allows potassium reabsorption coupled to proton excretion, whilst an apical proton pump transports hydrogen ions into the lumen. In states of potassium depletion, there is upregulation of the apical H^+K^+ATPase pump in alpha intercalated cells.

3. When hypokalemia may be the presentation of an inherited tubulopathy?

Physiological serum potassium levels are usually tightly maintained between 3.5-5.0 mmol/L. Hypokalemia represents a deviation from this regulation and may be defined as mild, moderate or severe. Mild hypokalemia (Serum K^+ 3.0-3.5 mmol/L) is usually asymptomatic whilst moderate hypokalemia (Serum K^+ 2.5-3.0 mmol/L) may present with muscle weakness, myalgia, arrhythmias, cramps and constipation. With severe hypokalemia, (K^+ <2mmol/L), hyporeflexia, flaccid paralysis and occasionally rhabdomyolysis occur. There are many causes of hypokalemia to be considered before a renal tubulopathy is suspected. These can be divided into an assessment of potassium intake, potassium distribution within tissues and potassium excretion (see Table 1). In order to assess this, a careful history including history of drugs and over the counter medications, and the presence of Gastrointestinal (GI) disturbance (vomiting or diarrhoea) should be sought. Clinical examination (including blood pressure (BP) and orthostatic changes in BP)) is also necessary. This, combined with serum and urine biochemistry (including osmolality) will help to assess the causes of hypokalemia. Occasionally, a high WBC count may be associated with a spurious low serum potassium level. Pseudohypokalemia has recently been reported in 2 patients with hereditary spherocytosis secondary to AE1 mutations (Norgett, et al., 2011).

Potassium is present in a wide variety of foods (citrus fruits, vegetables, meat). Therefore, examples of inadequate intake are limited to anorexia, bulimia, alcoholism and starvation. Certain factors may affect the distribution of potassium from extracellular to intracellular compartments, leading to hypokalemia. Endogenous or administered insulin, catecholamines, beta-agonists and metabolic alkalosis will all promote cellular uptake of potassium. Excretion of potassium may be grouped into extra renal loss and renal loss. Extra renal loss of potassium is mainly via the gastrointestinal tract (GI) and may occur with diarrhoea, GI fistulas, and laxative abuse. Renal loss of potassium may be associated with a variety of acquired and inherited tubular disorders and drugs. Amphotericin B, aminoglycosides and cisplatin all increase renal potassium losses. Many diuretics, apart from potassium-sparing ones, cause increased urinary losses of potassium. Magnesium depletion may also lead to renal potassium wasting. A 24 h urine collection can be used to assess renal potassium excretion in a hypokalemia patient. This should be < 15 mmol/24 h if there is extra renal potassium wasting. In a similar way, a spot urine for a potassium/creatinine ratio should be less than 1 in the presence of extra renal potassium wasting. Calculations of transtubular potassium gradient will give similar information. Urinary chloride will also be low in cases of significant GI volume losses (vomiting, diarrhoea, laxative abuse). If renal K wasting is suspected and confirmed then further thought regarding the blood pressure and acid base status of the patient aids the diagnosis of hypokalemia.

Extra-renal Hypokalemia		
Spurious	Extra-renal Loss	Redistribution
High WBC count	Diarrhoea	Acid-base disturbance
Hereditary spherocytosis	GI fistulas	Insulin excess
	Laxative abuse	Beta-adrenergic agonists
	Dietary insufficiency	Drugs / toxins e.g. Barium, catecholamines
	Cutaneous losses	Hypokalemic periodic paralysis (familial and thyrotoxic)

Table 1. Causes of extra-renal hypokalemia

Reasons to suspect an inherited tubulopathy may include evidence for a persistent electrolyte disturbance, the presence of renal impairment, nephrocalcinosis and renal stone formation (Sayer &Pearce, 2001). A detailed and extensive family history is necessary. In paediatric cases, faltering growth, abnormal growth patterns, developmental delay and deafness may all be clues to an inherited tubulopathy. Neonates may present with a salt-wasting crisis and are particularly sensitive to severe hypovolemia and electrolyte disturbance due to immature tubular physiology and low-salt intakes in standard feeds. With nephron maturation, the propensity to present with salt-wasting crises decreases. Individual tubular diseases can be differentiated by their serum and urine biochemical profiles (discussed below). Hypokalemia may be the only presenting feature of a tubulopathy and it is important to follow the diagnostic 'lead' to differentiate the many causes. Nephrocalcinosis should be thoroughly investigated and differential diagnosis such as hyperparathyroidism, vitamin D intoxication and sarcoidosis first excluded. Renal tubular disorders associated with nephrocalcinosis include Bartter's syndrome, Dent's disease, hypomagnesemic hypercalciuric nephrolithiasis, idiopathic hypercalciuria and distal renal tubular acidosis.

Renal tubulopathies are best investigated by urine pH and 24-hour urine collection for potassium, calcium, magnesium, citrate and phosphate along with serum biochemistry. Nevertheless, renal tubulopathies are rare and they should be considered only after careful drug and dietary histories are taken, together with urine electrolytes and serum biochemistry.

4. Inherited tubulopathies leading to hypokalemic alkalosis

4.1 Bartter's syndrome

Bartter's syndrome is an autosomal recessive renal disorder described by Bartter et al. in 1962 (Bartter, et al., 1962). It has estimated incidence of 1.2 per million (Rudin, 1988). Impaired salt (sodium chloride) reabsorption in the thick ascending loop of Henle (TAL) leads to renal salt wasting and a hypokalemic metabolic alkalosis. The majority of cases present in the early neonatal period with salt-losing crises. An antenatal diagnosis can also be suspected if a pregnancy is complicated by polyhydramnios or premature birth (Sieck &Ohlsson, 1984). Bartter's syndrome is also associated with short stature, growth retardation in infancy, muscle weakness, polyuria and polydipsia. Some children have characteristic facies that are triangular-shaped with a prominent forehead, large eyes, protruding ears and a drooping mouth. Blood pressure is normal. Bartter's syndrome should be suspected in patient presenting with the above symptoms and signs and the following laboratory findings: hypokalemic alkalosis, high urinary chloride and urinary potassium levels and normal or raised urinary calcium level. Serum magnesium levels are typically normal or mildly low.

The biochemical abnormalities are a consequence of renal salt wasting in the TAL. This stimulates the renin-angiotensin II-aldosterone system (RAAS) and causes hyperplasia of juxtaglomerular apparatus, a feature originally noted by Bartter (Bartter, et al., 1962). Raised RAAS increases sodium reabsorption in the distal nephron (via ENaC) in exchange for K^+ and H^+, which leads to hypokalemic alkalosis. Increases in prostaglandin E2 synthesis aggravate the salt wasting by its effect on ROMK1 and NKCC2. Despite raised RAAS, leading to hyperreninemia and hyperaldosteronism, patients with Bartter's syndrome remain normotensive. The various phenotypes of Bartter's syndrome are now more simply classified by their underlying genetic mutation.

Antenatal Bartter's syndrome (Type 1) is caused by homozygous or compound heterozygous mutation in the *SLC12A1* gene, encoding NKCC2 (Simon, et al., 1996a). NKCC2 is kidney specific, electroneutral transporter protein, located at the apical membrane of the TAL (Simon, et al., 1996a).

Type 1 is a severe form of Bartter's syndrome which may present in utero with marked polyhydramnios and premature birth. Amniocentesis shows high chloride (and aldosterone) levels. Analysis of a pregnant mother's urine may also suggest the diagnosis, demonstrating low Na^+, Cl^- and Ca^{2+} (Matsushita, et al., 1999). A definitive diagnosis may be made using mutational analysis of DNA from amniocytes (Konrad, et al., 1999).

Prenatal diagnosis is important as indomethacin may be a useful treatment for polyhydramnios (Smith et al., 1990). and early neonatal treatment may be life saving. Neonates typically present with severe salt-wasting crises, hypokalemic alkalosis, vomiting and diarrhoea. The latter two symptoms are due to renal activation of prostaglandin synthesis, as a consequence of hypokalemia. A feature that distinguishes this type from others is marked hypercalciuria, which causes nephrocalcinosis and osteopenia in infancy. Treatment is with potassium supplements, often combined with potassium-sparing diuretics (such as spironolactone and amiloride) and inhibitors of prostaglandin-stimulated renin release (such as indomethacin and specific cyclo-oxygensae (COX-2) inhibitors).

Antenatal Bartter's syndrome (Type 2) is clinically indistinguishable from Type 1. It is caused by loss-of-function mutations in the *KCNJ1* gene (alias *ROMK1*) encoding the ATP-sensitive potassium channel ROMK1, also located apically in the TAL (Simon, et al., 1996b). ROMK1 allows potassium recycling from the TAL cells back to the luminal filtrate, and is electrogenic driving paracellular reabsorption of sodium, calcium and magnesium. ROMK1 is a regulator of the NKCC2 co-transporter and functional coupling of ROMK1 with NKCC2 is essential for effective NaCl reabsorption. Therefore, functional defects in the ROMK1 protein severely disrupt electrogenic chloride reabsorption in TAL, resulting in a similar antenatal phenotype, although the hypokalemia may be less severe (Kurtz, 1998). The treatment of Bartter's syndrome Type 2 is the same as for Bartter's syndrome Type 1.

Classic Bartter's syndrome (Type 3) is caused by mutations in *CLCNKB* encoding the CLC chloride channel member CLC-KB. This channel protein is located on the basolateral membrane of TAL cells, where it co-localizes with Barttin. The presentation of Type 3 / Classic Bartter's syndrome tends to be with weakness and hypovolemia during early childhood, with a milder defect of urinary concentrating ability and normal urinary calcium levels. Hence, nephrocalcinosis or nephrolithiasis is rarely a feature. Severe and chronic hypokalemia may lead to medullary cyst formation (Ariceta &Rodriguez-Soriano, 2006). Hyperuricemia may occur due to volume contraction. Renal function is usually preserved initially but may decrease as a result of chronic hypokalemia and tubulointerstitial damage. The primary defect alters chloride reabsorption, with defective basolateral exit of chloride via CLC-KB in the TAL. Clinical features in Type 3 Bartter's syndrome include short stature and salt wasting. However, *CLCNKB* mutations may present with variable phenotype, ranging from neonatal salt losing crises to asymptomatic patients detected in adulthood by routine electrolyte testing (Konrad, et al., 2000). A milder phenotype may be confused with Gitelman's syndrome. Indeed, some patients with *CLCKNB* mutations have profound hypomagnesaemia and hypocalciuria, closely mimicking Gitelman's syndrome (Jeck, et al., 2000,Konrad, et al., 2000).

Bartter's syndrome Type 4A is a form of infantile Bartter's syndrome caused by a mutation in the gene *BSND* encoding Barttin (Estevez, et al., 2001). Barttin is two-transmembrane protein and an essential subunit of the CLC chloride channels CLC-KB and CLC-KA. Barttin modulates both membrane insertion and function of both CLC-KA and CLC-KB (Scholl, et al., 2006,Waldegger, et al., 2002). In the kidney Barttin is expressed in the thin limb and the TAL of Henle. This type of Bartter's syndrome is associated with congenital sensorineural deafness (termed BSND) which may explained by the localisation of Barttin protein as a subunit for CLC-KA in inner ear cells. Again, the phenotype can be severe neonatal salt wasting or a more mild adult presentation (Miyamura, et al., 2003).

Type 4B Bartter's syndrome is associated with simultaneous mutations in both chloride channel genes, *CLCNKA* and *CLCNKB* resulting in sensorineural deafness and renal salt wasting. This form of Bartter's syndrome is rare but should be considered when BSND mutations are not detected. Children from consanguineous parents with homozygous mutations in both genes (Schlingmann, et al., 2004) and non consanguineous parents with digenic compound heterozygous mutations have been described (Nozu, et al., 2008).

Bartter's syndrome Type 5 is better known as autosomal dominant hypocalcaemia with Bartter'syndrome. Mutations in the *CASR* gene encoding the Calcium-sensing receptor can occasionally be associated with a Bartter's like phenotype (Vargas-Poussou, et al.,

2002,Watanabe, et al., 2002). The mechanism leading to this phenotype is thought to be constitutive activation of the mutant CASR, located on the basolateral membrane of the TAL, by normal serum calcium levels, leading to a secondary inhibition of sodium chloride transport in the TAL, thus mimicking Bartter's syndrome. Of note, the degree of metabolic alkalosis in these patients was mild (Sayer &Pearce, 2003).

4.2 Pseudo Bartter's syndrome

Pseudo antenatal Bartter's syndrome has been reported in a preterm child with cyanotic heart disease treated with high dose prostaglandins (Langhendries, et al., 1989). The biochemical phenotype of Bartter's may also be mimicked by loop diuretic abuse. Hypokalemic metabolic alkalosis may also be seen in patients with cystic fibrosis, bulimia and laxative abuse. In such cases, urinary chloride levels are low, given the salt wasting is not secondary to a tubular defect.

4.3 Gitelman's syndrome

Gitelman's syndrome refers to an autosomal recessive congenital condition, which is characterized by a hypokalemic alkalosis with hypocalciuria and often hypomagnesaemia (Gitelman, et al., 1966). Gitelman's syndrome has incidence of 1:40,000, which makes it one of the commonest inherited tubulopathies. The electrolyte disturbance mimics that of chronic thiazide diuretic use. Patients with this syndrome have genetic defect in the *SLC12A3* gene encoding the thiazide-sensitive sodium-chloride cotransporter (NCCT) (Simon, et al., 1996a). This cotransporter is located in the apical membrane of distal convoluted tubular (DCT) cells. Defects in NCCT result in reduced sodium reabsorption in the DCT, leading to increased delivery of sodium to the CCD. This leads to increased absorption of sodium via ENaC, coupled with K excretion, leading to hypokalemia. Subsequent stimulation of K reabsorption via H^+K^+ATPase in intercalated cells results in a metabolic alkalosis. Within the DCT, transcellular absorption of magnesium (via the apical magnesium channel TRPM6 and a putative basolateral Na^+/Mg^{2+} exchanger) is also reduced. The exact mechanism of hypocalciuria has been the subject of speculation for some time. Evidence from studying thiazide treatment in murine models now suggests that as result of volume contraction enhanced proximal tubular sodium reabsorption occurs, and with it, an increase in proximal tubular paracellular absorption of calcium (Nijenhuis, et al., 2005).

Gitelman's syndrome is often asymptomatic into adult life, presenting with weakness, paraesthesia, fatigue and tetany. Salt craving may be a feature. Typically the patients are normotensive and may have polyarthritis and chondrocalcinosis secondary to severe and longstanding hypomagnesaemia (Cobeta-Garcia, et al., 1998). Clinical diagnostic features for Gitelman's syndrome include a low urinary calcium:creatinine ratio (typically <0.2), low serum magnesium (<0.65 mmol/L) and a hypokalemic metabolic alkalosis, once thiazide use is ruled out. Surreptitious ingestion of thiazide may be ruled out by screening the urine. Cisplastin nephrotoxicity may resemble Gitelman's syndrome as may some of the magnesium wasting tubulopathies (Knoers et al., 2003) discussed below. Treatment is with lifelong potassium and magnesium supplements and diet rich in sodium and potassium. Amiloride and spironolactone may also be useful treatments to ensure maintained serum potassium levels. Occasionally, a severe childhood onset phenotype may occur, mimicking Bartter's syndrome in terms of severity. Early replacement of electrolytes is important and in common with Bartter's syndrome, NSAIDs have been used to good effect to promote growth in these children (Liaw, et al., 1999). Patients with Gitelman's syndrome have very good long term prognosis, however sudden cardiac deaths associated with prolonged QT intervals and cardiac arrhythmias have been reported (Cortesi, et al., 2010). In keeping with this less than benign phenotype, Gitelman's patients may have severe symptoms which are debilitating. For example, weakness, tetany and cramps are often so severe that emergency admissions to hospitals are required for intravenous potassium and magnesium replacement. Indeed, following quality of life questionnaires, Gitelman's patients' scores were comparable to patients with congestive heart failure (Cruz, et al., 2001). As discussed previously, mutations in *CLCNKB* encoding the basolateral chloride channel can also cause a Gitelman's phenotype. CLC-KB is expressed in the DCT as well as the TAL, accounting for this phenotypic overlap. Indeed, patients within the same family with identical *CLCNKB* mutation may present with a spectrum of phenotypes including both Bartter's and Gitelman's syndrome (Zelikovic, et al., 2003). In a recent large cohort of 448 Gitelman's patients, *CLCNKB* mutations accounted for just 3% of cases (Vargas-Poussou, et al., 2011).

4.4 "Pseudo" Gitelman's syndrome and reverse phenotypes

The molecular basis for the syndrome of autosomal dominant hypomagnesemia has recently been made (Glaudemans, et al., 2009). This syndrome presents in childhood with recurrent muscle cramps, tetanic episodes, tremor, and muscle weakness. Patients have low serum Mg^{2+} levels, while serum K^{+} and Ca^{2+} levels and urinary Ca^{2+} excretion are not affected. This condition is therefore biochemically different from both Gitelman's syndrome and other forms of inherited hypomagnesemia. Mutations were identified in the *KCNA1* gene, encoding the Kv1.1 potassium channel, expressed in the apical membrane of the DCT and connecting tubule (Glaudemans, et al., 2009). This potassium channel is thought to work to stabilize the apical membrane, in the context of TRPM6 mediated magnesium reabsportion in these nephron segments. Loss of function mutations leads to a depolarisation of the membrane and defective magnesium reabsorption, resulting in hypermagnesuria and hypomagnesemia.

In contrast to Gitelman's, the biochemical phenotype of patients with familial hypomagnesemia with hypercalciuria and nephrocalcinosis secondary to mutations in the genes encoding claudin 16 and claudin 19 includes hypercalciuria rather than hypocalciuria. Isolated dominant hypomagnesemia caused by mutations in FXYD2 leads to hypocalciuria, and can resemble Gitelman's syndrome. Patient may be relatively symptom free as magneseium levels are mildly low, and may also have chondrocalcinosis (Geven, et al., 1987,Meij, et al., 2000). Recently a complex syndrome including epilepsy, ataxia, sensorineural deafness and a tubulopathy resulting in Gitelman's like biochemical derangement has been described (Bockenhauer, et al., 2009, Scholl, et al., 2009). The syndrome has been named both EAST syndrome (Bockenhauer, et al., 2009) and SeSAME syndrome (Scholl, et al., 2009). The biochemical defects are hypokalemia, metabolic alkalosis, hypomagnesemia and hypocalciuria. Mutations have been identified in the *KCJN10* gene encoding the renal Kir4.1 potassium channel, located on the basolateral membrane of the DCT. Loss of function mutations therefore disrupt DCT tubular handling of salts in a similar manner to NCCT defects, leading to secondary activation of the renin-angiotensin-aldosterone axis.

Recent molecular genetic studies have identified the basis of Gordon syndrome, also known as pseudohypoaldosteronism type II or chloride shunt syndrome, an autosomal dominant form of hypertension. It is noteworthy and mentioned here given that the diagnostic features resemble a mirror image of Gitelman's syndrome. This includes hyperkalemia, hypertension and hyperchloraemic metabolic acidosis. It can present in early neonatal period with hyperkalemic acidosis or later in life with hypertension. Additional clinical features include short stature, muscle weakness, intellectual impairment and dental abnormalities. Laboratory findings include low fractional excretion of sodium, low renin and aldosterone levels and normal renal function. This syndrome is caused by mutations in the gene encoding WNK4 (Lalioti, et al., 2006), which is a member of serine-threonine protein kinases. In humans, WNK4 is present exclusively in kidney. WNK4 acts as an inhibitor of thiazide-sensitive sodium-chloride co-transporter (NCCT). Mutations in WNK4 relieve this inhibition causing excess sodium retention and subsequent hypertension. Hyperkalemia is explained by inhibition of potassium ROMK channels. Treatment of Gordon syndrome is with low potassium diet and use of thiazide diuretics. Sodium loading should be avoided as it may worsen hypertension.

4.5 Liddle's syndrome

Liddle's syndrome, also called pseudoaldosteronism, is an autosomal dominant disorder which is characterized by early onset severe hypertension, suppressed renin and aldosterone levels and hypokalaemic metabolic alkalosis (Liddle, et al., 1963). This syndrome is a familial renal disorder simulating primary aldosteronism but with negligible aldosterone secretion and is caused by up regulation of epithelial Na channel (ENaC) located in the collecting duct. Up regulation leaves the ENaC in 'open' state which enhances sodium reabsorption and causes hypertension. ENaC is a heterotrimeric protein, its three subunits named alpha, beta and gamma. Mutations in the beta and gamma subunits can cause constitutive channel opening (Hansson, et al., 1995a, Hansson, et al., 1995b). The beta and gamma subunits of ENaC are encoded by *SCNN1B* and *SCNN1G* genes, respectively. A key regulator of ENaC is NEDD4L, which is able to ubiquitinate ENaC leading to its removal from the luminal cell membrane in the renal collecting ducts. It has been postulated that loss of function defects in NEDD4L or alternative splicing of NEDD4L may also lead to hypertension (Dunn, et al., 2002). Patients with Liddle's syndrome are often asymptomatic and they are usually investigated after incidental finding of hypertension. Affected children may have symptomatic polyuria and polydipsia and faltering growth. A strong family history of premature stroke may prompt investigations. Liddle's syndrome should be suspected in a young person with high blood pressure, a family history of hypertension and low serum potassium together with a metabolic alkalosis. However, Liddle's syndrome may mimic essential hypertension as hypokalemia may not always be present (Rossi, et al., 2011). Indeed, genetic variants in ENaC genes may be found in patients with presumed essential hypertension (Hannila-Handelberg, et al., 2005). In Liddle's syndrome, there is a high variability of penetration which appears to be dependent on environmental factors such as dietary salt intake. Because serum and urine aldosterone levels are low, differential diagnosis should include certain forms of congenital adrenal hyperplasia, syndrome of apparent mineralocorticoid excess, chronic liquorice ingestion and carbenoxolone therapy. Treatment of Liddle's syndrome consists of sodium restriction and potassium-sparing diuretics, like amiloride and triamterene, which directly inhibit the ENaC. There is no benefit of using mineralocorticoid antagonists, such as spironololactone, as in this syndrome the up regulation of ENaC is not mediated by aldosterone.

4.6 Syndrome of Apparent Mineralocorticoid Excess (AME)

This autosomal recessive syndrome is characterised by hypertension, hypokalemia, metabolic alkalosis, with suppressed renin and aldosterone levels. Hypercalciuria and nephrocalcinosis may occur. Typically, an affected child will have polyuria and polydipsia, low birth weight and faltering growth. The molecular basis for this syndrome is secondary to mutations in the *HSD11B2* gene encoding the enzyme 11-beta-hydroxysteroid dehydrogenase 2 (Wilson, et al., 1995). This enzyme normally inactivates cortisol to cortisone, preventing overstimulation of the mineralocorticoid receptor (MR). Mutations lead to an excess of cortisol which is able to have a mineralocorticoid-like affect and stimulate sodium retention, volume expansion and renin and aldosterone suppression.

This syndrome may be mimicked by licorice ingestion (Walker &Edwards, 1994). Licorice contains glycyrrhizinic acid, which inhibits 11-beta-HSD2. Carbenoxolone also inhibits this enzyme. The treatment of choice for AME is a mineralocorticoid receptor blocker such as spironolactone or epleronone.

4.7 Activating mutations of the mineralocorticoid receptor

In a family with familial hypertension, hypokalemia and suppressed aldosterone levels, heterozygous mutations were identified in the NR3C2 gene encoding the mineralocorticoid receptor (MR), resulting in a gain of function (Geller, et al., 2000). Additionally, the specificity of the MR was altered such that progesterone was able to bind to it and activate it. Thus pregnant females in this family presented with severe hypertension.

4.8 Glucocorticoid remediable hypertension

Glucocorticoid remediable hypertension (also known as familial hyperaldosteronism type I) is characterised by autosomal dominant hypertension, low plasma renin levels, normal plasma aldosterone levels and hypokalemia (McMahon &Dluhy, 2004). The age of onset of hypertension is usually in teenage years, but may be in adulthood. Hypertension is typically refractory to treatment. The molecular basis for disease is secondary to a chimeric gene, involving CYP11B1, encoding 11-beta-hydroxylase and CYP11B2, encoding aldosterone synthase. The chimeric gene results in aldosterone synthesis under the regulatory control of ACTH, resulting in hyperaldosteronism (Lifton, et al., 1992). Thus, the causative mutation affects the cortical collecting duct indirectly, and therefore this is not a "tubulopathy". Traditionally, diagnosis has been made by a dexamathasone suppression test, which results in reduced plasma aldosterone levels. A specific urinary profile of 18 oxotetrahydrocortisol and 18 hydrocortisol may be sought, but molecular genetic testing also allows a definitive diagnosis. Treatment with glucocorticoids (using shorter acting agents prednisone or hydrocortisone) is often effective, but additional antihypertensives may be needed as adjuncts.

5. Conclusions

The ability to provide a definitive molecular genetic diagnosis to a patient with an inherited tubulopathy allows a confidence in the diagnosis, despite phenotypic variabilities (which may be intrafamilial). A molecular genetic diagnosis also allows the targeted pharmacology to be employed to achieve normalization / improvement in symptoms, serum biochemistry and blood pressure. The discovery of renal tubular transporters and channels has allowed significant gains in our understanding of this group of renal diseases, with families with inherited tubulopathies providing the ultimate "animal model". Although perhaps uncommon, the discovery of the molecular players of salt and water handling within the nephron has allowed applications to be made to sufferers of "essential hypertension".

It is certainly true that a patient with hypokalemia / metabolic alkalosis, no matter how mild, warrants further evaluation to determine the underlying cause.

6. Acknowledgements

JAS is a GlaxoSmithKline clinician scientist and is also supported by Kidney Research UK and the Northern Counties Kidney Research Fund.

7. References

Ariceta, G. & Rodriguez-Soriano, J. (2006) Inherited renal tubulopathies associated with metabolic alkalosis: Effects on blood pressure. *Semin Nephrol*, Vol. 26, No. 6, (Nov), pp. (422-433), 0270-9295 (Print) 0270-9295 (Linking).

Bartter, F.C., Pronove, P., Gill, J.R., Jr. & Maccardle, R.C. (1962) Hyperplasia of the juxtaglomerular complex with hyperaldosteronism and hypokalemic alkalosis. A new syndrome. *Am J Med*, Vol. 33, No. (Dec), pp. (811-828), 0002-9343 (Print) 0002-9343 (Linking).

Bockenhauer, D., Feather, S., Stanescu, H.C., Bandulik, S., Zdebik, A.A., Reichold, M., Tobin, J., Lieberer, E., Sterner, C., Landoure, G., Arora, R., Sirimanna, T., Thompson, D., Cross, J.H., van't Hoff, W., Al Masri, O., Tullus, K., Yeung, S., Anikster, Y., Klootwijk, E., Hubank, M., Dillon, M.J., Heitzmann, D., Arcos-Burgos, M., Knepper, M.A., Dobbie, A., Gahl, W.A., Warth, R., Sheridan, E. & Kleta, R. (2009) Epilepsy, ataxia, sensorineural deafness, tubulopathy, and kcnj10 mutations. *N Engl J Med*, Vol. 360, No. 19, (May 7), pp. (1960-1970), 1533-4406 (Electronic) 0028-4793 (Linking).

Cappola, T.P., Matkovich, S.J., Wang, W., van Booven, D., Li, M., Wang, X., Qu, L., Sweitzer, N.K., Fang, J.C., Reilly, M.P., Hakonarson, H., Nerbonne, J.M. & Dorn, G.W. (2011), 2nd. Loss-of-function DNA sequence variant in the clcnka chloride channel implicates the cardio-renal axis in interindividual heart failure risk variation. *Proc Natl Acad Sci U S A*, Vol. 108, No. 6, (Feb 8), pp. (2456-2461), 1091-6490 (Electronic) 0027-8424 (Linking).

Cobeta-Garcia, J.C., Gascon, A., Iglesias, E. & Estopinan, V. (1998) Chondrocalcinosis and gitelman's syndrome. A new association? *Ann Rheum Dis*, Vol. 57, No. 12, (Dec), pp. (748-749), 0003-4967 (Print) 0003-4967 (Linking).

Cortesi, C., Lava, S.A., Bettinelli, A., Tammaro, F., Giannini, O., Caiata-Zufferey, M. & Bianchetti, M.G. (2010) Cardiac arrhythmias and rhabdomyolysis in bartter-gitelman patients. *Pediatr Nephrol*, Vol. 25, No. 10, (Oct), pp. (2005-2008), 1432-198X (Electronic) 0931-041X (Linking).

Cruz, D.N., Shaer, A.J., Bia, M.J., Lifton, R.P. & Simon, D.B. (2001) Gitelman's syndrome revisited: An evaluation of symptoms and health-related quality of life. *Kidney Int*, Vol. 59, No. 2, (Feb), pp. (710-717), 0085-2538 (Print) 0085-2538 (Linking).

Dunn, D.M., Ishigami, T., Pankow, J., von Niederhausern, A., Alder, J., Hunt, S.C., Leppert, M.F., Lalouel, J.M. & Weiss, R.B. (2002) Common variant of human nedd4l activates a cryptic splice site to form a frameshifted transcript. *J Hum Genet*, Vol. 47, No. 12), pp. (665-676), 1434-5161 (Print) 1434-5161 (Linking).

Estevez, R., Boettger, T., Stein, V., Birkenhager, R., Otto, E., Hildebrandt, F. & Jentsch, T.J. (2001) Barttin is a cl- channel beta-subunit crucial for renal cl- reabsorption and inner ear k+ secretion. *Nature*, Vol. 414, No. 6863, (Nov 29), pp. (558-561),

Fry, A.C. & Karet, F.E. (2007) Inherited renal acidoses. *Physiology (Bethesda)*, Vol. 22, No. (Jun), pp. (202-211), 1548-9213 (Print).

Geller, D.S., Farhi, A., Pinkerton, N., Fradley, M., Moritz, M., Spitzer, A., Meinke, G., Tsai, F.T., Sigler, P.B. & Lifton, R.P. (2000) Activating mineralocorticoid receptor mutation in hypertension exacerbated by pregnancy. *Science*, Vol. 289, No. 5476, (Jul 7), pp. (119-123), 0036-8075 (Print) 0036-8075 (Linking).

Geven, W.B., Monnens, L.A., Willems, H.L., Buijs, W.C. & ter Haar, B.G. (1987) Renal magnesium wasting in two families with autosomal dominant inheritance. *Kidney Int*, Vol. 31, No. 5, (May), pp. (1140-1144), 0085-2538 (Print) 0085-2538 (Linking).

Gitelman, H.J., Graham, J.B. & Welt, L.G. (1966) A new familial disorder characterized by hypokalemia and hypomagnesemia. *Trans Assoc Am Physicians*, Vol. 79, No.), pp. (221-235), 0066-9458 (Print) 0066-9458 (Linking).

Glaudemans, B., van der Wijst, J., Scola, R.H., Lorenzoni, P.J., Heister, A., van der Kemp, A.W., Knoers, N.V., Hoenderop, J.G. & Bindels, R.J. (2009) A missense mutation in the kv1.1 voltage-gated potassium channel-encoding gene kcna1 is linked to human autosomal dominant hypomagnesemia. *J Clin Invest*, Vol. 119, No. 4, (Apr), pp. (936-942), 1558-8238 (Electronic) 0021-9738 (Linking).

Hannila-Handelberg, T., Kontula, K., Tikkanen, I., Tikkanen, T., Fyhrquist, F., Helin, K., Fodstad, H., Piippo, K., Miettinen, H.E., Virtamo, J., Krusius, T., Sarna, S., Gautschi, I., Schild, L. & Hiltunen, T.P. (2005) Common variants of the beta and gamma subunits of the epithelial sodium channel and their relation to plasma renin and aldosterone levels in essential hypertension. *BMC Med Genet*, Vol. 6, No. (Jan 20), pp. (4), 1471-2350 (Electronic) 1471-2350 (Linking).

Hansson, J.H., Nelson-Williams, C., Suzuki, H., Schild, L., Shimkets, R., Lu, Y., Canessa, C., Iwasaki, T., Rossier, B. & Lifton, R.P. (1995a) Hypertension caused by a truncated epithelial sodium channel gamma subunit: Genetic heterogeneity of liddle syndrome. *Nat Genet*, Vol. 11, No. 1, (Sep), pp. (76-82), 1061-4036 (Print) 1061-4036 (Linking).

Hansson, J.H., Schild, L., Lu, Y., Wilson, T.A., Gautschi, I., Shimkets, R., Nelson-Williams, C., Rossier, B.C. & Lifton, R.P. (1995b) A de novo missense mutation of the beta subunit of the epithelial sodium channel causes hypertension and liddle syndrome, identifying a proline-rich segment critical for regulation of channel activity. *Proc Natl Acad Sci U S A*, Vol. 92, No. 25, (Dec 5), pp. (11495-11499), 0027-8424 (Print) 0027-8424 (Linking).

Jeck, N., Konrad, M., Peters, M., Weber, S., Bonzel, K.E. & Seyberth, H.W. (2000) Mutations in the chloride channel gene, clcnkb, leading to a mixed bartter-gitelman phenotype. *Pediatr Res*, Vol. 48, No. 6, (Dec), pp. (754-758), 0031-3998 (Print) 0031-3998 (Linking).

Knoers, N.V., de Jong, J.C., Meij, I.C., Van Den Heuvel, L.P. & Bindels, R.J. (2003) Genetic renal disorders with hypomagnesemia and hypocalciuria. *J Nephrol*, Vol. 16, No. 2, (Mar-Apr), pp. (293-296), 1121-8428 (Print) 1121-8428 (Linking).

Konrad, M., Leonhardt, A., Hensen, P., Seyberth, H.W. & Kockerling, A. (1999) Prenatal and postnatal management of hyperprostaglandin e syndrome after genetic diagnosis from amniocytes. *Pediatrics*, Vol. 103, No. 3, (Mar), pp. (678-683), 1098-4275 (Electronic) 0031-4005 (Linking).

Konrad, M., Vollmer, M., Lemmink, H.H., van den Heuvel, L.P., Jeck, N., Vargas-Poussou, R., Lakings, A., Ruf, R., Deschenes, G., Antignac, C., Guay-Woodford, L., Knoers, N.V., Seyberth, H.W., Feldmann, D. & Hildebrandt, F. (2000) Mutations in the chloride channel gene clcnkb as a cause of classic bartter syndrome. *J Am Soc Nephrol*, Vol. 11, No. 8, (Aug), pp. (1449-1459),

Kurtz, I. (1998) Molecular pathogenesis of bartter's and gitelman's syndromes. *Kidney Int*, Vol. 54, No. 4, (Oct), pp. (1396-1410), 0085-2538 (Print) 0085-2538 (Linking).

Lalioti, M.D., Zhang, J., Volkman, H.M., Kahle, K.T., Hoffmann, K.E., Toka, H.R., Nelson-Williams, C., Ellison, D.H., Flavell, R., Booth, C.J., Lu, Y., Geller, D.S. & Lifton, R.P. (2006) Wnk4 controls blood pressure and potassium homeostasis via regulation of mass and activity of the distal convoluted tubule. *Nat Genet*, Vol. 38, No. 10, (Oct), pp. (1124-1132), 1061-4036 (Print).

Langhendries, J.P., Thiry, V., Bodart, E., Delfosse, G., Whitofs, L., Battisti, O. & Bertrand, J.M. (1989) Exogenous prostaglandin administration and pseudo-bartter syndrome. *Eur J Pediatr*, Vol. 149, No. 3, (Dec), pp. (208-209), 0340-6199 (Print) 0340-6199 (Linking).

Liaw, L.C., Banerjee, K. & Coulthard, M.G. (1999) Dose related growth response to indometacin in gitelman syndrome. *Arch Dis Child*, Vol. 81, No. 6, (Dec), pp. (508-510), 1468-2044 (Electronic) 0003-9888 (Linking).

Liddle, G.W., Bledsoe, T. & Coppage, W.S. (1963) A familial renal disorder simulating primary aldosteronism but with negligible aldosterone secretion. . *Trans Assoc Am Physician*, Vol. 76, No.), pp. (199-213),

Lifton, R.P., Dluhy, R.G., Powers, M., Rich, G.M., Gutkin, M., Fallo, F., Gill, J.R., Jr., Feld, L., Ganguly, A., Laidlaw, J.C. & et al. (1992) Hereditary hypertension caused by chimaeric gene duplications and ectopic expression of aldosterone synthase. *Nat Genet*, Vol. 2, No. 1, (Sep), pp. (66-74), 1061-4036 (Print) 1061-4036 (Linking).

Matsushita, Y., Suzuki, Y., Oya, N., Kajiura, S., Okajima, K., Uemura, O. & Suzumori, K. (1999) Biochemical examination of mother's urine is useful for prenatal diagnosis of bartter syndrome. *Prenat Diagn*, Vol. 19, No. 7, (Jul), pp. (671-673), 0197-3851 (Print) 0197-3851 (Linking).

McMahon, G.T. & Dluhy, R.G. (2004) Glucocorticoid-remediable aldosteronism. *Cardiol Rev*, Vol. 12, No. 1, (Jan-Feb), pp. (44-48), 1061-5377 (Print) 1061-5377 (Linking).

Meij, I.C., Koenderink, J.B., van Bokhoven, H., Assink, K.F., Groenestege, W.T., de Pont, J.J., Bindels, R.J., Monnens, L.A., van den Heuvel, L.P. & Knoers, N.V. (2000) Dominant isolated renal magnesium loss is caused by misrouting of the na(+),k(+)-atpase gamma-subunit. *Nat Genet*, Vol. 26, No. 3, (Nov), pp. (265-266), 1061-4036 (Print) 1061-4036 (Linking).

Miyamura, N., Matsumoto, K., Taguchi, T., Tokunaga, H., Nishikawa, T., Nishida, K., Toyonaga, T., Sakakida, M. & Araki, E. (2003) Atypical bartter syndrome with sensorineural deafness with g47r mutation of the beta-subunit for clc-ka and clc-kb chloride channels, barttin. *J Clin Endocrinol Metab*, Vol. 88, No. 2, (Feb), pp. (781-786), 0021-972X (Print) 0021-972X (Linking).

Nijenhuis, T., Vallon, V., van der Kemp, A.W., Loffing, J., Hoenderop, J.G. & Bindels, R.J. (2005) Enhanced passive ca2+ reabsorption and reduced mg2+ channel abundance explains thiazide-induced hypocalciuria and hypomagnesemia. *J Clin Invest*, Vol. 115, No. 6, (Jun), pp. (1651-1658), 0021-9738 (Print) 0021-9738 (Linking).

Norgett, E., Su, Y., Cartwright, D., Blake-Palmer, K., Best, A., Horita, S., Fry, A., Al-Lamki, R., Norden, A. & Karet, F. (2011) Pseudohypokalaemia: A novel clinical phenomenon associated with hereditary spherocytosis due to ae1 mutations. *British Renal Society Abstract O58*, Vol. No.), pp.

Nozu, K., Inagaki, T., Fu, X.J., Nozu, Y., Kaito, H., Kanda, K., Sekine, T., Igarashi, T., Nakanishi, K., Yoshikawa, N., Iijima, K. & Matsuo, M. (2008) Molecular analysis of digenic inheritance in bartter syndrome with sensorineural deafness. *J Med Genet*, Vol. 45, No. 3, (Mar), pp. (182-186), 1468-6244 (Electronic) 0022-2593 (Linking).

Rossi, E., Farnetti, E., Nicoli, D., Sazzini, M., Perazzoli, F., Regolisti, G., Grasselli, C., Santi, R., Negro, A., Mazzeo, V., Mantero, F., Luiselli, D. & Casali, B. (2011) A clinical phenotype mimicking essential hypertension in a newly discovered family with liddle's syndrome. *Am J Hypertens*, Vol. No. (Apr 28), pp. 1879-1905 (Electronic) 0895-7061 (Linking).

Rudin, A. (1988) Bartter's syndrome. A review of 28 patients followed for 10 years. *Acta Med Scand*, Vol. 224, No. 2), pp. (165-171), 0001-6101 (Print) 0001-6101 (Linking).

Sayer, J.A. & Pearce, S.H. (2001) Diagnosis and clinical biochemistry of inherited tubulopathies. *Ann Clin Biochem*, Vol. 38, No. Pt 5, (Sep), pp. (459-470), 0004-5632 (Print).

Sayer, J.A. & Pearce, S.H. (2003) Extracellular calcium-sensing receptor dysfunction is associated with two new phenotypes. *Clin Endocrinol (Oxf)*, Vol. 59, No. 4, (Oct), pp. (419-421), 0300-0664 (Print).

Schlingmann, K.P., Konrad, M., Jeck, N., Waldegger, P., Reinalter, S.C., Holder, M., Seyberth, H.W. & Waldegger, S. (2004) Salt wasting and deafness resulting from mutations in two chloride channels. *N Engl J Med*, Vol. 350, No. 13, (Mar 25), pp. (1314-1319), 1533-4406 (Electronic) 0028-4793 (Linking).

Scholl, U., Hebeisen, S., Janssen, A.G., Muller-Newen, G., Alekov, A. & Fahlke, C. (2006) Barttin modulates trafficking and function of clc-k channels. *Proc Natl Acad Sci U S A*, Vol. 103, No. 30, (Jul 25), pp. (11411-11416), 0027-8424 (Print) 0027-8424 (Linking).

Scholl, U.I., Choi, M., Liu, T., Ramaekers, V.T., Hausler, M.G., Grimmer, J., Tobe, S.W., Farhi, A., Nelson-Williams, C. & Lifton, R.P. (2009) Seizures, sensorineural deafness, ataxia, mental retardation, and electrolyte imbalance (sesame syndrome) caused by mutations in kcnj10. *Proc Natl Acad Sci U S A*, Vol. 106, No. 14, (Apr 7), pp. (5842-5847), 1091-6490 (Electronic) 0027-8424 (Linking).

Sieck, U.V. & Ohlsson, A. (1984) Fetal polyuria and hydramnios associated with bartter's syndrome. *Obstet Gynecol*, Vol. 63, No. 3 Suppl, (Mar), pp. (22S-24S), 0029-7844 (Print) 0029-7844 (Linking).

Simon, D.B., Karet, F.E., Hamdan, J.M., DiPietro, A., Sanjad, S.A. & Lifton, R.P. (1996a) Bartter's syndrome, hypokalaemic alkalosis with hypercalciuria, is caused by mutations in the na-k-2cl cotransporter nkcc2. *Nat Genet*, Vol. 13, No. 2, (Jun), pp. (183-188), 1061-4036 (Print) 1061-4036 (Linking).

Simon, D.B., Karet, F.E., Rodriguez-Soriano, J., Hamdan, J.H., DiPietro, A., Trachtman, H., Sanjad, S.A. & Lifton, R.P. (1996b) Genetic heterogeneity of bartter's syndrome revealed by mutations in the k+ channel, romk. *Nat Genet*, Vol. 14, No. 2, (Oct), pp. (152-156), 1061-4036 (Print) 1061-4036 (Linking).

Smith, L.G., Jr., Kirshon, B. & Cotton, D.B. (1990) Indomethacin treatment for polyhydramnios and subsequent infantile nephrogenic diabetes insipidus. *Am J Obstet Gynecol*, Vol. 163, No. 1 Pt 1, (Jul), pp. (98-99), 0002-9378 (Print) 0002-9378 (Linking).

Vargas-Poussou, R., Dahan, K., Kahila, D., Venisse, A., Riveira-Munoz, E., Debaix, H., Grisart, B., Bridoux, F., Unwin, R., Moulin, B., Haymann, J.P., Vantyghem, M.C., Rigothier, C., Dussol, B., Godin, M., Nivet, H., Dubourg, L., Tack, I., Gimenez-Roqueplo, A.P., Houillier, P., Blanchard, A., Devuyst, O. & Jeunemaitre, X. (2011) Spectrum of mutations in gitelman syndrome. *J Am Soc Nephrol*, Vol. 22, No. 4, (Apr), pp. (693-703), 1533-3450 (Electronic) 1046-6673 (Linking).

Vargas-Poussou, R., Huang, C., Hulin, P., Houillier, P., Jeunemaitre, X., Paillard, M., Planelles, G., Dechaux, M., Miller, R.T. & Antignac, C. (2002) Functional characterization of a calcium-sensing receptor mutation in severe autosomal dominant hypocalcemia with a bartter-like syndrome. *J Am Soc Nephrol*, Vol. 13, No. 9, (Sep), pp. (2259-2266), 1046-6673 (Print) 1046-6673 (Linking).

Waldegger, S., Jeck, N., Barth, P., Peters, M., Vitzthum, H., Wolf, K., Kurtz, A., Konrad, M. & Seyberth, H.W. (2002) Barttin increases surface expression and changes current properties of clc-k channels. *Pflugers Arch*, Vol. 444, No. 3, (Jun), pp. (411-418), 0031-6768 (Print) 0031-6768 (Linking).

Walker, B.R. & Edwards, C.R. (1994) Licorice-induced hypertension and syndromes of apparent mineralocorticoid excess. *Endocrinol Metab Clin North Am*, Vol. 23, No. 2, (Jun), pp. (359-377), 0889-8529 (Print) 0889-8529 (Linking).

Watanabe, S., Fukumoto, S., Chang, H., Takeuchi, Y., Hasegawa, Y., Okazaki, R., Chikatsu, N. & Fujita, T. (2002) Association between activating mutations of calcium-sensing receptor and bartter's syndrome. *Lancet*, Vol. 360, No. 9334, (Aug 31), pp. (692-694), 0140-6736 (Print) 0140-6736 (Linking).

Wilson, R.C., Krozowski, Z.S., Li, K., Obeyesekere, V.R., Razzaghy-Azar, M., Harbison, M.D., Wei, J.Q., Shackleton, C.H., Funder, J.W. & New, M.I. (1995) A mutation in the hsd11b2 gene in a family with apparent mineralocorticoid excess. *J Clin Endocrinol Metab*, Vol. 80, No. 7, (Jul), pp. (2263-2266), 0021-972X (Print) 0021-972X (Linking).

Zelikovic, I., Szargel, R., Hawash, A., Labay, V., Hatib, I., Cohen, N. & Nakhoul, F. (2003) A novel mutation in the chloride channel gene, clcnkb, as a cause of gitelman and bartter syndromes. *Kidney Int*, Vol. 63, No. 1, (Jan), pp. (24-32), 0085-2538 (Print) 0085-2538 (Linking).

5

Variability of Biological Parameters in Blood Samples Between Two Consecutive Schedules of Hemodialysis

Aurelian Udristioiu[1], Manole Cojocaru[2], Alexandra Dana Maria Panait[3], Radu Iliescu[4], Victor Dumitrascu[5] and Daliborca Cristina Vlad[5]

[1]Emergency County Hospital Targu Jiu, Clinical Laboratory
[2]Titu Maiorescu University, Medicine Faculty, Physiology, Bucharest
[3]National Agency of Drugs, Department of Research, Bucharest
[4]Polytechnic Institute of New York University, Brooklyn, New York
[5]Hospital University of Timisoara
[1,2,3,5]Romania
[4]USA

1. Introduction

Epidemiologic studies have suggested that anemia may be associated with poorer outcomes in a variety of disorders. The WHO criteria define anemia by hemoglobin (HGB) concentration of < 130 g/L for adult men and<120 g/L for adult females. [1]
Nonetheless, recent evidence indicates that even mild anemia is independently associated with increased risk of recurrent falls, poorer physical function, hospitalization, and mortality in older adults. [2, 3]
A number of studies have reported differential distributions of anemia by age and sex, but less attention has been devoted to disparities in anemia by race. According to NHANES III estimates, older non-Hispanic blacks were 3 times more likely to have anemia compared to older non-Hispanic whites (27.8% vs 9.0%). [1]
Similar disparities in anemia prevalence have been observed in other population-based studies of older blacks and whites [4, 5]. These observations have led some to consider race-specific criteria for defining anemia. [6]
A recent study in Iceland defined mild anemia as a hemoglobin concentration between 10.0 and 11.9 g/dL in women and between 10.0 and 12.9 g/dL in men [7]. This cross sectional analysis provides evidence of anemia in 36.7% of hospitalized patients, and shows an association among anemia, poor nutritional status, and inflammation [8].
Future research on anemia in the elderly should focus on the age-related physiologic changes underlying this condition and whether anemia correction can reduce anemia-associated risks, and improve quality of life [9, 10].
Erythrocytes indices, derivatives from value of HGB and numbers of erythrocytes was used in correlation with serum iron to establish grades and types of anemia and was pathological results of these indices was noted as first signals of latent anemia in hematological diseases.
Mean corpuscular volume (MCV) measures the mean or average size of individual red blood cells. To obtain the MCV, the hematocrit is divided by the total RBC count.

$$MCV = \frac{Hematocrit\ 1/1x1000}{Number\ of\ erythrocytes\ (x10^{12}/L)}$$

The MCV is an indicator of the size of red blood cells. MCV is measured in cubic micrometers or fento-liters (Reference values: adult men: 80-94 fl, women: 81-99 fl).
Mean corpuscular hemoglobin (MCH) measures the amount, or the mass, of hemoglobin present in one RBC. The weight of hemoglobin in an average cell is obtained by dividing the hemoglobin by the total RBC count.

$$MCH = \frac{Hemoglobin\ (g/L)}{Number\ of\ erythrocytes\ (x10^{12}/L)}$$

MCH is expressed in picograms of hemoglobin per cell (pg/L, 1 pg = 10-12 g).
(Reference values: adult men; MCH = 27 - 31 pg, women = 27-30 pg). Mean corpuscular hemoglobin concentration (MCHC) measures the proportion of each cell taken up by hemoglobin.

$$MCHC = \frac{Hemoglobin\ (g/L)}{Hematocrit\ 1/1}$$

The results are reported in percentages, reflecting the proportion of hemoglobin in the RBC. The hemoglobin is divided by the hematocrit and multiplied by 100 to obtain the MCHC. (Reference values: adults: MCHC = 32- 36 %}
RDW (red cell distribution width) reflects the size distribution of the erythrocyte population. The hematological instrument calculates it as a coefficient of variation (CV),

$$RDW = \frac{Standard\ deviation\ of\ red\ blood\ cell\ size\ distribution}{MCV}$$

(Reference values: adults RDW = 11.5 - 15.5)
The aim of this study was to identify the values and changes of hematological and biochemical parameters in blood samples between two consecutive schedules of hemodialysis and assesses the effect of plasma osmolality on errors of platelets count, to the hospitalized patients admitted in hospital with diagnosis chronic renal diseases complicated with chronic renal failure.

2. Method

The prospective study of laboratory was performed on 90 known patients with chronic kidney diseases(CKD) complicated with chronic renal failure(CRF), admitted in hospital, prior to undergoing schedules of dialysis, (55 men and 35 women), in average ages 35-65 years (mean, age 50, SD= +_2).
The patients were analyzed once a month, all at the same day, to connection and after connection of hemodialysis schedules, in medical internal department.
For diagnosis of specific anemia of chronic renal diseases, laboratory tests included hemoglobin (HGB), hematocrit (HCT), white blood cells and platelets count, differential count and red cell indices (mean cell volume (MCV), mean cellular hemoglobin (MCH), mean corpuscular hemoglobin concentration (MCHC) red cell distribution width (RDW), being performed using an automated analyzer (Coulter HMX with 22 parameters) and for

specific biochemical parameters in chronic renal failure as serum iron, total iron binding capacity, and index saturation transferrin (IST), usually and specific biochemical tests:
Glucose, Urea nitrogen, Creatinine, Sodium, Potassium, E CO2, was used a dry chemistry analyzer Vitros 700(Ortho Diagnostics), Johnson $ Johnson.
Reticulocyte count (RET %) was calculated after microscopic analysis of brilliant cresyl blue stained slides, (normal ranges adult: 0.5 - 1.5%). To evaluate rate of erythropoiesis, the Reticulocyte Production Index (RPI) was calculated using the formula: [RPI = RET% x HCT patient /45 /reticulocyte time maturation], where maturation time (reticulocytes survival days in peripheral blood) was considered 1 day
for HCT 36-45%, 1.5 days for HCT 26-35%, 2 days for HCT 16- 25% and 2.5 days for HCT < 15%. Reference interval for RPI in healthy individuals is 1.0-2.0; and RPI < 2 in a person with anemia indicates ineffective erythropoiesis, while values > 2 indicate compensation for decreased red cell survival (bleeding, hemolysis) [11].
Three methods were used to assess platelet counts of hemodialysis patients: optical microscopy, peripheral blood smear and user of the cytometry principle with impedance principle (VIC) by Coulter HNX hematological analysis. For to avoid systematic errors during platelets count by optical microscopy, a method of direct counting in the Burker-Turk chamber(hemacytometer) has been recommended for use in parallel with determination of the number of platelets counted on peripheral blood smear, (by optical microscopy). Calculation of the platelets counted in the Burker-Turk chamber considers the height of the chamber and the surface of the middle square of the chamber to yield a value of $0.2mm^2$. [12].
The calculation formula for hemacytometer cell counts determines the number of cells within 1µL (1 mm^3) of blood. To make this determination, the total number of cells counted must be corrected for the initial dilution of blood and the volume of diluted blood used. The standard dilution of blood for platelet counts is 1:100; therefore the dilution factor is 100. The volume of diluted blood used is based on the area and depth of the counting area. The area counted is 2 mm^2 and the depth is 0.1 mm; therefore the volume factor is 0.2 mm^3. Total number of cells counted • dilution factor • 1/volume factor = cells/mm3 (cells/mm^3= cells/µL or cells/µL • 10^3µL /L = cells x 109/L).
Direct microscopy of the blood smear yields the number of thrombocytes count by counting those found between 1000 erythrocytes (5 microscopic fields of 200 red cells) multiplied by the number of erythrocytes/$mm.^3$ and then divided /1000) with the results expressed as platelets/ mm^3. The estimate of platelet count from slides uses a semiquantitative method, whereby 1 platelet / oil immersion field is equivalent with 20.000 plt/mm^3. Figure 1 In optical microscopy, one assesses a panoptic colored blood smear under the immersion objective(100 X). Most platelets have a dendritic aspect and fringe-like extension. Normal platelets have diameter of 2-4 microns on the blood smear with 70% alone, 20% in groups of 2 or 3 and 10% in larger groups or "big pools". Correctly executed blood smear reveal microscopic fields on the oil-immersion objective with an average of 10 platelets;as either isolated or grouped. Visualization of <5 platelets on the microscopic field connotes thrombocytopenia while >40 indicates thrombocythemia. [13].
Platelets are typically disk-shaped with a more dense central (granular) area and a peripheral (crystalline) area with functional dendritic fringes [14]. If activated by toxic metabolic factors, platelets become more spherical, which can yield a decrease in the intensity of the image in the microscopic lenses, due to light transmission and diffusion through samples. When platelets are activated, they become spherical with a hypogranular

cytoplasm and release small particles. This may lead to the erroneous detection of platelets when using the microscopy owing to their deformed morphology.

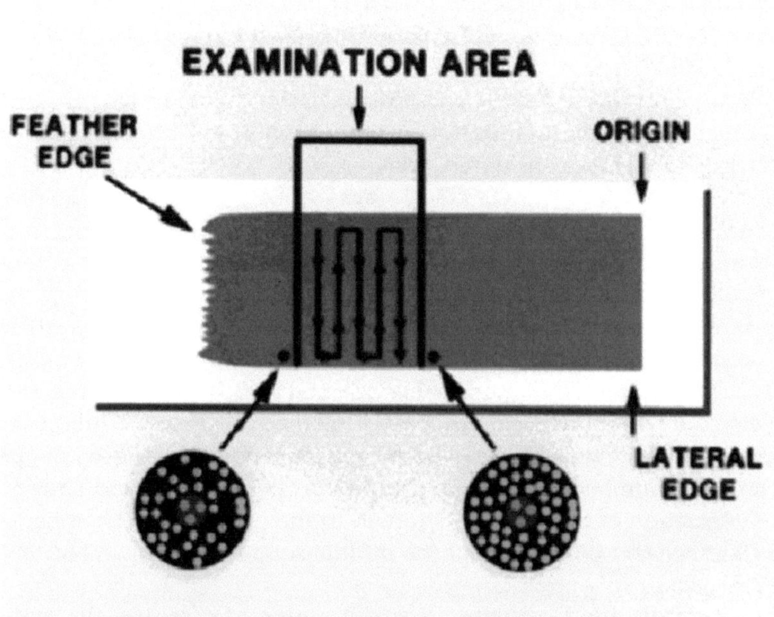

Fig. 1.

Recognizing erroneous results of platelet counts is especially critical for a consistent decision in the diagnosis of disseminated intravascular coagulation (DIC) and for clinical decision making regarding transfusion.

The platelet count is an indispensable parameter in the DIC scoring system proposed by the International Society on Thrombosis and Hemostasis Sub-Committee of the Scientific and Standardization Committee on DIC, in which platelet counts of less than 100 × 103/μL (100 × 109/L) and less than 50 × 103/μL (50 × 109/L) would score 1 and 2 points, respectively. [15, 16] The samples were assessed for platelet count by statistical parameters: [SD = (Xi- Xm)2 /n – 1; accuracy: (%Diff = X average – X target/ X mean x 100, with normal value until + − 25) and Z score(Z = X average-X target/SD, with normal value until +-2, R>0.95%), for average platelets 150-400 x10^3/μl, 95% CI.].

3. Results

From total patient in our study, a minority of patients, 36 patients (40%) had normal results for all hematological tests under monitoring treatment of specialty. In type of anemia from kidney chronic diseases, an additional 16 (18%) patients had normal HGB and HCT, but low MCV or MCH ((mean value 72 fL, SD= 2.1) or MCH (mean value 24.3pg, SD= 1.6). Other 28 patients (31%) had mild anemia (HGB decreased but > 106 g/L), while only 10 patients (11%) have had severe anemia. All individuals in the group with severe anemia had low RET (mean value 1.2%, range 0.5-1.5%), and RPI in mean value of <1.4, indicating a hypo-regenerative type of anemia.

To the 54 patients with anemia of chronic kidney diseases (ACKD) and chronic renal failure(CRF) were registered in 30.90% of cases normal TIBC values (mean value 282 microgram/ d L, SD=2.5), low RPI in mean value of 1.33, low IST in mean value of 7.62%, with middle ineffective erythropoiesis and moderate iron deficiency anemia (IDA) and to 19.10 % of patients with ACKD and CRF associated with renal inflammations, were calculated low RPI, in mean value of 1.21, high TIBC value (mean value 468 microgram/d L, SD =2.4) and low IST in mean value of 6.5%, with severe ineffective erythropoiesis and severe IDA.

In biochemical field, in this study on this cohort of hemodialysis patients, was obtained the variability of plasma osmolality past normal individual values (310 Osm/l), in the samples taken from the patients with chronic renal failure because of high values of Urea nitrogen (mean value 112 mg%; 40 mmol/L; SD = 2.40); Creatinine (mean value 5.5 mg/%; 4.85 mmol/L); SD=0.15); Sodium (mean value 170 mmol/L; SD=0.14); Potassium (mean value 14.5 mmol/l; SD=2.88); E CO2 (mean value 11 mmol/L; SD=0.26). Prevalence of anemia to patients admitted in hospital for undergoing schedules of hemodialysiss have been registered in percents: 60% of cases, with normochromic-normocytic anemia, 30% of cases with microcytic-hypochomic anemia and nutritional iron deficiency, 7% of cases with aplastic anemia and 3% with macrocytic and vitamin B12 deficiency.

In cases with microcytic-hypochomic anemia and nutritional iron deficiency were registered by this study that mean corpuscular volume (MCV) of red cells decreases below normal value before that the hemoglobin to be decreased under normal value. Iron deficiency anemia associated with ACKD was presented in three forms:

- Prevalent anemia with low serum ferritin (SF), when ferritin descends in early stages of iron deficiency, before changes of concentration of hemoglobin concentration, size of erythrocyte, level of iron serum value, with high TIBC (8%),
- Latent anemia with low SF and low circulating serum iron, TIBC is increased, urine iron is low and erythrocytes with low iron in content have aspect of hypochromic red blood cells (10%),
- Installed anemia with deficiency of erythropoiesis, low ferritin (< 50 microgram/L) in bone morrow, TSI < 16% in serum iron and hypochromic and microcytic erythrocytes (12%), [17,18]. When the aspect Iron/TIBC is less than 15%, we have had the certain diagnostic of ACKD associate with IDA. Low serum iron, serum ferritin increased and low TIBC means ACD. Low serum iron, low serum ferritin and TIBC increased means IDA [19].

In the two cases of study were registered suspect flags on Coulter HMX: neutropenia, lymphopenia and increased MCV erythrocyte index (109 f L). On blood smear from peripheral blood, in optic microscopy the reticulocyte count was decreased (0.4%), and neutrophil granulocytes showed multi-segmented nuclei, macrocytes (larger than normal RBCs) presence of ovalocytes (oval-shaped RBC) but Howell-Jolly bodies(chromosomal remnant) was absented. An elevated MCV should not be ignored because the patient is especially suspected of alcohol abuse. Blood chemistries will also showed: an increased lactic acid dehydrogenase (LDH) values of .increased of homocysteine, folic and vitamin B12 deficiency.

Bone marrow (checked in a patient suspected of megaloblastic anemia on hematological analyzer, in 3% from cases) showed megaloblastic hyperplasia~ 45%, ploycromathopil and acidophil erythroblasts with megaloblastic character, large metamielocytes and giant band forms. Biopsy results from gastric mucosa showed lesions of chronic gastritis, non-atrophic epithelium and the patient was receiving the recommendation from clinician doctor to assess B12 vitamin.

Diagnosis in all these patients has been established in collaboration with clinician doctors from department of hospitals in the system of evidence based medicine, on data encompassed in observation daily sheet of patients.

The suspect cases with hemolytic anemia were verified on biochemistry panel (unconjugated bilirubin, LDH) and in hematological field by Coombs test direct (DET) and indirect,reticulocytes presented in elevated number, haptoglobin levels decreased, also increased urobilinogen in urine analysis.

The bone marrow aspiration was performed by sternum bone puncture, to 7 patients with suspect chronic refractory anemia from myelodisplastic syndrome on evidence of aspect of peripheral smear with neutropenia, anemia and thrombocytopenia, (low cell counts of white and red blood cells, and platelets, respectively) with blast count <5% in the peripheral blood, beside macrocytosis and microcytosis. The morphological abnormality was observed in the granulocytes. These included bi-lobed or un-segmented nuclei (pseudo–Pelger-Huet abnormality) and granulation abnormalities in vary from.

After this aspect the clinician doctors recommended bone morrow puncture to National Institute of Reference Hematological Diseases, City Bucharest, (Romania). Was excluded the diagnosis of acute myeloid leukemia when < 20% blasts was observed on blood smear of bone morrow. In severe cases, red blood cells in eliptocytes forms accompanied microcytic and hypochromic cells on blood film. Low SI, IST%, and SF combined with elevated RDW, TIBC suggest IDA and this type of anemia must be differentiated from uncomplicated anemia from ACKD. An association between, HCT, HGB and RBC (Graphic 1) or HCT, TIBC, RPI and IST (Table 1) can be applied and in assessment of anemia from chronic diseases taken in this study.

HTC %	RPI	TIBC microgram/d L	IST %
35 - 30	1.52	225	29.1
29 - 25	1.33	282	7.62
24 - 18	1.21	468	6.5

Table 1. Correlation between Hematocrit (HTC), Reticulocytes Production Index (RPI) Total Iron Binding Capacity (TIBC) and Index Saturation Transferrin (IST) in Anemia of Chronic Renal Failure

The platelet count determined on the peripheral blood smear was used to complement data from the quantitative methods and provided morphological information.

The comparison between the platelet counts on the Coulter HMX (mean value $\bar{X}$ = 233 x 10^3µl; p=0.028; SD=2; % Diff=0.90; Z score = - 0.30) and by optical microscopy ($\bar{X}$ = 250 x 10^3µl; p=0.029; SD= 2.6; %Diff = -3.6; Z score =0.40) yielded similar values in a control group (120 male and female healthy subjects, ages 25-55 years(mean age 40).

For the dialysis patients, we found that results for platelet counts with the Coulter HMX, before and after hemodialysis were similar: (pre-dialysis mean $\bar{X}$ = 230 10^3 µl; p=0.024; SD=3.45; % Diff = -4.53; Z score =2.5; post dialysis mean $\bar{X}$ = 245 x 10^3µl; p=0.034; SD=2.1; %Diff = 6.34; Z score = 0.10) but differences appeared if counting was done using optical microscopy (pre-dialysis mean $\bar{X}$ =261 x 10^3µl; p = 0.020; SD=7.1; %Diff= 5.90; Z score=3.90); post-dialysis mean $\bar{X}$ = 167 x 10 ^{3}µl; p = 0.6; SD=4.2; %Diff= -7.10; Z score= -2.90). Table 2

The latter results may be attributable to the variability of plasma osmolality in the samples taken from the patients with chronic renal failure: Glucose (98mg%; 5.44mmol/L; SD=2.80); Urea nitrogen (112 mg%; 40 mmol/L; SD = 2.40); Creatinine (5.5 mg/%; 4.85 mmol/L);

SD=0.15); Sodium (170 mmol/L; SD=0.14); Potassium (14.5 mmol/l; SD=2.88); E CO2 (11 mmol/L; SD=0.26). (Table3. Graphic 2)

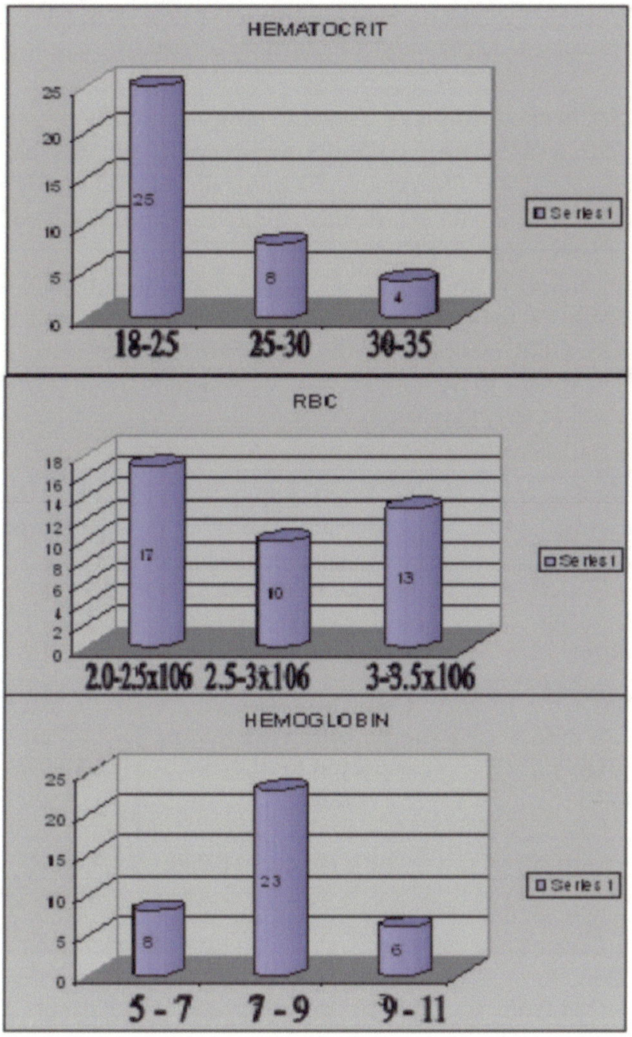

Graphic 1. Levels of HGB, RBC and HTC in chromic renal failure

The performance of devices used was assessed by **Z score = < 1 = optic performance; 1 < Z < 2 = good performance; 2 < Z < 3 = satisfactory performance and Z > 3 =unsatisfactory performance.** In parallel, we assessed platelet count using the peripheral blood smear and found that it provided information that was complentary to the other methods, especially with respect to morphological aspects of platelets.

Counting thrombocytes on slide from peripheral blood smear is necessary in quantitative platelet disorders, as isolated thrombocytopenia: immune versus nonimmune, thrombocytopenia associated with other hematological abnormalities or in differential diagnosis with platelet clump, thrombocytosis and qualitative disorders, as giant platelets (megathrombocytes), platelet inclusion or granule abnormalities, bizarre in shape and size.

The control group to 40 potential health persons (20 adult men and 20 adult females), on hematological analyzer Coulter HMX, was next results (mean value), form men: WBC=9700/dL, RBC=4500 000/dLHGB=13,9g/dL, MCV= 90 f L, RDW=13.5%, MCV = 29 f L, MCHC = 34%) and for women WBC=95/dL, RBC=4200 000/dL, HGB=12,5g/dL, MCV= 80 f L, RDW=14.5%, MCV = 27 f L, MCHC = 30%) [Sensitivity = (35/ 40) x 100 = 87.50%].

In biochemistry field, normal results of the same group control were registered next results: Creatinine, 1.2 mg/dl, with SD=0.15,CV%=29, accuracy [Z] =-1.36; Iron, 100 microgram/dl, SD=2.88, CV%=1.8, Z=-0.56; Phosphate, 27.mEq/dl, SD=0.14.CV%=2.2, Z=-0.8; Urea, 40mg/dl, SD=2.40, CV=2.2, Z=-0.13; Uric acid, 8mg/dl, SD=0.26; CV=3.2, Z=-0.79; [Normal Z = ±2 in Control of Levey Jennings Chart.].

The precision to our cohort in study was registered as next results: CV < 2% for RBC, CV < 1% for HGB and CV < 2% for HCT, (Accuracy: r > 0.95 for HGB and HCT, 95% CI), mean SD=2.2 and p=0.04 for HGB, mean SD = ± 2.5 and p < 0.05 for MCV in CBC, MCHC with CV =2%, MCH with CV=1.5%, RDW with CV = 3%. [Specificity = (124/140) x 100 = 88%]. Positive predictive value (107/124) = 86%.

Coulter HMX **Normal Patients;** $\bar{X}$ = 233 x 10^3µl; p=0.028; SD=2; %; Diff=0.90; Z score = - 0.30;	**Microscopy** **Normal Patients** $\bar{X}$ = 250 x 10^3µl; p=0.029; SD= 2.6; %; Diff = -3.6; Z score =0.40.	**Microscopy** **Normal slide blood** $\bar{X}$ = 240 x 10^3 µl;CV=5.3%, SD= 12.7; %; Diff= 8.30; Z score= 3.33;
Coulter HMX **Patients with CRF before connected to dialysis devices** $\bar{X}$ =230 x10^3 µl; p=0.024; SD=3.45; % Diff = -4.53; Z score =2.5),	**Optic Microscopy** **Patients with CRF before connected to dialysis devices** $\bar{X}$ =261 x 10^3µl; p = 0.020; SD=7.1; %; Diff= 5.90; Z score=3.90	**Microscopy slides** **Patients with CRF before connected to dialysis devices** $\bar{X}$ = 275 x 10^3 µl; CV=5%; SD= 13.75; %; Dif= 15.75; Z score = -3.46,
Coulter HMX **Patients disconnected from dialysis devices** $\bar{X}$ = 245 x 10^3 µl; p=0.034; SD=2.1; %; Diff = 6.34; Z score = 0.10),	**Optic Microscopy** **Patients disconnected from dialysis devices** $\bar{X}$ 167 x 10 ^{3} µl; p = 0.6; SD=4.2; %; Diff= -7.10; Z score= -2.90	**Microscopy slides** **Patients disconnected from dialysis devices** $\bar{X}$ =190 x10^3 µl;CV=4.6%; SD= 8.74; %Diff =18; Z score =7.60;

Table 2. Assessment of performances for methods used in platelets count to patients with Chronic Renal Failure, undergoing dialysis

Functional ID was closely related to the production of hypochromic red cells, and measurement of red cells hemoglobinization provides a sensitive method for determining the quantity of circulating iron incorporated into the red blood cells which, reflect recent changes in erythropoiesis.

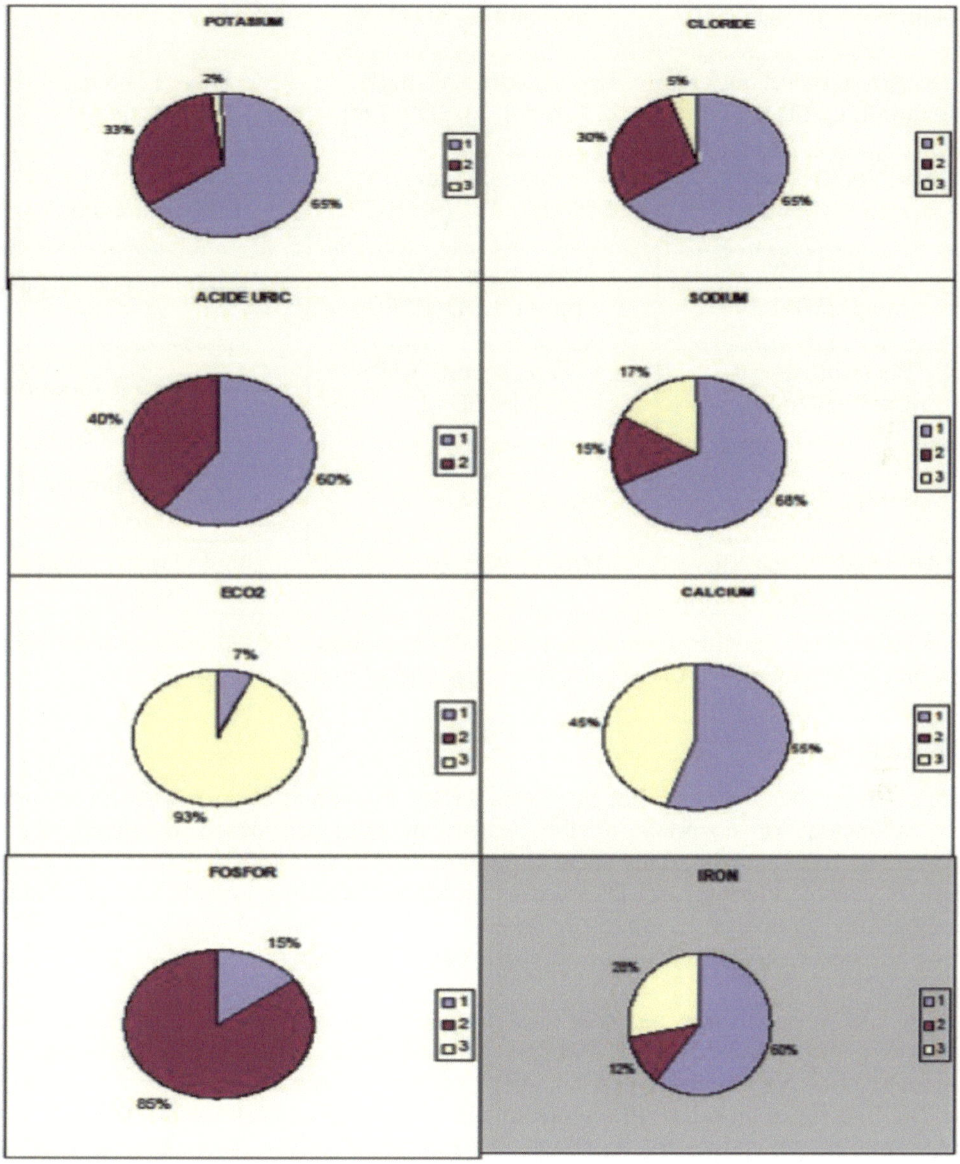

Graphic 2. Biochemical parameters of chronic renal failure which are frequently increased in Chronic Kidney Diseases (CKD)

Parameters in Chronic Renal Failure before schedules of Dialysis (mean value)	Parameters in Chronic Renal Failure after undergoing the schedules of Dialysis (mean value)	Normal Range of Blood Tests used in Diagnosis of CRF (laboratory reference)
Glucose: 98mg%; (5.44mmol/L); SD=2.80;	Glucose: 105 mg%; (5.76 mmol/L) SD=1.04;	Glucose: 65- 115 mg%; (3.9-6.1 mmol/L)
Urea nitrogen: 112 mg%; (40 mmol/L); SD = 2.40;	Urea nitrogen: 65 mg%; (23.2 mmol/L); SD = 1.60;	Urea: 17-45 mg%; (1.7-8.3 mmol/ L)
Creatinine; 5.5 mg/ %; (4.85 mmol/L); SD=0.15;	Creatinine; 1.8 mg/ %; (1.58mmol/)L; (SD=0.20;	Creatinine: 0.2-1.25; (0.07-0.12 mmol/L)
Sodium: 170 mmol/L;SD=0.14	Sodium: 145 mmol/L;SD=0.70	Sodium: 137-145 mmol/L;
Potassium14.5 mmol/l;SD=2.88	Potassium7.1 mmol/l;SD=2.90	Potassium: 3,6—5mmol/L
E CO2: 11 mmol/L;SD=0.26;	E CO2: 19 mmol/L;SD=2.29;	E CO2: 22-30mmol/L
Hb= 8.5g/- 9.2mg/dl; SD=2.20	Hb= 10.5- 11.2mg/dl SD= 2.45;	Hb=11.4-13.6mg/dl; SD=2.7

Table 3.Values of biochemical and hematological parameters in blood samples from patients with Chronic Renal Failure, undergoing the schedules of dialysis

4. Discussions

Diagnosis in all these patients has been established in collaboration with clinician doctors from department of hospitals in the system of evidence based medicine, on data encompassed in observation daily sheet of patients.

Anemia of chronic kidney (ACKD) diseases associated with the iron deficiency (IDA) was microcytic and hypochromic, especially once the HGB level fall below 100g/L and HCT are somewhat lower that seen in normochromic, normocytic anemia from chronic diseases(ACKD).

Proportion of hypochromic red cells is a time average marker, was similar in anemic patients like glucose, HbA1c in diabetes patients. The marker for IDA, hypochromic erythrocytes, has been investigated for every patient, on blood film slide, May Gunwald stain. The hypochromic cells >10% were considered functional ID, in correlation low with iron. Various cut off values for functional ID is reported in literature ranging from 2% to 10% of hypocromic cells [17]

Measuring of TIBC was made as an indirect method of assessing transferrin and provided comparable information [18]. TSI indicates the percent of iron binding sites on transferring that is carrying iron. TSI is derived from a calculation using the formula: [(SI/TIBC) x100] and TSI is generally considered to be the most sensitive laboratory test for detecting altered iron metabolism in hereditary hemochromatosis (HH). It may be elevated prior to

significant deposition of tissue iron. TS levels increase as additional iron is accumulated. A drawback to using the TS is that it is dependent on performing both the SI and TIBC.
Current guidelines from the American College of Physicians include a normal level of TSI encompassed between 20-40%, a cut off level of TSI >55% identifying iron overload and TSI < 15% meaning IDA. Red distribution width (RDW) is a mathematical expression of size variation used to quantify anisocytosis. The higher the RDW means the greater the anisocytosis. Increased RDW may be an early indication of iron deficiency, where it may precede the onset of microcytosis.
These measurements, known as erythrocyte or red blood cell indices, provide an important information about various types of anemia. If the MCV is low, the cells are microcytic or smaller than normal. Microcytic red blood cells have been seen in iron deficiency anemia and thalassemia minor. If the MCV is high, the cells are macrocytic, or larger than normal. Macrocytic red blood cells were associated with pernicious anemia or folic acid deficiencies. If the MCV is within the normal range, the cells are referred to as normocytic and nomocytic anemia was met with more frequency in chronic diseases/inflammation, small MCH under 27% show hypocromic erythrocytes, frequently encountered in IDA. In the same correlation with MCHC less than 32% indicates that the red blood cells are deficient in hemoglobin concentration.
This situation is most often seen with iron deficiency anemia. RDW is a measurement of anisocytosis. IDA and thalassemia are both microcytic-hypochromic anemia. As screening tests for discovery of anemia to elderly we used, beside additional tests, erythrocytes indexes such as MCV, MCH, and RBC number to distinguish this anemia types. MCH is just the equivalent of Retyculocites -Hemoglobin (Ret-He) that indicates the long term of life span of erythrocytes.
Both serum transferrin receptor and erythrocyte zinc protoporphyrin have been demonstrated to be useful in a variety of clinical situations. Serum transferrin receptor can be best used in diagnosing iron disorders, especially for patients with pathologies that may affect iron metabolism. Erythrocyte zinc protoporphyrin can be best used as a primary screening test for assessing iron status, especially in patients likely to have uncomplicated iron deficiency hemoglobin status and life span of erythrocytes [18].
Other anemia, most notably thalassemia, are also characterized by low MCV, MCH, MCHC and additional tests are needed for confirmation of thalassemia Patient with a ratio target cells/normal cells > 1% in low power field and with >20% microcytic red cells on blood film (magnification x 400), were suspicious for beta-thalssemia. RBC count result higher in thalassemia minor group in comparison with IDA. Microcytic, hypochromic and polyglobulia are more evident in thalassemia minor compared with IDA and hemoglobin and hematocrit can be normally but only MCV and MCH decreased in thalassemia silent carrier. (Graphic 3)
The bone morrow hemosiderrin and microscopic bone marrow examination have been recommended in clinical management in most elderly patients with anemia in Mielodysplastic Syndrome (MDS) The problems in diagnostic anemia occurs when the iron reserves are depleted and not.
The peptide hormone Hepcidin appears to play a central role in the pathogenesis of the anemia of chronic disease, but is extremely difficult to measure in the serum. Thus the "anemia of chronic disease" may include patients with a variety of patho-physiological mechanisms. The peptide hormone Hepcidin, secreted by the liver, controls plasma iron concentration by inhibiting iron export from macrophages cells(cut off, 15 ng/d L, Elisa

method). The effect of Hepcidin is to increase intracellular iron stores in ACD, decreased dietary iron absorption and decrease circulating iron concentration in chronic anemia from inflammations and infections [19].

Laboratory Test Results

Test	Patient Result	Reference Intervals (Adult female)
White blood cell (WBC) count	$3.7 \times 10^9/L$	$4.4 - 11.3 \times 10^9/L$
Red blood cell (RBC) count	$5.6 \times 10^{12}/L$	$4.1 - 5.1 \times 10^{12}/L$
Hemoglobin (Hb)	10.5 g/dL	12.3 - 15.3 g/dL
Hematocrit (HCT)	36.6%	35.9 - 44.6%
MCV	65.8 fL	80.0 - 96.0 fL
MCH	19.9 pg	27.5 - 33.2 pg
MCHC	26.7%	33.4 - 35.5%
RDW	14.0	<14.5
Platelets	$249.0 \times 10^9/L$	$100.0 - 450.0 \times 10^9/L$
Total serum iron	165 µg/dL	60 - 150 µg/dL
Iron-binding capacity	230 µg/dL	250 - 400 µg/dL

Graphic 3. The RBC count is increased for the amout of hemoglobin present. The concentration of hemoglobin in the RBCs is slighlty decreased (hypochromic) and the cells are small (microcytic). The varioation in RBC size (RDW) is whitin normal limits.

In chronic renal failure (CRF), the peripheral blood smear can reveal activated thrombocytes with fingers(burr cells) as isolated cells or organized in groups. By contrast, with diabetic ketoacidosis, one can see the reverse phenomenon, thrombocytes that are isolated, with round shape form and without activated fringes. Figure 2 It is interesting that platelet activation markers were associated with the severity of DIC and erroneous platelet counts, suggesting that platelet activation is a potential source for the inter-method variation in platelet counts. More attention needs to be given to improve the accuracy of platelet counts, especially in clinical conditions with high levels of platelet activation.

It is well known that white light is comprised of luminous waves with different wave lengths of 750-250 nm. Optical microscopy uses light diffraction but can have light reflection, refraction, diffusion and dispersion phenomena, especially through media with non-homogenous densities.

Thus, it has been recommended that one conduct platelet counts using phase-contrast microscopy, which helps eliminate such light interference phenomena because it the image is formed by a diffraction process in two stages: incident light diffraction and diffraction of the light refracted in the objective.

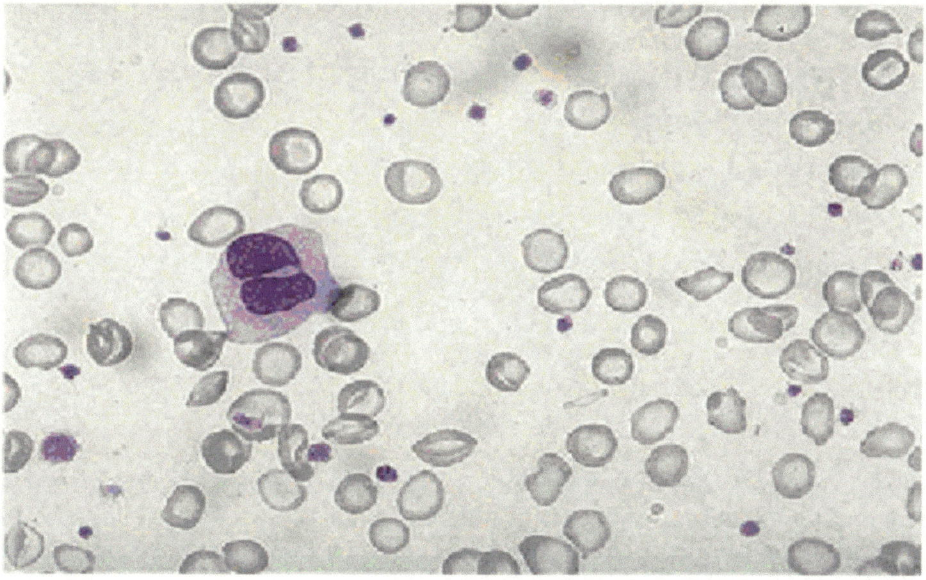

Fig. 2. Qualitative platelets disorders: platelets with abnormality bizarre in shape and size

The optical conventional techniques used for platelet counting have limits that are influenced by the human eye, especially for detection of objects <5 microns. Thus, the modern trend is to replace optical systems and introduce some electronic optical systems.

Electronic microscopy with Beta rays and wave lengths thousands of times smaller than the white light gives a higher power of resolution and thus, analyzers well-suited for platelet count in biological fluids are ones that use either of two methods: WCS technology of impedance (Volume, Conductivity and Scatter Light), {Graphic 4} and WOC analysis by laser ray (White Cell Optical Count) [20], Graphic 5. In WCS, the fat within the cell membrane behaves as an object that facilitates generation of an electronic impulse with an amplitude proportionate as the cell volume and helps create a potential difference next to the count cleft Since VCS technology includes a highly accurate measure of cell volume, we can use this information to correct the conductivity and scatter signals. The result of this volumetric compensation is a pair of measurements that are very powerful, and unique to Beckman Coulter. The HMX Coulter Analyzer utilizes the Coulter principle to provide cellular information for the complete WBC differential. The system measures the amount of light "lost" due to diffraction and absorbance as compared to full transmission when no cell is present.

The signals collected are converted into voltage pulses and are processed. The size and shape of the voltage pulses are equivalent to the unique nuclear and morphologic structure of the cells being analyzed conductivity offers information about opacity, which is directly proportional to cell density [21].

In WOC technology the laser light measures cellular elements in 4 specific angles and every angle of light scatter from 0° through 90° is influenced by cellular size. The low angles are the most affected, and are often used as an indirect estimation of cellular size. The zero angle measures the dimension of cells and impedance is used to count RBC corpuscles > 36 fL and platelets, corpuscles with the dimensions between 2-20 fL [22].

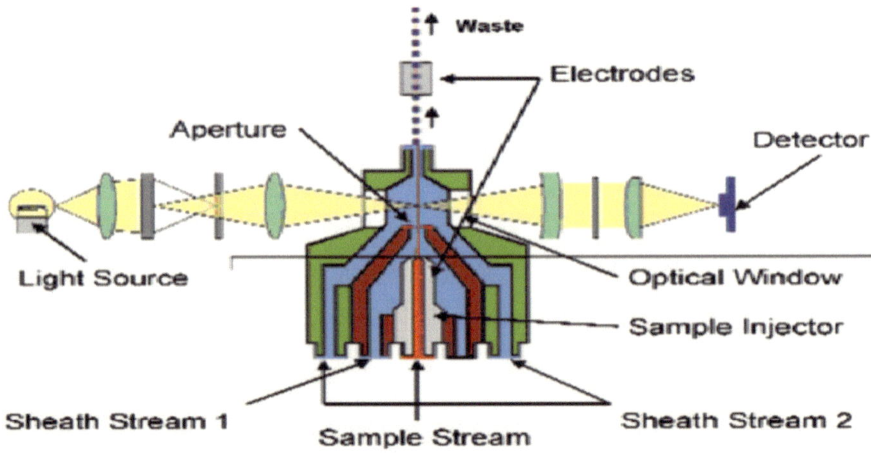

Graphic 4. VCS Technology includes a highly accurate measure of cell volume and this information is added to the Conductivity and Scatter signals. Every angle of light scatter from 0° through 90° is influenced by cellular size. The low angles are most affected, and are often used as an indirect estimation of cellular size.

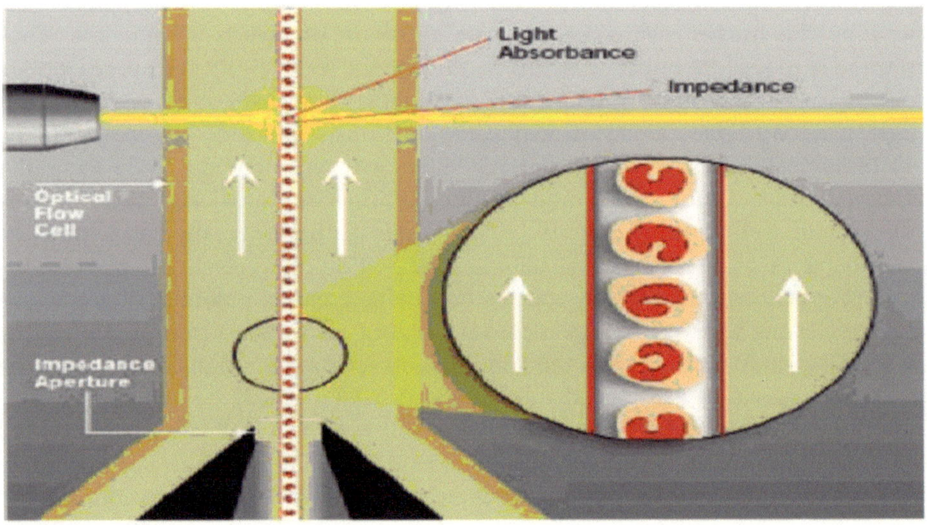

Graphic 5. WOC channel (White Cell Optical Count) is used for counting blood cells and differential count by laser technokigy. The result of this volumetric compensation is a pair od measurements that are very powerful, and unique to Beckman Coulter.

The main elements that maintain the plasma osmolality in normal values (310 Osm/l) are; Na, K, urea and glucose. Serum osmolality is normal whenever the osmotic pressure set by urea and glucose is negligible and the Na+ concentration can largely define osmolality [Osm = 2.1 x conc Na mEq/L).Whenever the level of plasma urea or glucose is high, the osmolality becomes: 2.1 (Na + K) mmol/L + urea mg% / 2.8 + glucose mg% /18.02), result expressed in Osm /L[23]. In metabolic states with high osmolality (e.g. from chronic renal failure), errors in platelet counts occur in optical microscopy due to the double refraction phenomenon.

This phenomenon occurs because particles <5μ create reflection, refraction, diffusion and diffraction of light through environments with different properties (ε) and in solutions with higher osmolality. The diffraction of rays by objects < 5μ are not sufficiently dispersed and only a part of the issued light falls on the object from the objective of microscope.

The angle comprised between the rays which delimit the light cone represents the numerical aperture(A) and the resolution power or the spectral separation power, dependent of light diffraction (D), light wave length (L) and numerical aperture (A) , (D = L / A), [24].

Optical instruments contain light separation media that are non-homogenous, including glass (ocular, objectives, prisms, air) and thus yield losses in the intensity of the incidence, reflection, refraction and diffraction rays through the media crossed by them. After the expression: $S = [n1 - n2/n1 \times n2]^2$, where "n" represent the refraction index from the environment, the losses of the incidental ray, because of interference, is 4% from the intensity of incidental fascicle [25].

Platelets with dimensions <2μ and are met by light rays, with a very high speed of propagation through liquid environments may not be seen in optical microscopy if increased osmolarity concentrations are present. In accordance with Huygens interference principle, clefts S1 and S2 become secondary oscillation sources. The sources of secondary vibration of the light generated waves can overlap between the interference areas and fringes, thus yielding what is termed the interference domain.

Thus, the average of the intensity values of the object light image in the ocular may has the range between 0 value and 4 'e" ($e= {}^1/4nS$) in the minimal, respectively, maximum interference phase.

The minimal intensity state of the light reflected on the object in order to create its reversed image in the ocular leads image loss for the human eye.

The normal thrombocytes having the diameter of 2-4 microns, create reflection, refraction, diffusion and diffraction of light through microscopy and become more less visible to manual counting.

There has been some debate over which counting principle, between the impedance and optical methods, measures platelet counts more accurately. Some studies suggested that the accuracy of the optical methods was superior for thrombocytopenic specimens, while recent studies demonstrated the impedance method to be more accurate for samples from patients undergoing cytotoxic chemotherapy [26].

5. Conclusions

The anemia of hospitalized patients with chronic or acute renal diseases undergoing hemodialysis exists in our study in 60% from studied cases and must be managed of laboratory medicine in collaborative with the clinician. A routine anemia screening should be recommended using HGB, HCT and erythrocytes indexes MCV, MCH, MCHC and must be redefined the anemia by these common parameters.

An iron panel (serum iron, TIBC, IST% and RPI) is useful in differentiating anemia of chronic disease from iron deficiency. By this study the anemia can be defined as a decrease of HGB and or hematological indexes with 10%from initial normal values, with cut of 117g/L HGB for men and 108g/L HGB for women.

The methods used to assess platelet counts of hemodialysis patients, optical microscopy, peripheral blood smear and use of the cytometry principle with impedance principle (VIC), yielded similar results with samples from normal subjects but the accuracy of the automatic method ensures a high quality count of hemodialysis patients.

The all three methods yielded similar results with samples from normal subjects and that the accuracy of the automatic method ensures a high quality count but apparently not so, for patients post-dialysis.

Examination of the peripheral blood smear appears to offer important advantages, in particular for dialysis patients, so as to assess for qualitative as well as quantitative changes in platelets in such patients We concluded that should be a clinical guideline for the management of anemia in the elderly with chronic renal diseases.

6. Abbreviations

ACD - Anemia of Chronic Disease;
CFR- Chronic Renal Failure;
CBC-complete blood count;
CHr -reticulocyte hemoglobin;
EPO -erythropoietin;
HGB-hemoglobin;
HCT - hematocrit;
IDA - iron deficiency anemia;
IST - index saturation transferrin;
MA -megaloblastic anemia;
MCV -mean cell volume;
MCH - mean cellular hemoglobin;
MCHC -mean cell hemoglobin concentration;
RPI-Reticulocyte Production Index;
TS - transferrin saturation;
RDW 0 red cell distribution width;
RET - reticulocyte count;
SI - serum iron;
sTR - soluble transferrin receptor;
TIBC - total iron binding capacity

7. References

Guralnik JM, Eisenstaedt RS, Ferrucci L, Klein HG, Woodman RC. Prevalence of anemia in persons 65 years and older in the United States: evidence for a high rate of unexplained anemia. Blood 2004; 104:2263–2268

Blanc B, Finch CA, Hallberg L, et al. Nutritional anemia: report of a WHO Scientific Group. WHO Tech Rep Ser 1968; 405:1–40.

Salive ME, Cornoni-Huntley J, Guralnik JM, et al. Anemia and hemoglobin levels in older persons: relationship with age, gender, and health status. J Am Geriatri Soc 1992; 40:489–4964

Zakai NA, Katz R, Hirsch C, et al. A prospective study of anemia status, hemoglobin concentration, and mortality in an elderly cohort: the Cardiovascular Health Study. Arch Intern Med 2005; 165:2214–2220

Pan WH and Habicht JP. The non-iron-deficiency-related difference in hemoglobin concentration distribution between blacks and whites and between men and women. Am J Epidemiol 1991; 134:1410–1416

Beutler E and Waalen J. The definition of anemia: what is the lower limit of normal of the blood hemoglobin concentration? Blood 2006; 107:1747–175

Riva E, Tettamanti M, Mosconi P, Apolone G, Gandini F et al. Association of mild anemia with hospitalization and mortality in the elderly: the Health and Anemia population-based study. Haematologica. 2009; 94(1):22-8

Ramel A, Jonsson PV, Bjornsson S, Thorsdottir I. Anemia, nutritional status, and inflammation in hospitalized elderly. Nutrition. 2008; 24(11-12):1116-22

Eisenstaedt R, Penninx BW, Woodman RC. Anemia in the elderly: current understanding and emerging concepts. Blood Rev. 2006; 20(4):213-26.

Adamson J W. Longo D L. Mc Graw H. Braunwald E. Anemia and polycythemia et all. Harrison's Principles of Internal Medicine. New York 2001; 15th Edition

ACP CPSC Tools: Reticulocyte Production Index. American College of Physicians. Internal Medicine/ Doctor1s for Adults 1999, 2000

Brecher G, Cronkite EP. Morphology and enumeration of human blood platelet. J Appl Physiol.1995; 3:365.

Moreno A, Menke D. Assessment of platelet numbers and morphology in the peripheral blood smear. Clin Lab Med 2002; 22(1): 193-213.

Bennett J M, Rogers G. Practical Diagnosis of Hematological Disorders, 2-th Edition. Let Thrombocytes. Chicago: ASCP Press 2006; p: 301 - 311.

Seon Young Kim, Ji-Eun Kim, Hyun Kyung Kim, ; Kyou-Sup Han, Cheng Hock Toh. Accuracy of Platelet Counting by Automated Hematologic Analyzers in Acute Leukemia and Disseminated Intravascular Coagulation: Potential Effects of Platelet Activation. American Journal of Clinical Pathology 2010; 134(4):634-647.

Segal HC, Briggs C, Kunka S, et al. Accuracy of platelet counting haematology analysers in severe thrombocytopenia and potential impact on platelet transfusion. *Br J Haematol.* 2005;128:520–525.

Steensma DP, Tefferi A. Anemia in the elderly: how should we define it, when does it matter, and what can be done?. Mayo Clin Proc 2007; 82(8): 958-66.

Labbé RF, Dewanji A. Iron assessment tests: transferrin receptor vis-à-vis zinc. ClinBiochem 2004; 37 [3]: 165-174.

Knezevic V. Differentiation of Anemia from Chronic Diseases (ACD) with Anemia from Iron Deficiency (IDA).[Abstract p136]. 10-16 Meeting of Balkan ClinicalLaboratory Federation 2008; p. 162.

Hennessy M, Buckley T. C, Leadon D, Scott C. S. Automated analysis of blood samples from thoroughbred horses with the Abbott cell DYN 3500 (CD3500) hematology analyzer. Comparative Hematology International 2006(3); 8

Hickerson DH, Bode AP. Flow cytometry of platelets for clinical analysis. *Hematol Oncol Clin North Am.* 2002;16: 421–454.

Hervig T, Haugen T, Liseth K, et al. The platelet count accuracy of platelet concentrates obtained by using automated analysis is influenced by instrument bias and activated platelet components. *Vox Sang.*2004; 87:196–203.

Mehdi R, Kiarash R. K. *Comparison of methods for calculating serum osmolality: multivariate linear regression analysis,* Clin. Chem.Lab *2005; 43*: 635-640.

David W Piston. Concepts in Imaging and Microscopy, Choosing Objective Lens: The importance of Numerical Aperture and Magnification in Digital Optical Microscopy Biol Bull 1998; (1); 4: 195:-199.

Sterian P. Fizica. Chap, Interferenta luminii. Ed Did si Ped Bucuresti 2008; p: 302-401.

Briggs C, Harrison P, Machin SJ. Continuing developments with the automated platelet count. Int J Lab Hematol 2007; 29(2): 77-97.

Part 2

Acute Kidney Injury

6

The Metamorphosis of Acute Renal Failure to Acute Kidney Injury

John W Pickering[1] and Zoltán H Endre[1,2]
[1]*Christchurch Kidney Research Group, University of Otago Christchurch*
[2]*Department of Nephrology, Prince of Wales Hospital, University of New South Wales, Sydney*
[1]*New Zealand*
[2]*Australia*

1. Introduction

Successive generations of scientists and nephrologists have failed to prevent or cure Acute Kidney Injury (AKI) and thousands every year die because of this. Recent innovations in proteomics and genomics have brought hope and renewed interest in preventing this blight. Motivated by high incidence and lack of effective treatments, researchers have focussed on how to detect AKI early in the disease process so as to provide the maximum opportunity for early intervention and positive outcomes. AKI Incidence is greatest in the intensive care, at about 11-52% in larger studies (n>500) (Ahlstrom et al. (2006); Bagshaw et al. (2008); Cruz et al. (2007)). Cardiac surgery and procedures involving radiocontrast pose smaller, but significant, risk of AKI with an incidence of 3-15% depending on cohort (Harjai et al. (2008); Lassnigg et al. (2008)). From 13 studies the mortality with AKI was 31.2% and was associated with an increase in relative risk of death from 2.40 to 6.15 depending on AKI severity (Ricci et al. (2008)). Stimulating much recent research has been the discovery of new kidney injury biomarkers, some of which appear to have sufficient sensitivity and specificity to be clinically useful.

This chapter will outline the history of the development of the concepts of clearance, acute renal failure, and acute kidney injury. This history provides the context for the current clearance based AKI diagnostic paradigm. The discovery of novel kidney injury biomarkers is challenging that paradigm. We will discuss the nature of that challenge and the opportunity it provides for development of early intervention treatments. All epidemiology, biomarker studies and clinical trials rely on tools to quantify AKI and assess efficacy of diagnostic or treatment efficacy. In section 3 we will discuss those tools before moving on to considering how they may best be applied in practice (section 4).

2. From ARF to AKI

2.1 Clearance and the rise and fall of creatinine

While suppression of urine flow, ischuria renalis, was recognised as a fundamental manifestation of renal disease from the 17th Century, clear metabolic manifestations of AKI were not documented until World War I in the German and World War II in the English literature (see Eknoyan (2002); McGrath (1852)). The term "Acute Renal Failure" first appeared in the literature in 1946 (Frank et al. (1946)), although it has been attributed to Homer Smith (Eknoyan (2002)). In keeping with a recent change in nomenclature we shall use the term "Acute Kidney Injury" (AKI) unless we are specifically referring to an historic use of ARF.

The historical development of clearance techniques and the relationship to glomerular filtration rate (GFR) are discussed by Berliner in his tribute to the great renal physiologist Homer Smith (Berliner (1995)). The term clearance was introduce in 1928 with reference to urea and to clearance of a defined volume of plasma in unit time (Moller et al. (1928)). The idea of creatinine clearance as a measure of glomerular filtration rate (GFR) was beautifully first demonstrated by Rehberg in experiments on himself (Rehberg (1926)). These also highlighted how variations in serum creatinine could be induced by diet: Rehberg ingested different quantities of creatinine to vary his serum creatinine. The utility of clearance as a technique was further established in the laboratory of Homer Smith, especially with para-amminohippuric acid clearance, a measure of secretion and renal blood flow (Smith et al. (1945)).

Creatinine is formed non-enzymatically from creatine in muscle, has a molecular weight of 113.12 Da, is freely filtered at the glomerulus and completely cleared by renal excretion when renal function is normal. The proximal tubules secrete creatinine, which accounts for 10 to 20% of the excreted load, and results in overestimation of GFR when measured by creatinine clearance (Perrone et al. (1992); Shemesh et al. (1985)). The contribution of tubular creatinine secretion to clearance, is increased when GFR is reduced and may reach 50%, but is highly variable amongst individuals (Perrone et al. (1992)). In contrast, the tubules reabsorb creatinine in some clinical settings such as decompensated heart failure and uncontrolled diabetes (Levinsky & Berliner (1959); Perrone et al. (1992)).

With creatinine clearance firmly established as a reasonable approximation to GFR, the next step was to estimate creatinine clearance based on the reciprocal relationship with plasma creatinine. This was popularized by the Cockroft-Gault equation which was derived by, firstly, a regression to estimate creatinine excretion/kg body weight according to age in hospitalised male patients; then clearance was calculated by multiplying by weight and dividing by the serum creatinine (Cockcroft & Gault (1976)). An untested 15% reduction for female gender was included, based on the observation that, on average, females had less fat and muscle mass than males (Cockcroft & Gault (1976)). This formula has been widely replaced by other estimates of GFR (eGFR), most notably by the Modification of Diet in Renal Disease (MDRD) equation originally developed in a population of CKD patients (Levey et al. (1999)).

Many alternative algorithms for creatinine-based eGFR have been developed, including those regularly in use for children; these equations are more accurate and precise than estimates from measurement of creatinine alone (*KDOQI Clinical Practice Guidelines for Chronic Kidney Disease: Evaluation, Classification, and Stratification* (2002)). The various iterations of the MDRD equation rely on plasma creatinine plus several other variables, including gender and race, and originally albumin and urea (as blood urea nitrogen) concentrations, but excluding mass although they do incorporate body surface area via the units; the latest version is more accurate than the MDRD equation for patients with GFR>60 ml/min (Levey et al. (2009)) but caveats remain (Rule (2010)) and drug dosing tends to be based on Cockroft-Gault (Ryzner (2010)).

Classical measurement of clearance with timed urine collection is cumbersome, so logically, the surrogate of clearance, the serum creatinine (actually measured in plasma), is usually the sole measure used to define renal status including development of AKI. However, serum creatinine increases slowly in response to a single step alteration in GFR. Serum creatinine has a half-life of approximately 4 hours when GFR is normal and 77 hours when GFR is reduced to 5% (Chiou & Hsu (1975); see section 3.1). As 3 to 5 half-lives are required after any change in GFR to obtain a new steady-state estimate, a reliable GFR based on the serum creatinine will require at least 12 hrs after even a minimal change in GFR. The current consensus definition (RIFLE: Risk, Injury, Failure, Loss, End-stage) of AKI requires at least a 33% decline in GFR, but a 25% reduction is traditionally accepted for diagnosis of contrast-induced AKI) (Bagshaw et al. (2008); Endre et al. (1989); Pickering & Endre (2009a)). Thus a new steady-state creatinine-based estimate of GFR will take from 24 to 72 hours. Obviously, the extent of increase in creatinine, which is determined by the extent of initial decrease in GFR and creatinine production, may allow diagnosis of AKI prior to the time needed to reach steady-state. However, the limited precision of creatinine measurement and the extent of intra-patient variation mean that a minimum 10% change in creatinine has traditionally been required by clinicians to demonstrate measurably significant change. An increase in serum creatinine has also been used as a major trigger for intervention (renal replacement therapy, RRT) in both AKI and chronic kidney disease (Gibney et al. (2008)).
The recognised imprecision in determining change in GFR led to removal of GFR from the new Acute Kidney Injury Network (AKIN) consensus classification of AKI so that an absolute or percentage increase in creatinine alone or in combination with oliguria has become the new consensus definition of AKI (Mehta et al. (2007)). Thus, despite many limitations, such as dependence on muscle mass, diet etc (Perrone et al. (1992)), serum creatinine became the accepted shorthand for estimating GFR and significant change in creatinine became the definition of AKI and marker of AKI severity.
Since there is an inverse relationship between serum creatinine and GFR, it is easy to forget that a small increase in serum creatinine represents a substantial decline in GFR. Consequently, prior to the now widespread reporting of eGFR estimated from creatinine, clinicians often ignored small increases in creatinine, and characterised these as "mild" or "moderate" increases. Combined with the uncertainty associated with the precision of measurement, years of ignoring such small increases in creatinine have impaired insight into how AKI is triggered. Even if an increase is observed, the delay required for diagnosis creates uncertainty regarding the timing of the renal insult leading to AKI. This represents a lost opportunity to investigate and identify the underlying pathophysiology of AKI in humans. Even mild grades of severity of AKI and transient (less than 24 hour increases in creatinine) are associated with increased hospital mortality (Chertow et al. (2005); Uchino et al. (2010; 2006)).
Inevitably, much of our interpretation of the pathophysiology of AKI is based on an animal model; the classical model utilises temporary cessation of renal blood flow to induce injury, usually through bilateral renal artery clamping. While this model may parallel human AKI after aortic surgery or renal transplantation, it greatly exaggerates the degree of tubular injury compared with that in the limited number of available human renal biopsies and is probably less relevant to AKI that does not follow hypoperfusion (Heyman et al. (2010)). Even in this model there is limited understanding of how major pathophysiological events in AKI are integrated, for example, the mechanism and timing of the switching "off" and "on" of

glomerular filtration. With few exceptions (Alejandro et al. (1995); Myers et al. (1984)), most of our experimental interventions have been validated only in this and nephrotoxic animal models (Vaidya et al. (2010)).

While there is a great deal of information about a large number of cellular (tubular and endothelial) events and the autonomic, inflammatory and renal vascular responses in experimental ischemia-reperfusion injury (Devarajan (2006); Heemskerk et al. (2009)), there is little corroborative and time-relevant clinical pathophysiological data. Usually, the clinical diagnosis of ischemic AKI is a diagnosis of exclusion. Thus, the potential delay imposed by reliance on creatinine is further delayed by investigations (eg exclusion of urinary outflow obstruction) or interventions (fluid loading to treat underlying "pre-renal" AKI) designed to exclude rather than confirm the diagnosis of ischemic AKI. Other investigations such as measurement of global or parenchymal renal blood flow, or renal biopsy, which might provide insight into human AKI, are delayed, difficult to interpret in the absence of baseline data, and usually not performed.

Since diagnosis is delayed it is not surprising, that there has been failure of pharmacological intervention in clinical trials, which are largely based on experimental interventions to prevent rather than treat AKI (Jo et al. (2007)). However, pharmacologic prevention of AKI has also largely failed, even when the apparent aetiology is known, eg parenteral administration of iodinated radiocontrast (Fishbane (2008); Nigwekar et al. (2009); Zoungas et al. (2009)). The failure to translate apparently effective pharmacologic preventive measures in animal models into clinical practice, suggests that the serum creatinine-inspired delay in diagnosis, merely complements a lack of fundamental understanding of pathophysiology in human AKI.

2.2 The rise and rise of injury

The change in nomenclature from acute renal failure to acute kidney injury recognised that an acute decline in renal function is usually secondary to injury (*American Society of Nephrology Renal Research Report* (2005); Mehta et al. (2007)). The need for a renal-specific biomarkers of injury akin to a troponin was presaged in the late 1990s (Star (1998)) and the discovery of such proteins was later accorded highest priority by The American Society of Nephrology (*American Society of Nephrology Renal Research Report* (2005)) with the expectation that such biomarkers would: "Diagnose AKI before the rise in serum creatinine; Stratify patients with respect to severity of injury and; Provide prognostic indicators." The term "secondary prevention" was introduced to highlight that biomarker detection would lead to early intervention ideally prior to loss of GFR (Pickering & Endre (2009c)).

Some urinary proteins, notably α_1-microglobulin, β_1-microglobulin, and N-acetyl-β-D-glucosaminidase (NAG), were already known to be associated with acute tubular injury (Yu et al. (1983)), whilst others awaited discovery. In 1998 Kidney Injury Molecule-1 (KIM-1) was identified as being upregulated in the proximal tubule cells after ischemic/reperfusion (I/R) injury (Ichimura et al. (1998)) and soon discovered in the urine of patients with I/R injury (Han et al. (2002)). Around the same time a small study of ICU patients identified urinary tubular injury makers, α and π-glutathone S-transferase (α and π-GST), and the bursh border enzymes, γ-glutamyl-transpeptidase (GGT) and alkaline phosphatase (AP), as diagnostic of AKI (Westhuyzen et al. (2003)). A transcriptome wide interrogation study to identify genes induced early after I/R injury identified neutrophil gelatinase-associated lipocalin (NGAL) to be upregulated in a mouse model (Mishra et al. (2003)). Plasma and urinary NGAL quickly showed spectacular success as diagnostic markers. The first, a trial of 71 children undergoing cardiopulmonary bypass of whom 20 developed AKI showed urinary and plasma NGAL to increase 10-fold in AKI 2-h post surgery (Mishra et al. (2005)). Similarly, interluekin-18, IL-18, first identified as being released into the urine following I/R injury in mice (Melnikov et al. (2001)) was found to appear in large quantities in the urine of patients with acute tubular necrosis (Parikh et al. (2004)). Proteomic and genomic approaches continue to be a rich source of new urinary proteins which may predict AKI (Bennett & Devarajan (2011); Devarajan (2008)).

AKI Biomarker discovery has followed the well trodden path of "early promise" with some highly sensitive and specific biomarkers in demographically homogeneous populations (eg paediatric cardiopulmonary bypass surgery), followed by a more tempered response as studies evaluated candidate biomarkers in demographically heterogeneous populations with multiple causes of AKI and co-morbidities. There is no one biomarker which will successfully diagnose or predict a decline in renal function in all situations. Three factors have emerged which are likely to become determinant factors in the choice of biomarker for a particular clinical context, namely: *(i)* likely aetiology of AKI, *(ii)* pre-existing renal function, *(iii)* time from renal insult. IL-18 is an example of a biomarker which has been shown to be elevated following ischaemic/repurfusion injury (Hall et al. (2010); Parikh et al. (2006)), but possibly not following radiocontrast induced nephrotoxic injury (Bulent Gul et al. (2008)). Mcilroy et al demonstrated that in a cohort of 426 adult cardiac surgery patients urinary NGAL concentrations post-operatively did not differ between those who developed and those who did not develop AKI when their estimated baseline GFR (eGFR) was less than 60 ml/min, yet for those with a normal baseline eGFR (90-120 ml/min) NGAL was significantly elevated in the AKI cohort (Mcilroy et al. (2010)). In our own head to head comparison of 6 urinary biomarkers (GGT, AP, NGAL, Cystatin C, IL-18, and KIM-1) in 529 adult patients on entry to an intensive care unit, we demonstrated that the performance of biomarkers is critically dependent on both baseline renal function and time from renal insult (Endre et al. (2011)). Peak diagnostic performance at a level that may be considered clinically useful was limited to patients with eGFR 90-120 ml/min within 12-h of insult for GGT, 6-h for NGAL and from 6 to 12-h for Cystatin C, IL-18 and KIM-1, and to patients with eGFR < 60 ml/min from 12 to 36-h for GGT, Cystatin C, NGAL and IL-18.

There are many excellent recent reviews of biomarkers of AKI. The pathophysiology of AKI in relation to potential biomarkers has been reviewed and discussed specifically in relation to AKI following cardiopulmonary bypass (Haase et al. (2010)), AKI with varying aetiology (Vaidya et al. (2008)), and AKI involving biomarker mediators of inflammation (Akcay et al. (2009)). Reviews of biomarker performance specific to nephrotoxic injury (Bonventre et al. (2010); Ferguson et al. (2008)), septic AKI (Bagshaw et al. (2007)), ischemic injury following cardiopulmonary bypass (Haase et al. (2010)), acute allograft rejection and ischemic injury (Alachkar et al. (2010)) as well as broader reviews across aetiologies (Coca et al. (2008); Edelstein & Faubel (2010); Endre & Westhuyzen (2008); Malyszko (2010)) have been published within the last 4 years. We have published a more specialist review considering biomarkers in the early phase of injury (Pickering & Endre (2009c)) and there has been one meta-analysis of the performance of NGAL (Haase et al. (2009)).

2.3 Paradigm lost and paradigm found

The relationship between clearance (the function paradigm) and injury has, to date, been studied in humans primarily in sample populations of about 20 to 600 in which a biomarker's ability to diagnose a subsequent rise in a surrogate marker of function (normally creatinine) is assessed. However, we need to explore the early stages of, and prior to, loss of renal function in order to understand the relevant pathophysiology of clinical AKI. We can conceptualise this as an evaluation of the evolution of injury phase which leads to loss of GFR and the early loss of function phase immediately following a GFR decrease (Figure 1). Detection and characterisation of this very early phase in man appears essential for progress. This highlights the need for quantifying the time course of injury biomarkers in relation to change in GFR and for real-time assessment of renal function. Two promising techniques are under development. The ambulatory renal monitor (ARM) is a shielded detector which monitors extracellular excretion of ^{99m}TcDTPA over up to 24 hours following injection and relates this to GFR (Rabito et al. (2010)). The ratiometric fluorescence approach monitors the plasma disappearance of both a rapidly filtered and a poorly filtered fluorescent marker introduced by a single bolus infusion, changes in the ratio of which enable a calculation of GFR (Wang et al. (2010)). Both techniques allow a rapid (5 to 15 min) measure of GFR. Ideally these or similar techniques would allow monitoring of kidney function from prior to the time of insult through the evolution time until change of GFR and beyond.

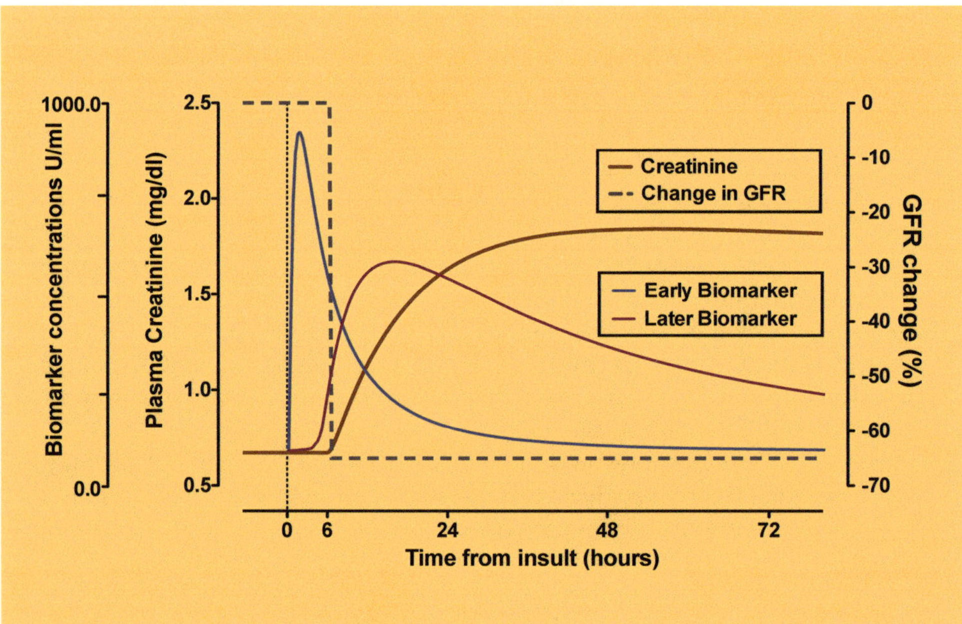

Fig. 1. The paradigm of function compared with the paradigm of injury. Following injury the early injury biomarker is elevated prior to change in function (here, a 65% loss of GFR, approximately 6 hours post-injury). The later biomarker takes takes longer to be elevated. Creatinine is only elevated following loss of GFR (following equation 6)

Much of the literature describes a biomarker as "predicting" AKI when it precedes an increase in plasma creatinine. However, a biomarker is only truly predictive if it precedes a decrease in GFR. If it is elevated shortly after such a decrease, then it should be described as *diagnostic* rather than predictive of AKI even though it may predict the latter increase in plasma creatinine.

3. Defining AKIs

In its broadest sense renal failure is simply the rapid loss of renal filtration (ie decrease in GFR). As discussed, current clinical diagnosis of AKI and evaluation of novel biomarkers of kidney injury are largely dependent on observation of changes in creatinine as a surrogate for a change in GFR. An understanding of the kinetics of the relationship between creatinine and GFR provides a basis for understanding the definitions of AKI and their limitations. Plasma cystatin C, an alternative to creatinine (Nejat et al. (2010); Westhuyzen (2006)), follows similar kinetics.

3.1 Creatinine and cystatin C kinetics

Creatinine and cystatin C are generated in tissue outside of the plasma compartment, diffuse into the plasma compartment from where they are lost by renal and non-renal excretion. Because both creatinine and cystatin C are not bound to plasma proteins the exchange between the extravascular and plasma compartments is rapid (compared with rates of production and elimination) allowing us to conflate the two compartments into one compartment with volume of distribution, V (Figure 2).

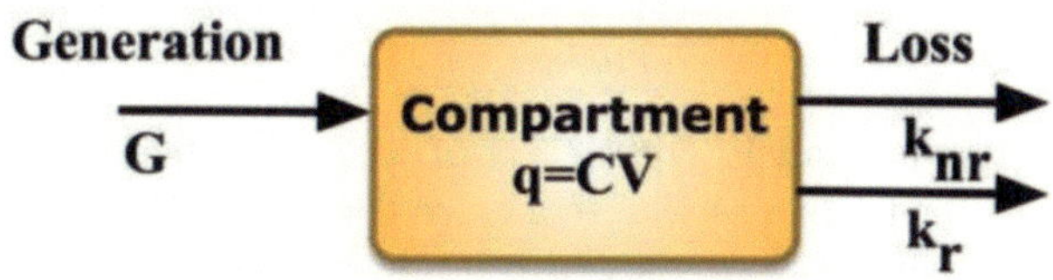

Fig. 2. One compartment pharmacokinetics model

The change in total mass (q) of creatinine/cystatin C depends on the rate at which it is entering and the rate at which it is leaving the compartment:

$$\frac{dq}{dt} = \text{gain from generation} - (\text{renal loss} + \text{non-renal loss}) \tag{1}$$

Under normal circumstances non-renal losses are much less than renal losses and may be ignored. The renal loss is the product of the renal elimination rate constant, k_r, and the total mass, q. As the total mass is the product of the concentration C and volume of distribution V, equation 1 becomes:

$$C\frac{dV}{dt} + \frac{dC}{dt}V = G - k_r CV \tag{2}$$

where G is the generation rate of creatinine/cystatin C (see Box 3.1). The volume of distribution of creatinine is equal to the total body water (TBW) and that of cystatin C to the extracellular fluid (about one third of TBW)(see Box 3.2). If this is assumed not to change then equation 2 becomes:

$$\frac{dC}{dt} = \frac{G}{V} - k_r C \tag{3}$$

At equilibrium ($dC/dt = 0$ at $t = 0$), prior to any change in GFR the renal elimination rate constant may be determined from equation 3:

$$k_{r0} = \frac{G}{C_b V} \tag{4}$$

where C_b is the baseline concentration (at time $t = 0$). k_{r0} may also be estimated from the renal clearance (Cl) which is simply the product k_{r0} and V. For creatinine, this may be measured in critically ill paitients using a short duration creatinine clearance and an estimate of an individual's volume of distribution (see below). From the EARLYARF study (Endre et al. (2010)) where 4-h creatinine clearances were measured on entry to ICU in 484 patients we were able to calculate a median (interquartile range) for k_{r0} of 0.11 (0.07-0.17) h^{-1}.
Following a loss in GFR (Δg%), the renal elimination rate constant becomes:

$$k_r = (1 - \frac{\Delta g}{100})k_{r0} \tag{5}$$

and equation 3 may be solved numerically, or, if we assume of G, V, or k_r are not varying, may be integrated to give the concentration as a function of time (Chiou & Hsu (1975); Chow (1985)):

$$C(t) = \frac{G}{k_r V}(1 - e^{-k_r t}) + C_b e^{-k_r t} \tag{6}$$

As $t \to \infty$ the concentration asymptotically approaches a new steady state, C_{ss} which from equation 6 is:

$$C_{ss} = \frac{G}{k_r V} \tag{7}$$

Mathematically the concentration is within 5% of the new steady state in 4.4 half lives (Half life: $t_{1/2} = ln(2)/k_r$). In practice this is well within the uncertainty in creatinine measurements. The new steady state may also be determined by substituting equations 5 and 4 into equation 7:

$$C_{ss} = \frac{C_b}{(1 - \frac{\Delta g}{100})} \tag{8}$$

From this equation we may determine the equivalences between a decline in GFR and a rise in creatinine used in the RIFLE definition of AKI (Table 1).

Box 3.1. Creatinine and Cystatin C production rates

Creatinine production (Bjornsson (1979)):

Male ($r^2 = 0.919$): $G_0 = (27 - 0.173 \times age) \times weight/24 \quad (mg/h)$
Female ($r^2 = 0.966$): $G_0 = (25 - 0.175 \times age) \times weight/24 \quad (mg/h)$

Creatinine production may decrease during critical illness (Griffiths (1996)). If the reduction is at constant rate m%, (eg 2% per day as suggested by Griffiths) then:

$$G(t) = G_0 e^{-mt} \quad \text{and} \quad \frac{dG}{dt} = -mG$$

Cystatin C production
Only one study has measured the rate constant of Cystatin C (Sjostrom et al. (2005)). There was no significant difference with age, sex or lean body mass. The rate constant per $1.73m^2$ of body surface area was:

$$G_{CysC} = 7.44 \quad (mg/h/1.73m^2)$$

Box 3.2. Estimating the volume of distribution

The volume of distribution of creatinine is equal to the total body water (TBW) and of cystatin C to the volume of the extracellular fluid which is about $1/3^{rd}$ of the TBW (Hansen (2002)). TBW is often estimated from the body weight as:

$$TBW = 0.6 \times Body\ weight \quad (L)$$

More accurate formulae have been derived from population studies (Watson et al. (1980)):

$$\text{Male } (r^2 = 0.704): \quad TBW = 2.447 - 0.09516 \times age + 0.1074 \times height + 0.3662 \times weight \quad (L)$$
$$\text{Female } (r^2 = 0.736): \quad TBW = 2.097 + 0.1069 \times height + 0.2466 \times weight \quad (L)$$

where *height* is measured in cm, *weight* in kg, and *age* in years.

Where height is not available, the slightly less robust equations may be used:

$$\text{Male } (r^2 = 0.689): \quad TBW = 20.03 - 0.1183 \times age + 0.3626 \times weight \quad (L)$$
$$\text{Female } (r^2 = 0.717): \quad TBW = 14.46 + 0.2549 \times weight \quad (L)$$

3.2 Categorical consensus

In 2004 the Acute Dialysis Quality Initiative Group (ADQI) developed a consensus definition for AKI and severity staging (RIFLE: Risk, Injury, Failure, Loss, End Stage) (Bellomo et al. (2004)). The scheme involved both a creatinine based classification and a urine output based classification (Table 1). A decrease in GFR of more than 25% or increase in serum creatinine of 50% was deemed sufficient to diagnose AKI. Unfortunately, there was an error in calculating this relationship which was not identified until 2009 (Pickering & Endre (2009a)). A 50% increase in creatinine is equivalent to a one third decrease in GFR (see equation 8) not a 25% decrease. Similarly, for RIFLE stage F a 200% increase in creatinine is equivalent to a two thirds decrease in GFR not a 75% decrease. Whilst plasma creatinine rather than a GFR measure, or an estimation with creatinine clearance, is the analyte of choice in AKI studies, creatinine is but a surrogate for GFR and GFR should remain the principal diagnostic parameter of AKI (Pickering & Endre (2009b)). The ADQI group recommended AKI be defined as "sustained" (lasting at least 24hrs) and "abrupt" (1-7 days) (http://www.ccm.upmc.edu/adqi/ADQI2/ADQI2g1.pdf). Whilst duration did not appear in the seminal RIFLE publication it was included in later publications (Hoste et al. (2006); Lameire et al. (2006)).

On the back of new evidence that even minor changes in serum creatinine are associated with poor outcomes (eg Chertow et al. (2005); Lassnigg et al. (2004)), the Acute Kidney Injury Network modified the RIFLE definition to include a small absolute rise in creatinine (0.3 mg/dl or 26.4 μmol/l). Further modifications included requiring the change to occur within 48 hours for the definition of AKI, and removing RIFLE stages L and E in preference to all patients requiring renal replacement therapy to be assigned to severity stage III (Table 1).

Both definitions have received broad support and there is considerable evidence for an association of increased mortality with increased RIFLE or AKIN stages (Bagshaw et al. (2008); Ricci et al. (2008)). More recently, duration of AKI (using the AKIN criteria) has been shown to be independently associated with long-term mortality (Brown et al. (2010); Coca et al. (2010); Goldberg et al. (2009)). KDIGO (Kidney Disease for Improving Global Outcomes:

www.kdigo.org) has recently reviewed the use of the AKIN and RIFLE criteria and is shortly to release a new consensus definition which combines the two definitions.

RIFLE			AKIN		RIFLE and AKIN
Stage	Creatinine increase	GFR decrease	Stage	Creatinine increase	Urine output
Risk (R)	$\geqslant 50\%$	$> 33.3\%^*$	I	$\geqslant 0.3$ mg/dl or $\geqslant 50\%$	< 0.5 mg/kg/h for 6 h
Injury (I)	$\geqslant 100\%$	$> 50\%$	II	$\geqslant 100\%$	< 0.5 mg/kg/h for 12 h
Failure (F)	$\geqslant 200\%$ or $\geqslant 0.5$ mg/dl and above 4.0 mg/dl	$> 66.7\%^{**}$	III	$\geqslant 200\%$ or $\geqslant 0.5$ mg/dl and above 4.0 mg/dl	< 0.3 mg/kg/h for 24 h or anuria for 12 h

*,** corrected from 25% and 75% see Pickering & Endre (2009a)

Table 1. Severity Staging: Consensus definitions

3.3 A continuum needing continuous variables

One of the intentions of ADQI in setting up RIFLE was that it would provide common outcomes in clinical trials. During the four year period (2005-08) only 36% of published AKI (non Contrast Induced Nephropathy, CIN) trials used RIFLE or AKIN as an outcome variable, and the use was not consistent in terms of timing and duration of injury (Endre & Pickering (2010)). Amongst CIN intervention trials only 13% used RIFLE or AKIN, whereas most continued to use an increase in creatinine of $\geqslant 25\%$ and/or $\geqslant 0.5$ mg/dl (44.2 μmol/l) to diagnose CIN. This later definition is slightly anomalous as only those with pre-existing kidney disease (creatinine > 2.0 mg/dl) can have a greater than 0.5 mg/dl elevation in creatinine that is less than 25%. We have recommended that all CIN studies adopt the AKIN or RIFLE definition of AKI (Endre & Pickering (2010)).

We investigated whether a continuous variable measure of kidney function, the Relative Average Creatinine (RAVC), performed better than the RIFLE and AKIN categorical definitions as an outcome variable in AKI prevention or intervention trials. The RAVC is the integral of the area under the plasma creatinine curve above baseline creatine divided by the total time and baseline creatinine:

$$RAVC(\%) = \frac{100}{C_b t} \int_0^t (C(t) - C_b) dt \tag{9}$$

which in practice is calculated using the trapezoidal rule (Figure 3):

$$RAVC(\%) = \frac{100}{C_b(t_N - t_1)} \sum_{0<n<N-1} \frac{(C_{n+1} - C_b) + (C_n - C_b)}{2} (t_{n+1} - t_n) \tag{10}$$

where N is the number of creatinine measurements.

We created a population of 10,000 Virtual-In-Patients (VIPs) whose baseline creatinine and changes in GFR were based on real ICU populations. Placebo controlled trials were simulated by randomly assigning half the VIPs to treatments which ameliorated loss of renal

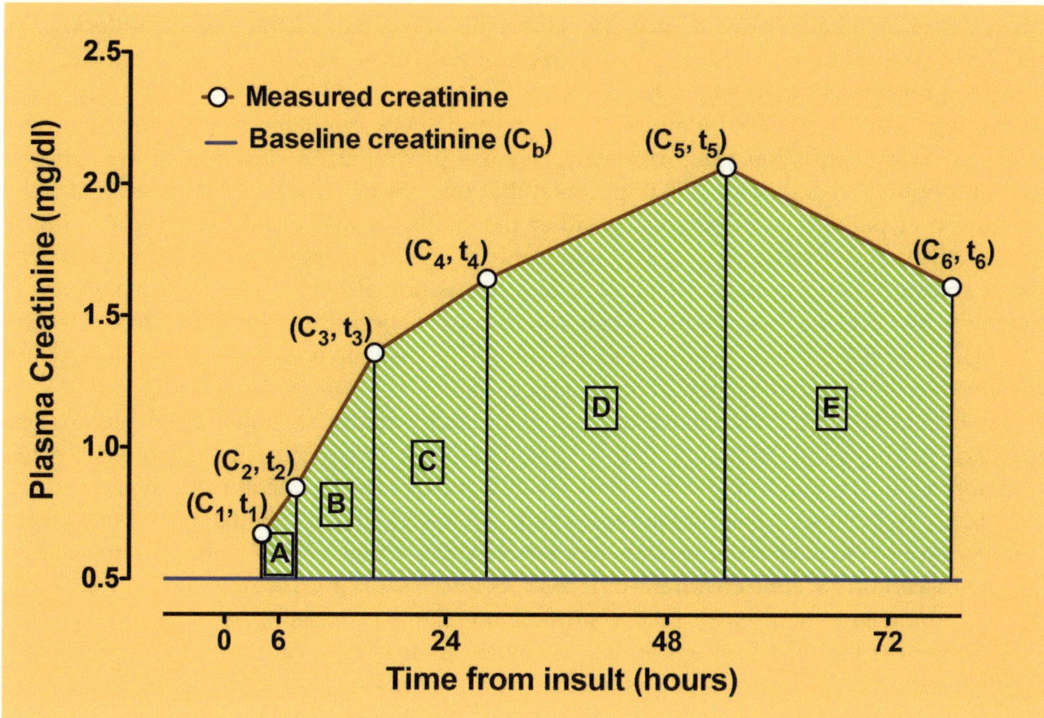

Fig. 3. The Relative Average Creatinine by the trapezoidal rule is the sum of the areas A to E divided by $(t_6 - t_1)$(following equation 10).

function (ie reduced the reduction in GFR). The more efficacious the treatment, the less the decrease in GFR. Creatinine profiles were calculated using equation 6 (Pickering et al. (2009)). AKIN, RIFLE and RAVC as outcome variables were compared. At low treatment efficacy, the categorical outcomes underestimated and at high treatment efficacy overestimated the effect of treatment. These effects were exaggerated when the population contained a high proportion of patients with more severe AKI. The RAVC, on the other hand, responded in an almost linear fashion across treatment efficacies. Importantly, when the efficacy was low it was best able to distinguish between placebo and treatment arms. The advantage of the RAVC over the categorial metrics is two fold, first it includes the effect of treatment on those patients who had mild kidney injury which in normal circumstances would not exceed the diagnostic threshold for AKI according to a categorical definition, but which may result in a small increase (eg 20-30%) in creatinine and, second, it measures function over a (pre-determined) time period. As discussed previously, the length of time creatinine is elevated is independently of the maximum elevation associated with mortality. The RAVC captures both severity *and* duration of injury and was used as the primary outcome in the EARLYARF trial, which was the first randomised control trial to use an injury biomarker to triage patients to placebo or high-dose erythropoietin (Endre et al. (2010)).

3.4 The baseline issue

All creatinine based definitions of AKI and the RAVC depend on knowing the normal, or "baseline", plasma creatinine for each individual. For patients undergoing elective surgery

this is easily obtainable prior to surgery. However, about half of the patients entering the ICU have no previous record of plasma creatinine to serve as a baseline. For trials this requires a retrospective determination of renal function. The ADQI recommend assuming a normal (eg 75 ml/min) GFR for all these patients and "back-calculating" a plasma creatinine using the MDRD equation. Unfortunately, this has proved erroneous. We showed that in our VIP population and in an ICU population that this approach seriously overestimates the proportion of patients with AKI using either the AKIN or RIFLE definitions (Pickering & Endre (2010); Pickering et al. (2009)). Randomly assigning a baseline creatinine produced just as accurate results as back-calculation. In a population already with AKI the presence of patients with CKD was seen to be driving the overestimation (Bagshaw et al. (2009)). Using the emergency department creatinine as an alternative baseline underestimated AKI (AKIN) and lowered the sensitivity (Siew et al. (2010)).
In the EARLYARF trial we overcame this problem by using an adjudicated hierarchical approach to choose in each patient the measured plasma creatinine that best represented normal renal function. Outpatient plasma creatinine prior to admission were considered the most likely to represent true baseline function. Whilst CKD can be diagnosed over three months, up to twelve months appears to be a reasonable time period prior to admission in which to ascertain baseline creatinine as it reduces misclassification of AKI (Lafrance & Miller (2010)). Amongst patients with no pre-admission creatinine measurement, a post-discharge measurement is the next best option if it is stable. Increasing creatinine may be indicative of developing CKD. Hence, it is preferable that a post-discharge creatinine is within three months of the insult. As a last resort the lower of the first hospital or final hospital (when there is recovery) may be used. We have presented our recommended hierarchical approach in table 2. This differs from the earlier approach in that we now consider that for cardiac arrest and trauma patients where there is no baseline prior to admission available the first hospital sample is likely to be the best estimate of baseline function if it is measured close to the time of renal insult. In our experience this is less than 2-h for most cardiac arrest and trauma patients. For the creatinine to have increased considerably in this time frame the loss of GFR would have had to have been substantial.

3.5 Quantifying function in a dilute environment

Fluid resuscitation dilutes plasma creatinine concentrations, which in turn may lead to delayed diagnosis or severity underestimation. This may explain why the only successful AKI intervention in the ICU has been early consultation with a nephrologist (Mehta et al. (2002)). The effect of fluids may be estimated by adjusting plasma creatinine for fluid balance (Macedo et al. (2010)):

$$C_{adjusted} = C_{measured} \times \frac{\text{admission weight (kg)} \times 0.6 + \sum \text{daily cumulative fluid balance (L)}}{\text{admission weight (kg)} \times 0.6} \quad (11)$$

3.6 Injury meets function

Current evaluation of novel biomarkers of renal injury is largely confined to evaluation of their performance to predict increases in plasma creatinine which lead to a diagnosis of AKI according to RIFLE or AKIN. This runs the risk of missing significant injury because creatinine did not increase beyond the diagnostic threshold of 50% or 0.3 mg/dl. In a large series

Situation	Timing of baseline creatinine sample
1 Elective surgery	Prior to surgery
2 All	Pre-hospital outpatient or prior admission Preferably this is between 7 and 90 days prior to admission. 7 days avoids a period which may reflect changing renal function. Less than 90 days is preferable because 90 days is the period usually used to diagnose CKD. Up to 365 days may be used if there is little likelihood of CKD having developed during that period.
3 Cardiac Arrest	First hospital If a pre-hospital value is not available and the time between insult and the first measurement is short (< 2h). Within a short time frame the creatinine will not (yet) have become elevated.
4 Trauma	First hospital If a pre-hospital value is not available and the time between insult and the first measurement is short (< 2h) and crush-injuries are not involved.
5	Post ICU discharge Within 90 days of admission to avoid capturing the development of CKD.
6	Lowest of first hospital or final ICU

Table 2. Hierarchical determination of baseline creatinine

of experimental studies of nephrotoxic AKI biomarkers, serum creatinine and blood urea nitrogen (BUN) were the poorest predictors of histologically determined injury compared with numerous urinary biomarkers (Dieterle et al. (2010); Ozer et al. (2010); Vaidya et al. (2010); Yu et al. (2010)). In what may turn out to be a seminal publication Haase et al. (2011) demonstrated that across 10 studies patients with a positive NGAL, yet negative plasma creatinine, for AKI had worse outcomes (mortality, need for dialysis, and ICU length of stay) than those with both negative NGAL and negative creatinine.

Biomarker clinical utility is most often quantified by the area under the receiver operator characteristic curve (AUC or c-statistic, see Box 3.3). The AUC is crude estimation of the ability of the biomarker to distinguish between those with and without AKI. However, a high AUC does not necessarily imply clinical utility. Clinical utility depends on what alternative biomarkers there are, what treatments are available, and the risks and costs involved with false negatives or false positives. The calculation of the sensitivity, specificity and particularly the negative and positive predictive values at either an established cut-off from the literature, or a cut-off chosen for clinical reasons, or derived mathematically from the ROC. The latter is usually either the cut-off closest to a Sensitivity and Specificity of 1 or the Youden index.

Comparing AUCs between different studies is problematical. AUCs for AKI are highly dependent on the AKI definition. Typically a definition requiring greater injury (eg RIFLE sustained for 24-h, compared with an increase of 0.3 mg/dl within 48-h) will result in higher AUCs. Within a study when more than one biomarker is being measured they should be compared using the method of DeLong (DeLong et al. (1988)). One biomarker should not be described as "better" than another unless the difference between the two is statistically significant at $p < 0.05$.

Box 3.3. The Area Under the Curve (AUC)

The receiver operator characteristic curve (ROC) is a plot of sensitivity verse 1-specificity. An AUC of 1 means the biomarker always discriminates between patients with and without the disease (no false negatives and no false positives). An AUC of 0.5 is equivalent to a coin toss. Whilst an AUC of less than 0.5 means the reciprocal of the biomarker is diagnostic. Some statistics packages, however, will always express the AUC as greater than 0.5 by inverting the biomarker concentration where necessary. The AUC from a study is strictly speaking an estimate of the AUC of the population, therefore it should **always** be presented with appropriate confidence intervals (usually 95%). The 95% confidence interval is ± 1.96 times the standard error of a proportion:

$$\widehat{AUC} - 1.96\sqrt{\widehat{AUC}(1-\widehat{AUC})/n} \quad \text{to} \quad \widehat{AUC} + 1.96\sqrt{\widehat{AUC}(1-\widehat{AUC})/n}$$

where n is the sample size and $\widehat{AUC}$ the estimated AUC. This is equation is adequate for sample sizes > 30, but for smaller sample sizes a bootstrapping should be used. Only an AUC for which the lower limit of its 95% confidence interval is greater than 0.5 may be described as diagnostic (or prognistic).

Figure 4 is an example of a ROC from the EARLYARF trial (Endre et al. (2011)). It shows the ability of NGAL to diagnose AKI when the sample was taken between 12 and 36 hours following renal insult. The AUC lower limit of the 95% confidence interval, 0.62, is greater than 0.5, therefore it is diagnostic.

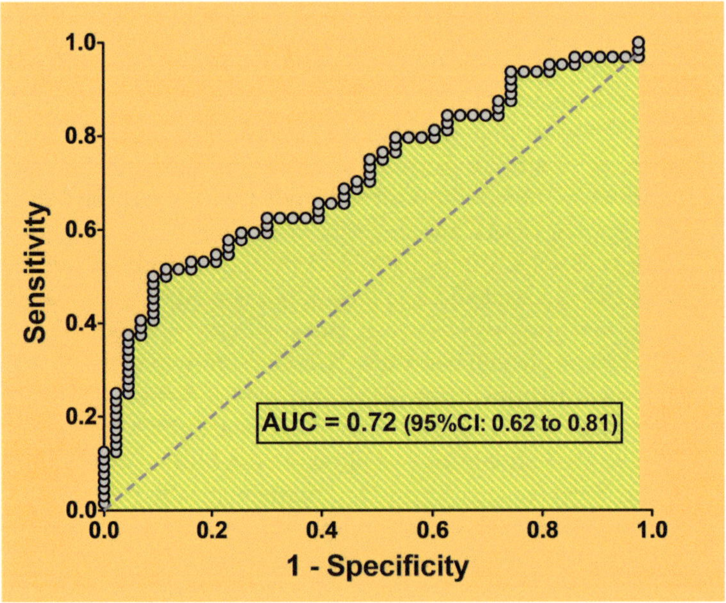

Fig. 4. An example of a receiver operator characteristic curve

It is anticipated that panels of biomarkers will be needed to diagnose AKI in heterogeneous populations with multiple AKI aetiologies. Attempts to assess a panel of biomarkers usually involve logistic regression models with two or more biomarkers measured at the same time point. The EARLYARF trial has demonstrated that the efficacy of any one particular biomarker is very much time dependent, and that each biomarker has its own "window of opportunity" during which it has have diagnostic utility (Endre et al. (2011)). Logistic regression models are not a suitable approach for assessment of biomarker panels because of this. Until we know the time courses of biomarkers much better, an "either and/or" approach is likely to yield greater results. For example, in an ICU population either an elevated GGT and/or an elevated NGAL may be considered diagnostic.

There is a need to move away from assessing injury biomarkers only in relation to function. All trials should report mortality data, even if the incidence is too low for statistical analysis. This will facilitate later meta-analysis of the relationship between a biomarker and mortality.

The EARLYARF trial paved the way for future trials of early intervention based on an elevated biomarker. Since the inception of that trial new biomarkers with rapid assay turn-around (necessary in an early intervention trial) have become available. Plasma and urinary NGAL, and KIM-1 head the list along with urinary Cystatin C and GGT which are already routinely available in many hospital laboratories. It is anticipated that the next early intervention trial will use one or more of these biomarkers.

3.7 Quantifying injury in a dilute environment

Changes in GFR and water handling will change urinary biomarker concentrations independent of injury. Normalising biomarkers to urinary creatinine has been proposed to account for these effects. This process also amplifies the signal soon after a decline in function (Waikar et al. (2010)). This may be advantageous in an early intervention trial if the threshold for intervention is set high enough, but it may distort the analysis of biomarker performance in a biomarker performance study. Whilst there is no consensus on whether biomarkers should or should not be normalised to urinary creatinine we recommend reporting both normalised and non-normalised results.

4. Practical considerations

Table 3 presents a summary of practical measures to take into account when planning AKI epidemiology, biomarker efficacy studies or prevention or intervention trials.

4.1 Epidemiology

Most epidemiological studies are retrospective and face the difficulty of missing data, particularly baseline creatinine data. This was discussed in section 3.4. It is important to quantify the severity of AKI, as more severe AKI is likely to have greater long term impact on health resources. Where possible, data on the duration of AKI as well as severity should be captured as this is an independent predictor of outcome. Three areas of epidemiology lack data. First, there are comparatively few good epidemiology studies in countries other than in Europe, North America or Australasia (Cerda et al. (2008)). The incidence of AKI in countries with large populations such as China, India, Indonesia, Nigeria has significance beyond their own borders. Some countries have numbers of particular AKI aetiologies which, if well studied, could provide useful data world-wide. For example, with anti-retroviral therapy reducing mortality in HIV patients, the incidence of AKI in this population may be increasing (Lopes et al. (2011)). In South-East Asia, AKI is a prominent complication of paraquat (a contact herbicide) self-poisoning (Roberts et al. (2011)). In both these cases epidemiology in countries with relevant populations would help identify the extent of risk in other countries where incidence of HIV or paraquat poisoning is relatively low. Second, there are few studies that have investigated AKI on CKD (Ali et al. (2007)). The growing world wide epidemic of CKD demands epidemiology that quantifies the additional risk CKD has for AKI and the effects of AKI on the progression of CKD. Third, there are few studies on CKD induced by AKI that have comparable control groups of hospitalised non-AKI patients (Coca et al. (2009)).

4.2 Biomarker studies

It is important to report the timing of sampling for biomarker measurements in relation to putative onset of injury. As we have seen, different biomarkers are likely to have different time profiles. A weakness of many studies is that samples are taken only at one or two time points, and even then they may be outside the temporal "window of opportunity" of the biomarker, possibly rendering the study results misleading. Temporal profiles are available for many biomarkers following the time of injury which can be used to plan sampling (eg Endre et al. (2011)) . For novel biomarkers, frequent sampling will be necessary to establish their time course. The first 12 hours following injury are crucial as this is the window for early intervention. There is also a need to discover and assess injury biomarkers with slightly longer (~24 to 36-h) time courses as samples may not be able to be taken earlier in many critically ill patients. Very few studies have measured biomarker profiles beyond a two or three days, yet there is tantilising evidence that some biomarkers (eg KIM-1) may become elevated during a repair phase which in some patients may not begin until several days following injury.

The choice of outcome variable is particularly important. Despite the caveats discussed with respect to using creatinine changes as a surrogate for change in GFR and the issue of comparing injury to function, we are still in a period where a functional definition of AKI is likely to be the outcome of choice for biomarker studies. Use of non-standard AKI definitions are unhelpful and should be avoided in preference to the AKIN, RIFLE and, potentially, new KDIGO AKI definitions. The duration as well as severity of creatinine increase is also of importance. The AKIN definition requires only one time point at which plasma creatinine may be elevated. This allows for mild and transient changes in function to equally be recorded as AKI. We have shown that transient increases in creatinine are associated with injury biomarkers (Nejat et al (2011b)), although not to the extent of more sustained increases. We recommend evaluating biomarkers in relation to duration of increase of creatinine as well as the increase itself.

Most biomarker studies are underpowered. The number of participants are rarely calculated *a priori*. Typically we want to ascertain if a biomarker is clinically useful. At a minimum we would want an AUC of 0.7, more likely 0.85 or greater. Given an expected incidence (proportion), I, in the population, how many participants (N) will we need in the study? Hanley and McNeil provide a general equation which we may adapt as we are interested in the difference between the true AUC and 0.5 (Hanley & McNeil (1982)):

$$N = \frac{1}{I}\left[\frac{0.5773Z_{\alpha} + Z_{\beta}\sqrt{0.1667 + \frac{AUC}{2-AUC} + \frac{2AUC^2}{1+AUC} - 2AUC^2}}{AUC - 0.5}\right]^2 \tag{12}$$

where Z_α is the Z coefficient for a Type I error and Z_β for a Type II error. In order to detect a true AUC of 0.7 with p<0.05 ($Z_\alpha = 1.96$ (two sided)) and at 80% power ($Z_\beta = 0.84$) in a population with a 30% incidence 212 participants would be needed. A population with a much lower incidence, say 5%, would need a much greater sample ($N = 1269$). If we were comparing a known biomarker with an AUC of 0.7 and wanting to know if another biomarker was better (AUC of 0.8 or more), then at p<0.05, 80% power and 30% incidence we would need 676 participants. This highlights the importance of knowing *a priori* the AKI incidence, what a clinically relevant AUC would be, and choosing a sample size appropriately.

In larger studies it is possible to assess the biomarker's ability to predict premature death or need for renal replacement therapy. In both cases, it is important to assess the risk relative to known risk factors. A useful technique is to use logistic regression models and compare a model of known risk factors with one with the same risk factors plus the biomarker. The integrated discrimination improvement (IDI) is a useful technique which, along with the AUC, allows for analysis of biomarker performance across the whole range of biomarker concentrations (Pencina et al. (2008)).

Studies in heterogeneous populations with multiple aetiologies and timing of injury are particularly difficult. Given the recent findings with respect to biomarker dependency on pre-existing renal function it is important that study size is sufficient to allow for cohort analysis, in particular cohorts of CKD and sepsis. In studies with CKD patients it is important to measure urinary albumin. Albumin is a possible AKI biomarker in its own right, but also competes for reabsorption in the proximal tubules with cystatin C and NGAL, IL-18 and possibly other markers (Nejat et al (2011a)).

The quality of reporting of biomarker studies varies widely. The Standards of Reporting of Diagnostic Accuracy (STARD) statement provides minimum standards and is worth referring to in the planning of the study (Bossuyt et al. (2003)). Biomarker concentrations should almost always be presented as median with inter-quartile range as they are usually non-normal distributions. With the jury still out on "normalising" urinary biomarkers to urinary creatinine we have recommended that both normalised and non-normalised results be presented.

4.3 Clinical trials

Clinical trial design follows one of three paradigms: (i) Prevention, namely treatment prior to a procedure which may cause injury; (ii) Early intervention following following a raised biomarker, but prior to observation of functional change (eg Endre et al. (2010)); (iii) Late intervention following an elevation of creatinine (Pickering & Endre (2009c); Pickering et al. (2011)). Whilst it may be anticipated that if successful prevention or early intervention treatments are developed there will be less need for late intervention treatments, late intervention treatments will still be needed either where prevention or early intervention fails, or where it is not possible to administer it. Injury biomarkers will play a role in all three paradigms. Some are being identified as risk factors, prior to a procedure (Bennett et al. (2008)), whilst others will be elevated early enough after injury to allow early intervention, finally others will serve as outcome variables. As with plasma creatinine as an outcome variable, analogous to the RAVC, it is likely that a continuous measurement of the biomarker over a pre-specified duration will serve best as an outcome variable.

		Epidemiology	Biomarker Studies	Clinical Trials
1	Use a continuous outcome variable (eg RAVC)	n/a	possibly	✔
2	Use RIFLE, AKIN or KDIGO definition as outcome variables (including for CIN trials)	✔	✔	✔
3	Use a hierarchical-adjudicated approach to determine baseline creatinine	✔	✔	✔
4	Include hard outcomes (RRT, Death)	✔	✔	✔
5	Include plasma cystatin C as an outcome	n/a	✔	✔
6	For subcohort analysis use KDIGO guidelines for CKD staging (Levey et al. (2003))	✔	✔	✔
7	Measure 2 to 4-h creatinine clearance	n/a	✔	✔
8	Use corrected $\Delta GFR(\%)$ for RIFLE classes R or F (Pickering & Endre (2009a))	n/a	✔	✔
8	Apply treatment within the time window following insult determined by experimental &/or pilot data	n/a	n/a	✔
9	Measure biomarkers within the time window following insult determined by experimental &/or pilot data	n/a	✔	n/a
10	Report urinary biomarker concentrations & concentrations normalised to urinary creatinine	n/a	✔	n/a
11	Report median and inter-quartile range for biomarker concentrations	n/a	✔	n/a
12	Report times and duration for which plasma outcomes were determined	✔	✔	✔

Table 3. Practical considerations

5. Conclusion

The discovery of many early biomarkers of kidney injury has begun to shift the paradigm from assessment of change in filtration function to measurement of direct injury. Lest we throw the baby out with the bathwater we must recognise the complementary role of assessing both renal injury and renal function. Our techniques for assessing injury are still in their infancy, but show much promise. Our techniques for assessing function have a long history, yet, as we have shown, have room for improvement. In particular, we are learning to use appropriate surrogates of function, categorical or continuous, depending on the type of study we are conducting. We await the development of rapid, near "real-time" measures of function which are the missing link in enabling us to understand the temporal profile of injury in relation to functional change. We also look forward to an era of clinical trials which utilise the injury biomarkers discovered to date so as to properly test of drugs found to be effective soon after injury in experimental models.

6. Acknowledgements

Dr Pickering is supported by an Australia and New Zealand Society of Nephrologists enabling and infrastructure grant and the Marsden Fund Council from government funding, administered by the Royal Society of New Zealand.

7. References

Ahlstrom, A., Kuitunen, A., Peltonen, S., Hynninen, M., Tallgren, M., Aaltonen, J. & Pettila, V. (2006). Comparison of 2 acute renal failure severity scores to general scoring systems in the critically ill, *Am J Kid Dis* 48(2): 262–268.

Akcay, A., Nguyen, Q. & Edelstein, C. L. (2009). Mediators of inflammation in acute kidney injury, *Mediat Inflamm* 2009: 137072.

Alachkar, N., Rabb, H. & Jaar, B. G. (2010). Urinary Biomarkers in Acute Kidney Transplant Dysfunction, *Nephron Clin Pract* 118(2): c173–c181.

Alejandro, V., Scandling, J., Sibley, R., Dafoe, D., Alfrey, E., Deen, W. & Myers, B. D. (1995). Mechanisms of filtration failure during postischemic injury of the human kidney. A study of the reperfused renal allograft, *J Clin Invest* 95(2): 820–831.

Ali, T., Khan, I., Simpson, W., Prescott, G., Townend, J., Smith, W. & Macleod, A. (2007). Incidence and outcomes in acute kidney injury: a comprehensive population-based study, *J Am Soc Nephrol* 18(4): 1292–1298.

American Society of Nephrology Renal Research Report (2005). 16(7): 1886–1903.

Bagshaw, S. M., George, C., Dinu, I. & Bellomo, R. (2008). A multi-centre evaluation of the RIFLE criteria for early acute kidney injury in critically ill patients., *Nephrol Dial Transpl* 23(4): 1203–1210.

Bagshaw, S. M., Langenberg, C., Haase, M., Wan, L., May, C. N. & Bellomo, R. (2007). Urinary biomarkers in septic acute kidney injury, *Intens Care Med* 33(7): 1285–1296.

Bagshaw, S. M., Uchino, S., Cruz, D., Bellomo, R., Morimatsu, H., Morgera, S., Schetz, M., Tan, I., Bouman, C., Macedo, E., Gibney, N., Tolwani, A., Oudemans-van Straaten, H. M., Ronco, C., Kellum, J. A. & Beginning and Ending Supportive Therapy for the Kidney (BEST Kidney) Investigators (2009). A comparison of observed versus estimated baseline creatinine for determination of RIFLE class in patients with acute kidney injury., *Nephrol Dial Transpl* 24(9): 2739–2744.

Bellomo, R., Ronco, C., Kellum, J. A., Mehta, R. L., Palevsky, P. M. & workgroup, A. D. Q. I. (2004). Acute renal failure - definition, outcome measures, animal models, fluid therapy and information technology needs: the Second International Consensus Conference of the Acute Dialysis Quality Initiative (ADQI) Group, *Crit Care* 8(4): R204–12.

Bennett, M. R. & Devarajan, P. (2011). Proteomic analysis of acute kidney injury: Biomarkers to mechanisms, *Proteom Clin Appl* 5(1-2): 67–77.

Bennett, M. R., Ravipati, N., Ross, G., Nguyen, M. T., Hirsch, R., Beekman, R. H., Rovner, L. & Devarajan, P. (2008). Using proteomics to identify preprocedural risk factors for contrast induced nephropathy, *Proteom Clin Appl* 2(7-8): 1058–1064.

Berliner, R. (1995). Homer Smith: His contribution to physiology, *J Am Soc Nephrol* 5(12): 1988–1992.

Bjornsson, T. (1979). Use of serum creatinine concentrations to determine renal-function, *Clin Pharmacokinet* 4(3): 200–222.

Bonventre, J. V., Vaidya, V. S., Schmouder, R., Feig, P. & Dieterle, F. (2010). Next-generation biomarkers for detecting kidney toxicity, *Nat Biotechnol* 28(5): 436–440.

Bossuyt, P., Reitsma, J., Bruns, D., Gatsonis, C., Glasziou, P., Irwig, L., Moher, D., Rennie, D., de Vet, H. & Lijmer, J. (2003). The STARD statement for reporting studies of diagnostic accuracy: Explanation and elaboration, *Clin Chem* 49(1): 7–18.

Brown, J. R., Kramer, R. S., Coca, S. G. & Parikh, C. R. (2010). Duration of Acute Kidney Injury Impacts Long-Term Survival After Cardiac Surgery, *Ann Thorac Surg* 90(4): 1142–1149.

Bulent Gul, C., Gullulu, M., Oral, B., Aydinlar, A., Oz, O., Budak, F., Yilmaz, Y. & Yurtkuran, M. (2008). Urinary IL-18: a marker of contrast-induced nephropathy following percutaneous coronary intervention?, *Clin Biochem* 41(7-8): 544–547.

Cerda, J., Lameire, N., Eggers, P., Pannu, N., Uchino, S., Wang, H., Bagga, A. & Levin, A. (2008). Epidemiology of acute kidney injury, *Clin J Am Soc Nephro* 3(3): 881–886.

Chertow, G. M., Burdick, E., Honour, M., Bonventre, J. V. & Bates, D. (2005). Acute kidney injury, mortality, length of stay, and costs in hospitalized patients, *J Am Soc Nephrol* 16: 3365–3370.

Chiou, W. L. & Hsu, F. H. (1975). Pharmacokinetics of creatinine in man and its implications in the monitoring of renal function and in dosage regimen modifications in patients with renal insufficiency, *J Clin Pharmacol* 15(5-6): 427–434.

Chow, M. S. (1985). A method for determining the pharmacokinetics of endogenous creatinine without exogenous creatinine administration, *Biopharm Drug Dispos* 6(2): 201–208.

Coca, S. G., King, J. T., Rosenthal, R. A., Perkal, M. F. & Parikh, C. R. (2010). The duration of postoperative acute kidney injury is an additional parameter predicting long-term survival in diabetic veterans, *Kidney Int* 78(9): 926–933.

Coca, S. G., Yalavarthy, R., Concato, J. & Parikh, C. R. (2008). Biomarkers for the diagnosis and risk stratification of acute kidney injury: A systematic review, *Kidney Int* 73: 1001–1016.

Coca, S. G., Yusuf, B., Shlipak, M. G., Garg, A. X. & Parikh, C. R. (2009). Long-term Risk of Mortality and Other Adverse Outcomes After Acute Kidney Injury: A Systematic Review and Meta-analysis, *Am J Kid Dis* 53(6): 961–973.

Cockcroft, D. & Gault, M. (1976). Prediction of creatinine clearance from serum creatinine, *Nephron* 16(1): 31–41.

Cruz, D. N., Bolgan, I., Perazella, M. A., Bonello, M., de Cal, M., Corradi, V., Polanco, N., Ocampo, C., Nalesso, F., Piccinni, P., Ronco, C. & on Acute Kidney Injury NEiPHROS-AKI Investigators, N. E. I. P. H. R. O. S. (2007). North East Italian Prospective Hospital Renal Outcome Survey on Acute Kidney Injury (NEiPHROS-AKI): targeting the problem with the RIFLE Criteria, *Clin J Am Soc Nephro* 2(3): 418–425.

DeLong, E., DeLong, D. & Clarke-Pearson, D. (1988). Comparing the areas under 2 or more correlated receiver operating characteristic curves - a nonparametric approach, *Biometrics* 44(3): 837–845.

Devarajan, P. (2006). Update on mechanisms of ischemic acute kidney injury, *J Am Soc Nephrol* 17(6): 1503–1520.

Devarajan, P. (2008). Proteomics for the investigation of acute kidney injury, *Contrib Nephrol* 160: 1–16.

Dieterle, F., Perentes, E., Cordier, A., Roth, D. R., Verdes, P., Grenet, O., Pantano, S., Moulin, P., Wahl, D., Mahl, A., End, P., Staedtler, F., Legay, F., Carl, K., Laurie, D., Chibout, S.-D., Vonderscher, J. & Maurer, G. (2010). Urinary clusterin, cystatin C, beta2-microglobulin and total protein as markers to detect drug-induced kidney injury, *Nat Biotechnol* 28(5): 463–469.

Edelstein, C. L. & Faubel, S. (2010). Chapter 5, *Biomarkers in Acute Kidney Injury*, Elsevier Inc., pp. 177–232.

Eknoyan, G. (2002). Emergence of the concept of acute renal failure, *Am J Nephrol* 22(2-3): 225–230.

Endre, Z. H., Allis, J. & Radda, G. (1989). Toxicity of dysprosium shift-reagents in the isolated perfused rat kidney, *Magnet Reson Med* 11: 267–274.

Endre, Z. H. & Pickering, J. W. (2010). Outcome definitions in non-dialysis intervention and prevention trials in acute kidney injury (AKI)., *Nephrol Dial Transpl* 25(1): 107–118.

Endre, Z. H., Pickering, J. W., Walker, R. J., Devarajan, P., Edelstein, C. L., Bonventre, J. V., Frampton, C. M., Bennett, M. R., Ma, Q., Sabbisetti, V. S., Vaidya, V. S., Walcher, A. M., Shaw, G. M., Henderson, S. J., Nejat, M., Schollum, J. B. W. & George, P. M. (2011). Improved performance of urinary biomarkers of acute kidney injury in the critically ill by stratification for injury duration and baseline renal function., *Kidney Int* 79(10): 1119–1130.

Endre, Z. H., Walker, R. J., Pickering, J. W., Shaw, G. M., Frampton, C. M., Henderson, S. J., Hutchison, R., Mehrtens, J. E., Robinson, J. M., Schollum, J. B. W., Westhuyzen, J., Celi, L. A., McGinley, R. J., Campbell, I. J. & George, P. M. (2010). Early intervention with erythropoietin does not affect the outcome of acute kidney injury (the EARLYARF trial)., *Kidney Int* 77(11): 1020–1030.

Endre, Z. H. & Westhuyzen, J. (2008). Early detection of acute kidney injury: Emerging new biomarkers (Review Article), *Nephrology* 13(2): 91–98.

Ferguson, M. A., Vaidya, V. S. & Bonventre, J. V. (2008). Biomarkers of nephrotoxic acute kidney injury, *Toxicology* 245(3): 182–193.

Fishbane, S. (2008). N-acetylcysteine in the prevention of contrast-induced nephropathy, *Clin J Am Soc Nephro* 3(1): 281–287.

Frank, H. A., Seligman, A. M. & Fine, J. (1946). Treatment of uremia after acute renal failure by peritoneal irrigation., *J Am Med Assoc* 130: 703–705.

Gibney, N., Hoste, E., Burdmann, E. A., Bunchman, T., Kher, V., Viswanathan, R., Mehta, R. L. & Ronco, C. (2008). Timing of initiation and discontinuation of renal replacement therapy in AKI: Unanswered key questions, *Clin J Am Soc Nephro* 3(3): 876–880.

Goldberg, A., Kogan, E., Hammerman, H., Markiewicz, W. & Aronson, D. (2009). The impact of transient and persistent acute kidney injury on long-term outcomes after acute myocardial infarction, *Kidney Int* 76(8): 900–906.

Griffiths, R. (1996). Muscle mass, survival, and the elderly ICU patient, *Nutrition* 12(6): 456–458.

Haase, M., Bellomo, R., Devarajan, P., Schlattmann, P., Haase-Fielitz, A. & NGAL Meta-analysis Investigator Group (2009). Accuracy of neutrophil gelatinase-associated lipocalin (NGAL) in diagnosis and prognosis in acute kidney injury: a systematic review and meta-analysis., *Am J Kid Dis* 54(6): 1012–1024.

Haase, M., Bellomo, R. & Haase-Fielitz, A. (2010). Novel biomarkers, oxidative stress, and the role of labile iron toxicity in cardiopulmonary bypass-associated acute kidney injury, *J Am Coll Cardiol* 55(19): 2024–2033.

Haase, M., Devarajan, P., Haase-Fielitz, A., Bellomo, R., Cruz, D. N., Wagener, G., Krawczeski, C. D., Koyner, J. L., Murray, P., Zappitelli, M., Goldstein, S. L., Makris, K., Ronco, C., Martensson, J., Martling, C.-R., Venge, P., Siew, E., Ware, L. B., Ikizler, T. A. & Mertens, P. R. (2011). The outcome of neutrophil gelatinase-associated lipocalin-positive subclinical acute kidney injury a multicenter pooled analysis of prospective studies., *J Am Coll Cardiol* 57(17): 1752–1761.

Hall, I., Yarlagadda, S., Coca, S. G., Wang, Z., Doshi, M., Devarajan, P., Han, W., Marcus, R. & Parikh, C. R. (2010). IL-18 and Urinary NGAL Predict Dialysis and Graft Recovery after Kidney Transplantation, *J Am Soc Nephrol* 21(1): 189–197.

Han, W. K., Bailly, V., Abichandani, R., Thadhani, R. & Bonventre, J. V. (2002). Kidney Injury Molecule-1 (KIM-1): a novel biomarker for human renal proximal tubule injury., *Kidney Int* 62(1): 237–244.

Hanley, J. A. & McNeil, B. J. (1982). The meaning and use of the area under a receiver operating characteristic (ROC) curve, *Radiology* 143(1): 29–36.

Hansen, J. T. (2002). *Netter's Atlas of Human Physiology*, Icon Learning Systems, Teterboro, NJ, USA.

Harjai, K. J., Ralzada, A., Shenoy, C., Sattur, S., Orshaw, P., Yaeger, K., Boura, J., Aboufares, A., Sporn, D. & Stapleton, D. (2008). A comparison of contemporary definitions of contrast nephropathy in patients undergoing percutaneous coronary intervention and a proposal for a novel nephropathy grading system, *Am J Cardiol* 101(6): 812–819.

Heemskerk, S., Masereeuw, R., Russel, F. G. M. & Pickkers, P. (2009). Selective iNOS inhibition for the treatment of sepsis-induced acute kidney injury, *Nat Rev Nephrol* 5(11): 629–640.

Heyman, S. N., Rosenberger, C. & Rosen, S. (2010). Experimental ischemia-reperfusion: biases and myths-the proximal vs. distal hypoxic tubular injury debate revisited, *Kidney Int* 77(1): 9–16.

Hoste, E. A. J., Clermont, G., Kersten, A., Venkataraman, R., Angus, D. C., de Bacquer, D. & Kellum, J. A. (2006). RIFLE criteria for acute kidney injury are associated with hospital mortality in critically ill patients: a cohort analysis, *Crit Care* 10(3): R73.

Ichimura, T., Bonventre, J. V., Bailly, V., Wei, H., Hession, C., Cate, R. & Sanicola, M. (1998). Kidney injury molecule-1 (KIM-1), a putative epithelial cell adhesion molecule containing a novel immunoglobulin domain, is up-regulated in renal cells after injury, *J Biol Chem* 273(7): 4135–4142.

Jo, S. K., Rosner, M. H. & Okusa, M. D. (2007). Pharmacologic treatment of acute kidney injury: why drugs haven't worked and what is on the horizon, *Clin J Am Soc Nephro* 2(2): 356–365.

KDOQI Clinical Practice Guidelines for Chronic Kidney Disease: Evaluation, Classification, and Stratification (2002).

Lafrance, J.-P. & Miller, D. R. (2010). Defining acute kidney injury in database studies: the effects of varying the baseline kidney function assessment period and considering CKD status., *Am J Kid Dis* 56(4): 651–660.

Lameire, N. H., van Biesen, W. & Vanholder, R. (2006). The changing epidemiology of acute renal failure, *Nat Clin Pract Nephrol* 2(7): 364–377.

Lassnigg, A., Schmid, E. R., Hiesmayr, M., Falk, C., Druml, W., Bauer, P. & Schmidlin, D. (2008). Impact of minimal increases in serum creatinine on outcome in patients after cardiothoracic surgery: do we have to revise current definitions of acute renal failure?, *Crit Care Med* 36(4): 1129–1137.

Lassnigg, A., Schmidlin, D., Mouhieddine, M., Bachmann, L., Druml, W., Bauer, P. & Hiesmayr, M. (2004). Minimal changes of serum creatinine predict prognosis in patients after cardiothoracic surgery: A prospective cohort study, *J Am Soc Nephrol* 15(6): 1597–1605.

Levey, A., Bosch, J., Lewis, J., Greene, T., Rogers, N. & Roth, D. (1999). A more accurate method to estimate glomerular filtration rate from serum creatinine: A new prediction equation, *Ann Intern Med* 130(6): 461–470.

Levey, A., Coresh, J., Balk, E., Kausz, A., Levin, A., Steffes, M., Hogg, R., Perrone, R., Lau, J. & Eknoyan, G. (2003). National kidney foundation practice guidelines for chronic kidney disease: Evaluation, classification, and stratification, *Ann Intern Med* 139(2): 137–147.

Levey, A. S., Stevens, L. A., Schmid, C. H., Zhang, Y., Castro, A. F., Feldman, H. I., Kusek, J. W., Eggers, P., van Lente, F., Greene, T. & Coresh, J. (2009). A New Equation to Estimate Glomerular Filtration Rate, *Ann Intern Med* 150(9): 604–613.

Levinsky, N. & Berliner, R. (1959). Changes in composition of the urine in ureter and bladder at low urine flow, *Am J Physiol* 196(3): 549–553.

Lopes, J. A., Melo, M. J., Viegas, A., Raimundo, M., Camara, I., Antunes, F. & Gomes da Costa, A. (2011). Acute kidney injury in hospitalized HIV-infected patients: a cohort analysis, *Nephrol Dial Transpl* .

Macedo, E., Bouchard, J., Soroko, S. H., Chertow, G. M., Himmelfarb, J., Ikizler, T. A., Paganini, E. P., Mehta, R. L. & Program to Improve Care in Acute Renal Disease Study (2010). Fluid accumulation, recognition and staging of acute kidney injury in critically-ill patients., *Crit Care* 14(3): R82.

Malyszko, J. (2010). Biomarkers of acute kidney injury in different clinical settings: a time to change the paradigm?, *Kidney Blood Press Res* 33(5): 368–382.

McGrath, J. (1852). Case of Ischuria Renalsis, *Am J Med Sci* 48(October): 390–392.

Mcilroy, D. R., Wagener, G. & Lee, H. T. (2010). Neutrophil gelatinase-associated lipocalin and acute kidney injury after cardiac surgery: the effect of baseline renal function on diagnostic performance., *Clin J Am Soc Nephro* 5(2): 211–219.

Mehta, R. L., Kellum, J., Shah, S., Molitoris, B. A., Ronco, C., Warnock, D., Levin, A. & the Acute Kidney Injury Network (2007). Acute Kidney Injury Network: report of an initiative to improve outcomes in acute kidney injury, *Crit Care* 11(2): R31.

Mehta, R., McDonald, B., Gabbai, F., Pahl, M., Farkas, A., Pascual, M., Zhuang, S., Kaplan, R. & Chertow, G. (2002). Nephrology consultation in acute renal failure: Does timing matter?, *Am J Med* 113(6): 456–461.

Melnikov, V. Y., Ecder, T., Fantuzzi, G., Siegmund, B., Lucia, M. S., Dinarello, C. A., Schrier, R. W. & Edelstein, C. L. (2001). Impaired IL-18 processing protects caspase-1-deficient mice from ischemic acute renal failure., *J Clin Invest* 107(9): 1145–1152.

Mishra, J., Dent, C. L., Tarabishi, R., Mitsnefes, M. M., Ma, Q., Kelly, C., Ruff, S. M., Zahedi, K., Shao, M., Bean, J., Mori, K., Barasch, J. M. & Devarajan, P. (2005). Neutrophil gelatinase-associated lipocalin (NGAL) as a biomarker for acute renal injury after cardiac surgery, *Lancet* 365(9466): 1231–1238.

Mishra, J., Ma, Q., Prada, A., Mitsnefes, M., Zahedi, K., Yang, J., Barasch, J. M. & Devarajan, P. (2003). Identification of neutrophil gelatinase-associated lipocalin as a novel early urinary biomarker for ischemic renal injury, *J Am Soc Nephrol* 14: 2534–2543.

Moller, E., McIntosh, J. & van Slyke, D. (1928). Studies of urea excretion II Relationship between urine volume and the rate of urea excretion by normal adults, *J Clin Invest* 6(3): 427–465.

Myers, B. D., MIller, D., Mehigan, J., Olcott, C., Golbetz, H., Robertson, C., Derby, G., Spencer, R. & Friedman, S. (1984). Nature of the renal injury following total renal ischemia in man, *J Clin Invest* 73(2): 329–341.

Nejat, M., Hill, J. V., Pickering, J. W., Edelstein, C. L., Devarajan, P. & Endre, Z. H. (2011). Albuminuria increases cystatin C excretion: implications for urinary biomarkers, *Nephrol Dial Transpl* .

Nejat, M., Pickering, J. W., Devarajan, P., Bonventre, J. V., Edelstein, C. L. & Endre, Z. H. (2011). Acute Kidney Injury (AKI) biomarkers are increased in prerenal AKI, *World Congress of Nephrology*.

Nejat, M., Pickering, J. W., Walker, R. J. & Endre, Z. H. (2010). Rapid detection of acute kidney injury by plasma cystatin C in the intensive care unit., *Nephrol Dial Transpl* 25(10): 3283–3289.

Nigwekar, S., Navaneethan, S., Parikh, C. R. & Hix, J. (2009). Atrial natriuretic peptide for preventing and treating acute kidney injury, *Cochrane Db Syst Rev* (4): Art. No.: CD006028.

Ozer, J. S., Dieterle, F., Troth, S., Perentes, E., Cordier, A., Verdes, P., Staedtler, F., Mahl, A., Grenet, O., Roth, D. R., Wahl, D., Legay, F., Holder, D., Erdos, Z., Vlasakova, K., Jin, H., Yu, Y., Muniappa, N., Forest, T., Clouse, H. K., Reynolds, S., Bailey, W. J., Thudium, D. T., Topper, M. J., Skopek, T. R., Sina, J. F., Glaab, W. E., Vonderscher, J., Maurer, G., Chibout, S.-D., Sistare, F. D. & Gerhold, D. L. (2010). A panel of urinary biomarkers to monitor reversibility of renal injury and a serum marker with improved potential to assess renal function, *Nat Biotechnol* 28(5): 486–494.

Parikh, C. R., Jani, A., Melnikov, V., Faubel, S. & Edelstein, C. L. (2004). Urinary interleukin-18 is a marker of human acute tubular necrosis, *Am J Kid Dis* 43: 405–414.

Parikh, C. R., Mishra, J., Thiessen-Philbrook, H., Dursun, B., Ma, Q., Kelly, C., Dent, C. L., Devarajan, P. & Edelstein, C. L. (2006). Urinary IL-18 is an early predictive biomarker of acute kidney injury after cardiac surgery, *Kidney Int* 70: 199–203.

Pencina, M. J., D'Agostino, R. B. & Vasan, R. S. (2008). Evaluating the added predictive ability of a new marker: From area under the ROC curve to reclassification and beyond, *Stat Med* 27(2): 157–172.

Perrone, R., Madias, N. & Levey, A. (1992). Serum creatinine as an index of renal-function - new insights into old concepts, *Clin Chem* 38(10): 1933–1953.

Pickering, J. W. & Endre, Z. H. (2009a). GFR shot by RIFLE: errors in staging acute kidney injury, *Lancet* 373(9672): 1318–1319.

Pickering, J. W. & Endre, Z. H. (2009b). RIFLE and AKIN–maintain the momentum and the GFR!, *Crit Care* 13(5): 416.

Pickering, J. W. & Endre, Z. H. (2009c). Secondary prevention of acute kidney injury., *Current opinion in critical care* 15(6): 488–497.

Pickering, J. W. & Endre, Z. H. (2010). Back-calculating baseline creatinine with MDRD misclassifies acute kidney injury in the intensive care unit., *Clin J Am Soc Nephro* 5(7): 1165–1173.

Pickering, J. W., Frampton, C. M. & Endre, Z. H. (2009). Evaluation of Trial Outcomes in Acute Kidney Injury by Creatinine Modeling, *Clin J Am Soc Nephro* 4(11): 1705–1715.

Pickering, J. W., Md Ralib, A., Nejat, M. & Endre, Z. H. (2011). New considerations in the design of clinical trials of acute kidney injury, *Clin Invest* 1(5): 637–650.

Rabito, C., Halpern, E. F., Scott, J. & Tolkoff-Rubin, N. (2010). Accurate, fast, and convenient measurement of glomerular filtration rate in potential renal transplant donors, *Transplantation* 90(5): 510–517.

Rehberg, P. B. (1926). Studies on Kidney Function: The Rate of Filtration and Reabsorption in the Human Kidney., *Biochem J* 20(3): 447–460.

Ricci, Z., Cruz, D. & Ronco, C. (2008). The RIFLE criteria and mortality in acute kidney injury: A systematic review, *Kidney Int* 73(5): 538–546.

Roberts, D. M., Wilks, M. F., Roberts, M. S., Swaminathan, R., Mohamed, F., Dawson, A. H. & Buckley, N. A. (2011). Changes in the concentrations of creatinine, cystatin C and NGAL in patients with acute paraquat self-poisoning., *Toxicol. Lett.* 202(1): 69–74.

Rule, A. D. (2010). The CKD-EPI equation for estimating GFR from serum creatinine: real improvement or more of the same?, *Clin J Am Soc Nephro* 5(6): 951–953.

Ryzner, K. L. (2010). Evaluation of Aminoglycoside Clearance Using the Modification of Diet in Renal Disease Equation Versus the Cockcroft-Gault Equation as a Marker of Glomerular Filtration Rate, *Ann Pharmacother* 44(6): 1030–1037.

Shemesh, O., Golbetz, H., Kriss, J. P. & Myers, B. D. (1985). Limitations of creatinine as a filtration marker in glomerulopathic patients., *Kidney Int* 28(5): 830–838.

Siew, E. D., Matheny, M. E., Ikizler, T. A., Lewis, J. B., Miller, R. A., Waitman, L. R., Go, A. S., Parikh, C. R. & Peterson, J. F. (2010). Commonly used surrogates for baseline renal function affect the classification and prognosis of acute kidney injury, *Kidney Int* 77(6): 536–542.

Sjostrom, P., Tidman, M. & Jones, I. (2005). Determination of the production rate and non-renal clearance of cystatin C and estimation of the glomerular filtration rate from the serum concentration of cystatin C in humans, *Scand J Clin Lab Inv* 65(2): 111–124.

Smith, H., Finkelstein, N., Alimnosa, L., Crawford, B. & Graber, M. (1945). The renal clearances of substituted hippuric acid derivatives and other aromatic acids in dog and man, *J Clin Invest* 24(3): 388–404.

Star, R. A. (1998). Treatment of acute renal failure, *Kidney Int* 54: 1817–1831.

Uchino, S., Bellomo, R., Bagshaw, S. M. & Goldsmith, D. (2010). Transient azotaemia is associated with a high risk of death in hospitalized patients, *Nephrol Dial Transpl* 25(6): 1833–1839.

Uchino, S., Bellomo, R., Goldsmith, D., Bates, S. & Ronco, C. (2006). An assessment of the RIFLE criteria for acute renal failure in hospitalized patients, *Crit Care Med* 34: 1913–1917.

Vaidya, V. S., Ferguson, M. A. & Bonventre, J. V. (2008). Biomarkers of acute kidney injury, *Annu Rev Pharmacol* 48: 463–493.

Vaidya, V. S., Ozer, J. S., Dieterle, F., Collings, F. B., Ramirez, V., Troth, S., Muniappa, N., Thudium, D., Gerhold, D., Holder, D. J., Bobadilla, N. A., Marrer, E., Perentes, E., Cordier, A., Vonderscher, J., Maurer, G., Goering, P. L., Sistare, F. D. & Bonventre,

J. V. (2010). Kidney injury molecule-1 outperforms traditional biomarkers of kidney injury in preclinical biomarker qualification studies, *Nat Biotechnol* 28(5): 478–485.

Waikar, S. S., Sabbisetti, V. S. & Bonventre, J. V. (2010). Normalization of urinary biomarkers to creatinine during changes in glomerular filtration rate, *Kidney Int* 78(5): 486–494.

Wang, E., Sandoval, R. M., Campos, S. B. & Molitoris, B. A. (2010). Rapid diagnosis and quantification of acute kidney injury using fluorescent ratio-metric determination of glomerular filtration rate in the rat, *Am J Physiol-Renal* 299(5): F1048–55.

Watson, P., Watson, I. & Batt, R. (1980). Total-body water volumes for adult males and females estimated from simple anthropometric measurements, *Am J Clin Nutr* 33(1): 27–39.

Westhuyzen, J. (2006). Cystatin C: a promising marker and predictor of impaired renal function, *Ann Clin Lab Sci* 36(4): 387–394.

Westhuyzen, J., Endre, Z. H., Reece, G., Reith, D., Saltissi, D. & Morgan, T. (2003). Measurement of tubular enzymuria facilitates early detection of acute renal impairment in the intensive care unit, *Nephrol Dial Transpl* 18: 543–551.

Yu, H., Yanagisawa, Y., Forbes, M. A., Cooper, E. H., Crockson, R. A. & MacLennan, I. C. (1983). Alpha-1-microglobulin: an indicator protein for renal tubular function., *J Clin Pathol* 36(3): 253–259.

Yu, Y., Jin, H., Holder, D., Ozer, J. S., Villarreal, S., Shughrue, P., Shi, S., Figueroa, D. J., Clouse, H., Su, M., Muniappa, N., Troth, S. P., Bailey, W., Seng, J., Aslamkhan, A. G., Thudium, D., Sistare, F. D. & Gerhold, D. L. (2010). Urinary biomarkers trefoil factor 3 and albumin enable early detection of kidney tubular injury, *Nat Biotechnol* 28(5): 470–477.

Zoungas, S., Ninomiya, T., Huxley, R., Cass, A., Jardine, M., Gallagher, M., Patel, A., Vasheghani-Farahani, A., Sadigh, G. & Perkovic, V. (2009). Systematic Review: Sodium Bicarbonate Treatment Regimens for the Prevention of Contrast-Induced Nephropathy, *Ann Intern Med* 151(9): 631–638.

7

Acute Kidney Injury in Pregnancy

Manisha Sahay
Department of Nephrology
Osmania Medical College and General Hospital, Hyderabad, Andhra Pradesh
India

1. Introduction

Acute kidney injury (AKI) is a life threatening complication of pregnancy.The incidence of AKI has sharply declined from 0.5 per 1000 pregnancies to one in 20,000 births in developed countries. (Beaufilis,2005) On the other hand, pregnancy is still responsible for 15–20% of AKI in developing countries. (Naqvi, 1996)Pregnancy related AKI (PRAKI) is on the decline from 14.5% reported in 1987 to 4.3% in 2005 in India(Chugh,1987).

1.1 Physiological changes in pregnancy

1.1.1Renal function during pregnancy

The kidney undergoes monumental physiologic and anatomic changes during a normal pregnancy. Renal plasma flow increases by 50-70%. Plasma volume increases by 50% and there is hemodilutional anemia. Cardiac output increases by 40%.Glomerular Filtration Rate (GFR) is maximum around the 13th week of pregnancy and can reach levels up to 150% of normal. Despite increased GFR the intraglomerular pressure remains normal. Serum creatinine falls by an average of 0.4 mg/dl to a pregnancy range of 0.4 to 0.8 mg/dl. Hence, a serum creatinine of 1.0 mg/dl, although normal in a non pregnant individual, reflects renal impairment in a pregnant woman. Serum creatinine rises near term and value of 1 mg/dl is considered normal. In the initial part of pregnancy there is decreased peripheral vascular resistance with a blood pressure fall of approximately 10 mm Hg in the first 24 weeks. The blood pressure gradually returns to prepregnancy level by term. Glycosuria occurs due to decrease in transport maximum for glucose(TMG) and high GFR. Aminoaciduria (2 g/d) may be seen. Increased uric acid clearance results in low uric acid level (2.5-5.5 mg/dl) but levels increase later and reach prepregnancy values at term. A value of >6 mg/dl reflects pregnancy induced hypertension (PIH). Potassium and almost 900 meq of sodium are retained. Calcium excretion increases but stone formation is not increased as there is increased excretion of inhibitors of stone formation. A reset in the osmostat occurs, resulting in increased thirst and decreased serum sodium levels (by 5 mEq/L) and low plasma osmolality (10 m0sm/kg less). Clearance of ADH is increased by placental vasopressinase and may result in transient Diabetes insipidus of pregnancy which may respond to DDAVP. On the other hand there are some reports of transient SIADH in pregnancy. Urine concentration and dilution are adequate. There is mild respiratory alkalosis and blood gas of 7.42-7.44/30 pCO2/HCO318-22 is representative (Chris Baylis,2007).

1.1.2 Anatomic changes

A dilatation of ureters and pelvis occurs till pelvic brim (iliac sign) with dilatation more pronounced on right secondary to dextrorotation of uterus and dilatation of right ovarian venous plexus. This leads to urinary stasis and an risk of urinary tract infections (UTIs). There is an increase in kidney size by 1-1.5 cm. As a rule, all the physiologic changes maximize by the end of the second trimester and then start to return to the prepartum level, whereas changes in the anatomy take up to 3 months postpartum to subside.(Hou, S . 1998, Chris Baylis, 1987)

1.1.3 Hormones

There is increase in aldosterone, desoxycorticosterone, progesterone, relaxin, oxytocin and vasodilating prostaglandins and a decrease in vasopressin (due to vasopressinase) and also resistance to action of aldosterone and renin.(August, P 1995)

1.1.4 Renal function tests

Urine examination- Microscopic hematuria may be seen in 20% but is not persistent and disappears after delivery. Proteinuria glycosuria, and hypercalciuia may be seen.

Glomerular filtration rate (GFR) -

MDRD formula- Creatinine-based formulae are inaccurate in pregnancy. The Modification of Diet in Renal Disease (MDRD) formula underestimates GFR by 40ml/min. Among pregnant women with preeclampsia or CKD, MDRD formula is slightly better, underestimating GFR by 23.3 and 27.3 ml/min respectively.

Creatinine clearance by24-h urine collection closely approximates GFR by inulin clearance among healthy pregnant women and is the gold standard in pregnancy.

Weight-based formulas such as Cockroft-Gault formulae overestimate GFR by approximately 40 ml/min.

Estimating of proteinuria during pregnancy

Urine protein excretion increases in pregnancy and upto 300 mg /day is normal. Albumin excretion is also increased .These values return to normal by 6th month post partum. Twenty-four-hour urine collection, although the gold standard for proteinuria quantification is cumbersome, inaccurate and result is delayed. The use of the protein to creatinine ratio (P:C ratio) to estimate24-h protein excretion is controversial in pregnancy though it has become the preferred method for the quantification of proteinuria in non pregnant population, because of high accuracy, reproducibility, and convenience. Most misclassifications occur in women with borderline proteinuria (250 to 400 mg/d). Hence, it is reasonable to use urine P:C ratio for diagnosis , with 24-h collection undertaken when result is equivocal.

Renal biopsy in pregnancy - Indications include severe symptomatic nephrotic syndrome and rapidly progressive renal failure. Biopsy can be done in 2nd trimester with patient in lateral position.

2. Acute kidney injury in pregnancy

Certain renal diseases are common in pregnancy. (Ananth Karumanchi,S 2007, Schrier RW 1997). Incidence of AKI in pregnancy is 1:20,000 and comprises 25% of AKI in developing countries with substantial mortality . Acute renal failure in pregnancy can be induced by any of the disorders leading to renal failure in the general population, such as acute tubular necrosis due to infection, glomerulonephritis related to lupus, or drug toxicity. There are, however, pregnancy complications characteristic of each trimester that can result in renal failure.

2.1 Causes of renal failure in pregnancy

Can be divided into

i. *Early pregnancy-* Hyperemesis gravidarum , Septic abortion .
ii. *Late pregnancy-*PIH and its complications, Hemolytic anemia ,elevated liver enzymes and low platelets (HELLP), Post partum Hemolytic uremic syndrome (HUS), Acute fatty liver of pregnancy, Volume loss -Antepartum hemorrhage (APH), Post partum hemorrhage (PPH), Sepsis

In a study carried out at Osmania General hospital ,Hyderabad ,India over a period of 8 years Obstetric renal failure accounted for 12.1% with PIH as the commonest cause accounting for 39.3%, PPH 20.7% ,Puerperal sepsis 10.6%, APH-9.2%.Septic abortion-4.9%,HUS-3.4% and 11.7% were undetermined .

Early pregnancy causes

2.1.1 Hyperemesis gravidarum

Severe vomiting in early pregnancy can lead to volume depletion and acute kidney injury. Metabolic alkalosis can be seen. Vomiting can be aggravated by certain triggers which include strong smells, postures which delay gastric emptying, hot foods etc. The patient may need hospitalization and volume replacement. Antiemetic drugs can be used to control vomiting. These include pyridoxine-doxylamine succinate combination therapy for initial pharmacologic treatment of nausea of pregnancy, antihistaminics, domperidone, metaclopramide, and ondensetron. Glucocorticoids have been used in refractory cases. Hyperemesis may recur in subsequent pregnancies. (ACOG, 2004)

2.1.2 Septic abortion

The commonest causative organism is Clostridium. It manifests few hours to 1-2 days after abortion with fever, vomiting and pain abdomen. Progression to shock and death is rapid. Jaundice due to hemolysis and cutaneous vasodilatation contribute to bronze skin coloration. Anemia, leucocytosis and thrombocytopenia with associated disseminated intravascular coagulation may be seen. Management consists of antibiotics and volume resuscitation. Other therapies include hysterectomy, hyperbaric oxygen, antitoxin and exchange transfusion.

Late pregnancy causes

2.1.3 Hypertensive disorders of pregnancy

Hypertensive disorders are the commonest cause of renal failure in pregnancy. These are seen in two settings: young primigravidas and older multiparous women.

2.1.3.1 Classification

Terminology of hypertensive disorders varies, but following 5 entities have been described by National High Blood Pressure Education Program (NHBPEP, 2000):

Gestational hypertension/ Transient hypertension - is defined as blood pressure of 140/90 mm Hg or greater with no hypertension before pregnancy. It usually affects nulliparous females mostly in third trimester. Preeclampsia does not develop and blood pressure returns to normal levels within 12 weeks postpartum. Patients are usually asymptomatic or have symptoms or signs like preeclampsia. It is a retrospective diagnosis and is confused with preeclampsia at the time of onset and with essential hypertension postpartum until the blood pressure returns to normal. Proteinuria does not occur, serum uric acid is normal. It may predict the development of hypertension later in life. It should be managed as preeclampsia when first diagnosed.

Chronic hypertension- is associated with underlying or preexisting hypertension. The diagnosis is established by a blood pressure of 140/90 mm Hg or greater before pregnancy or before 20 weeks' gestation, or by persistent hypertension after delivery. Renal biopsy shows nephrosclerosis rather than preeclampsia. Complications of chronic hypertension include superimposed preeclampsia and renal failure, abruptio placentae, growth restriction and fetal death. Methyldopa is the preferred treatment agent, but in mild cases, no therapy may be necessary. In women whose blood pressure is well controlled when they enter pregnancy, the same therapy should be continued. However, angiotensin II receptor blocking (ARB) agents and angiotensin converting enzyme inhibitors (ACEIs) are contraindicated in pregnancy due to the risk of fetal renal agenesis.

Preeclampsia - It is the leading cause of acute kidney injury in the last trimester and occurs in 7% of all pregnancies mostly in primigravidas. However it can be seen in multigravidas if the interpregnancy interval is prolonged. It is the leading cause of maternal and fetal mortality in the world. It is associated with intrauterine growth retardation and small for gestational age (SGA) babies. It is a triad of hypertension, proteinuria and oedema occurring after the 20th week of gestation with few cases developing postpartum within hours, usually in the first 24 to 48 hours. Preeclampsia does not occur before twenty weeks gestation except in molar pregnancies and in the presence of antiphospholipid antibody syndrome. Hypertension is defined as rise in systolic BP >30 mmHg and diastolic BP >15 mmHg. Proteinuria is defined as >300mg protein in urine per day. Oedema is not essential for diagnosis but sudden oedema and weight gain are common presenting features. Oedema is due to overfill with reduced GFR as in nephritic illnesses with suppressed renin and aldosterone and differs from oedema of CHF, cirrhosis and neprhotic syndrome which is associated with underfilling of vascular bed with high renin and aldosterone. Though increased capillary permeability and hypoalbuminemia may be seen they are not the sole contributing factors for oedema. The risk factors associated with the development of preeclampsia include age older than 35 years or younger than 16 years, chronic hypertension, obesity, preexisting diabetes , renal disease, insulin resistance, Anti phospholipid antibody syndrome, African American race and pregnancy with a new partner. Fetal risk factors may be twin or multiple gestations, trisomy 13 and hydatidiform mole. Some genetic factors contribute to the development of preecclampsia. It is four times more common if there is history of precclampsia in mother or sister. Polymorphisms of genes associated with control of blood pressure or coagulation system have been implicated. Some mutations described involve Endothelial nitric oxide synthetase (e NOS), renin angiotensinogen (T235), Leyden factor V, Prothrombin and Methyl tetra hydrofolate reductase(MTHFR) genes. A locus on 2p was described in Icelandic and Australian families. A Dutch study reported linkage to 12 q locus in HELLP syndrome which shows the genetic factors responsible for Preclampsia and HELLP may be different. Association with trisomy 13 indicates a linkage to chromosome 13. An activating mutation of mineralocorticoid receptor was described in patients with PIH but no proteinuria. Preclampsia is more commonly seen in women at high altitude or in third world countries suggesting the possible role of hypoxia or environmental pollution in genesis . HELLP syndrome

(Hemolysis, ELevated liver enzymes, and Low Platelets) is observed when severe preeclampsia or eclampsia is accompanied by significant liver involvement. Acute renal failure (ARF) may develop.(Lindheimer, 1991)

Eclampsia-is the occurrence of seizure activity with no other explainable cause in setting of preeclampsia.

Preeclampsia superimposed on chronic hypertension- defined as new-onset proteinuria (ie, >300 mg/d) after 20 weeks' gestation in a hypertensive patient or as a sudden increase in proteinuria or blood pressure in a patient with hypertension and proteinuria before 20 weeks' gestation.

2.1.3.2 Pathophysiology

Utero-placental ischemia: A combination of genetic and environmental factors results in inadequate invasion of uterine spiral arteries by placental trophoblasts resulting in inability of uterine vessels to transform from high resistance channels to a low resistance system. This results in utero-placental ischemia. In normal pregnancy Vascular endothelial growth factor (VEGF) and Placental induced growth factor (PIGF) are made by placenta and circulate in high concentrations in the blood. VEGF is also synthesized by glomerular podocytes and vascular endothelial cells. VEGF and PIGF induce synthesis of nitric oxide and vasodilating prostacylin in endothelial cells decreasing vascular tone and blood pressure. In PIH the utero-placental ischemia results in oxidative stress and release of a soluble cytokine, the sFlt-1 (soluble fms-like tyrosine kinase-1). sFlt-1 is a potent antagonist of VEGF and PIGF. In PET concentrations of sFlt-1 rise in the 2nd trimester with a decrease in VEGF and PIGF. Overproduction of sFlt-1 explains increased susceptibility to PET in multiple gestation, hydantidiform mole, trisomy 13 and first pregnancy. In addition, increased concentration of circulating pre-ecclamptic factors-angiotensin 1 /Bradykinin B2 receptor heterodimers, agonistic antibodies to angiotensin I receptor(AT 1 receptor antibody) and soluble endoglin are seen in PET. (Maynard,S 2003; Venkatesha,S 2006; Zhou,C.C,2008; Levine, RJ 2006)

There is an imbalance of vasoconstrictors and vasodilator substances hence there is a state of generalized vasoconstriction in preeclampsia. The levels of prorenin, angiotensin, thromboxane and endothelin are high while the levels of vasodilator prostaglandin ie Prostacyclin, PGE2, nitric oxide and bradykinin are low. In normal pregnancy there is less sensitivity of vascular bed to the hypertensive effects of angiotensin but this is lost in preeclampsia.

A myriad of markers for generalized endothelial dysfunction are seen in preeclampsia which include von Willebrand factor, Platelet activating factor (PAF-1), Endothelin and cellular fibronectin.

The increase in blood volume, increased GFR and vasodilatation seen in normal pregnancy are lost in preeclampsia. Though the blood volume in preeclampsia is decreased there is an increase in effective circulating volume with suppressed renin and aldosterone with elevation of brain natriuretic peptide.

2.1.3.3 Screening tests

Laboratory evaluation helps to determine disease severity by characterizing the extent of end organ involvement.

Hematocrit — Hemoconcentration supports the diagnosis of preeclampsia but hemolysis, if present, can decrease the hematocrit.

Platelet count — Preeclampsia accounts for 21% of cases of maternal thrombocytopenia. Thrombocytopenia is usually moderate and platelet count rarely decreases to < 20,000/µL. Thrombocytopenia in patients with preeclampsia always correlates with the severity of the disease. It is considered a sign of worsening disease and is an indication for delivery.
Quantification of protein excretion — Excretion of 300 mg or more in 24 hours is necessary for diagnosis. It is suggested by at least 1+ protein on dipstick of two urine specimens collected at least four hours apart. A dipstick of 3+ or greater or 5 g or more per day is a criterion of severe disease.
Serum creatinine concentration — An elevated or rising level suggests severe disease.
Serum alanine and aspartate aminotransferase concentrations (ALT and AST) — Elevated or rising levels suggest hepatic dysfunction indicative of severe disease.
Serum lactate dehydrogenase (LDH) concentration — Microangiopathic hemolysis is suggested by an elevated LDH level and red cell fragmentation (schistocytes or helmet cells) on peripheral blood smear. Elevation of total bilirubin may also suggest hemolysis. Microangiopathic hemolysis is present in severe disease or HELLP syndrome (Hemolysis, Elevated Liver function tests, Low Platelets).
Serum uric acid concentration — It is often elevated in preeclampsia, but not diagnostic. High uric acid levels may be due to hypoxia or due to reduced GFR.
Fetal well-being is evaluated by a nonstress test or biophysical profile. In addition, the fetus is examined by ultrasound to evaluate growth and amniotic fluid volume. Assessment of umbilical artery Doppler flow may also aid in evaluation of the fetal condition.
Coagulation function tests (eg, prothrombin time, activated partial thromboplastin time, fibrinogen concentration) are usually normal if there is no thrombocytopenia or liver dysfunction, and therefore do not need to be monitored routinely.
Recently, urinary PlGF values and sFlt-1 values have shown great promise as a means of identifying preclinical preeclampsia .

2.1.3.4 Management

The definitive treatment of preeclampsia is delivery to prevent development of maternal or fetal complications from disease progression. Several groups have formulated guidelines for diagnosis, evaluation, and management of hypertensive disorders of pregnancy (NHBPEP. Report of the National High Blood Pressure Education Program Working Group on High Blood Pressure in Pregnancy (2000), ACOG 2002).
Laboratory follow-up — The minimum laboratory evaluation should include platelet count, serum creatinine, and serum AST. These tests should be repeated once or twice weekly in women with mild preeclampsia to assess for disease progression, and more often if clinical signs and symptoms suggest worsening disease(ACOG 2000).The value of other tests is less clearly defined. A rising hematocrit can be useful to look for hemoconcentration, which suggests contraction of intravascular volume and progression to more severe disease, while a falling hematocrit may be a sign of hemolysis. An elevated serum LDH concentration is also a sign of hemolysis, and a marker of severe disease or HELLP syndrome. Hemolysis can be confirmed by observation of schistocytes and helmet cells on a blood smear .Quantification of protein excretion can be performed to determine whether the threshold for severe preeclampsia (5 g/24 hours) has been reached. Since several clinical studies have shown that neither the rate of increase nor the amount of proteinuria affects maternal or perinatal outcome in the setting of preeclampsia, repeated 24-hour urinary protein estimations are not useful once the threshold of 300 mg/24 hours for the diagnosis of

preeclampsia has been exceeded. Serum creatinine alone can be used to monitor renal function.

Treatment of hypertension – Nonpharmacologic treatments include bed rest and alcohol avoidance. Weight loss and salt restriction are not recommended. ACE inhibitors are contraindicated. Diuretics in pregnancy lead to intravascular volume depletion, organ and placental hypoperfusion. They may be used with caution in presence of significant edema. If preeclampsia develops diuretics must be discontinued. Beta-blockers have no major contraindications, although neonatal bradycardia, hypoglycemia, and respiratory depression can occur. Labetalol is not associated with neonatal bradycardia and is used for hypertensive emergencies. Alpha-methyldopa is the drug of choice for hypertension. Clonidine is also used. Calcium channel blockers may cause tocolysis in 3rd trimester hence should be used only if hypertension is unresponsive to other medications. Hydralazine is a first-line agent for hypertensive emergencies. Experience with minoxidil and prazosin is limited. The use of antihypertensive drugs to control mildly elevated blood pressure in the setting of preeclampsia does not alter the course of the disease or diminish perinatal morbidity or mortality. Novel therapies are under investigation. L-arginine is the physiologic precursor for nitric oxide, which has been implicated in the pathogenesis of preeclampsia and is being tested. Another randomized trial showed that plasma volume expansion did not improve maternal or fetal outcome.

Assessment of fetal well-being – A minimum of daily fetal movement counts and twice weekly fetal non stress testing with assessment of amniotic fluid volume, or biophysical profile is recommended. Early fetal growth restriction may be the first manifestation of preeclampsia or a sign of severe preeclampsia. Sonographic estimation of fetal weight should be performed to look for growth restriction and oligohydramnios at the time of diagnosis of preeclampsia and then repeated serially. Doppler velocimetry is useful for assessing fetal status if fetal growth restriction is present.

Delivery- The decision to deliver the fetus is based upon gestational age, maternal and fetal condition, and the severity of preeclampsia.

Mild PIH- Patients at term (>37 weeks) are delivered. Most experts advise that delivery should not be postponed beyond 40 weeks of gestation in any preeclamptic woman. Vaginal delivery is preferred at term if there are no contraindications. Cervical ripening agents should be considered in women with unfavorable cervices. Women with mild PIH with period of gestation <37 weeks can be managed expectantly. However maternal end-organ dysfunction and non reassuring tests of fetal well-being may be indications for delivery at any gestational age. Outpatient care is a cost-effective option for some women with mild preeclampsia. However these patients should comply with frequent maternal and fetal evaluations (every one to three days) and have ready access to medical care. Restricted activity is recommended; however, complete bed rest is not required. Hospitalization is needed in the event of fulminant progression to eclampsia, hypertensive crisis, abruptio placentae, or HELLP syndrome. Patients should be hospitalized immediately if they develop severe or persistent headache, visual changes, right upper quadrant or epigastric pain, nausea or vomiting, shortness of breath, or decreased urine output (ACOG 2000). As with any pregnancy, decreased fetal movement, vaginal bleeding, abdominal pain, rupture of membranes, or uterine contractions should be reported immediately.

Severe preeclampsia – Severe preeclampsia is generally regarded as an indication for delivery, regardless of gestational age, to minimize the risk of development of maternal and fetal complications. Prolonged antepartum management at a tertiary care setting or in consultation with a maternal-fetal medicine specialist may be considered in few women under 32 to 34 weeks of gestation. However, women who develop severe preeclampsia at or beyond 32 to 34 weeks of gestation should be delivered at an institution with appropriate facilities. Hyaline membrane disease is common in preterm infants of preeclamptic women. Therefore, antenatal corticosteroids (betamethasone) to promote fetal lung maturity should be administered to women less than 34 weeks of gestation since preterm delivery is common. Even in preterm delivery vaginal delivery may be attempted. Cervical ripening agents may be used prior to induction if the cervix is not favorable. However, a prolonged induction should be avoided. Some authors recommend cesarean delivery for women with severe preeclampsia who are under 30 weeks of gestation . Management of severe preeclampsia- or eclampsia-related pulmonary edema includes treatment of the severe preeclampsia or eclampsia, supplemental oxygen, and fluid restriction. Diuresis is indicated if there is fluid overload but care should be taken to avoid further intravascular volume depletion. Mechanical ventilation may be necessary. Close, continuous maternal-fetal monitoring is indicated intrapartum to identify worsening hypertension, deteriorating maternal hepatic, renal, cardiopulmonary, or hematologic function, and uteroplacental insufficiency or abruptio placentae (often manifested by fetal bradycardia/or vaginal bleeding). The vitals should be monitored every hour and preeclampsia laboratory tests should be repeated every six hours. Epidural anaesthesia should be avoided in presence of thrombocytopenia. Invasive hemodynamic monitoring can be useful in complicated patients. Anticonvulsant therapy is generally initiated during labor or while administering corticosteroids or prostaglandins prior to planned delivery. Therapy is continued for 24 hours postpartum (range 12 to 48 hours). Magnesium sulfate is the drug of choice for the prevention of eclampsia and prevention of recurrent eclamptic seizures. It is more effective than Phenytoin or Nimodipine or lytic cocktail (mixture of chlorpromazine, promethazine and pethidine) . Magnesium causes vasodilatation of the cerebral vasculature, inhibition of platelet aggregation, protection of endothelial cells from damage by free radicals, prevention of calcium ion entry into ischemic cells, decreasing the release of acetylcholine at motor end plates within the neuromuscular junction, and as a competitive antagonist to the glutamate N-methyl-D-aspartate receptor (which is epileptogenic). Anticonvulsant therapy is also used for prevention of seizures in women with mild preeclampsia, but its role in this setting is controversial. The magnesium sulfate dose is 4 g intravenously as a loading dose then 1 g/h, or 5 g intramuscularly into each buttock followed by 5 g intramuscularly every four hours. Hypotension is the major concern from regional anesthesia since preeclamptic women have depleted intravascular volumes.

Outcome – The major adverse outcomes associated with preeclampsia are related to maternal central nervous system, hepatic, and renal dysfunction (eg, cerebral hemorrhage, hepatic rupture, renal failure), bleeding related to thrombocytopenia, preterm delivery, fetal growth restriction, abruptio placentae, and perinatal death. Factors that influence outcome include gestational age at onset and delivery, severity of disease, and whether there are coexisting conditions present, such as multiple gestation, diabetes mellitus, renal disease, thrombophilia, or preexisting hypertension. There is approximately one maternal death due to preeclampsia-eclampsia per 100,000 live births, with a case-fatality rate of 6.4 deaths per 10,000 cases in US. In mild preeclampsia neonatal outcomes are generally good and comparable to those of normotensive women. Risk of recurrence in subsequent pregnancy depends upon severity of disease, gestational age at onset and gestational age at delivery.

Postpartum course -Vital signs are monitored every two hours while the patient remains on magnesium sulphate and laboratory tests are repeated until two consecutive sets of data are normal. Hypertension and proteinuria due to preeclampsia resolve postpartum, often within a few days, but sometimes take few weeks or rarely a year or more. Antihypertensive medications can be discontinued when blood pressure returns to normal levels. Elevated blood pressures that remain 12 weeks postpartum are unlikely to be related to preeclampsia and may require long-term treatment. Vasoconstriction and endothelial dysfunction resolve over a few days.

Postpartum preeclampsia Pre eclampsia /eclampsia occurring more than two days and less than six weeks after delivery. It is important to exclude other diagnoses, especially when symptoms suggest the possibility of central nervous system pathology. Late postpartum eclampsia is defined as eclamptic seizures developing greater than 48 hours, but less than four weeks postpartum). Controversial prevention strategies include calcium supplementation, fish oils, sodium restriction, low-dose aspirin and antioxidants.

2.1.4 Hemolysis, elevated liver enzymes, low platelets –HELLP syndrome

HELLP syndrome is a variant of severe preeclampsia, first described by Dr. Louis Weinstein in 1982. About 15 to 20 percent of affected patients do not have antecedent hypertension or proteinuria, leading some experts to believe that HELLP is a separate disorder from preeclampsia [Sibai BM1986, Reubinoff BE, 1991]. Both severe preeclampsia and HELLP syndrome may be associated with other hepatic manifestations, including infarction, hemorrhage, and rupture. HELLP develops in approximately 1 to 2 per 1000 pregnancies overall and in 10 to 20 percent of women with severe preeclampsia/ eclampsia. The majority of cases are diagnosed between 28 and 36 weeks of gestation with 70 percent occurring prior to delivery [Sibai BM, Ramadan MK 1993]. Of these patients, approximately 80 percent are diagnosed prior to 37 weeks of gestation and fewer than 3 percent develop the disease between 17 and 20 weeks of gestation. The disease presents postpartum in 30 percent, usually within 48 hours of delivery, but occasionally as long as seven days after birth. Only 20 percent of postpartum patients with HELLP have evidence of preeclampsia antepartum.

Diagnosis and classification of HELLP syndrome

There is no consensus regarding the degree of laboratory abnormality diagnostic of HELLP syndrome. Some studies use AST (and/or ALT) and LDH values above the upper limit of normal, while others require elevations of at least two standard deviations above the mean. Due to differences in assays used to measure these enzymes, an elevated value in one hospital may be near normal in another.HELLP syndrome and severe preeclampsia are probably part of a disease spectrum. A precise definition of HELLP is necessary for research purposes and for predicting maternal complications. We require the presence of all of the following criteria to diagnose HELLP.

Microangiopathic hemolytic anemia with characteristic schistocytes (also called helmet cells) on blood smear. Other signs suggestive of hemolysis include an elevated LDH or indirect bilirubin and a low serum haptoglobin concentration (≤25 mg/dL).

Platelet count ≤100,000 cells/microL .HELLP syndrome accounts for 21% of maternal thrombocytopenia in pregnancy.

Serum LDH ≥600 IU/L or total bilirubin ≥1.2 mg/dL

Serum AST ≥70 IU/L. Some investigators obtain ALT levels instead of, or in addition to, AST levels. An advantage of the AST is that it is a single test that reflects both hepatocellular necrosis and red cell hemolysis.

Women who do not meet all of the above laboratory abnormalities are considered to have partial HELLP syndrome. These patients may progress to complete expression of HELLP syndrome.

Approximately 50% of patients have complete HELLP (all components present), and 50% have incomplete HELLP (at least 1 components present: EL, HEL, ELLP, LP). Some physicians subclassify HELLP based on the severity of thrombocytopenia, as follows: Class 1 - Platelet count < 50,000/µL, Class 2 - Platelet count 50,000-100,000/µL, Class 3 - Platelet count 100,000-150,000/µL

Clinical manifestations

Clinical manifestations are nonspecific (nausea, vomiting, headache in 50%, epigastric or right upper quadrant pain in 50%).Early HELLP syndrome is often misdiagnosed as heartburn, hence a high index of suspicion for HELLP syndrome is important. All patients with HELLP syndrome do not meet the strict criteria for preeclampsia. Hypertension (blood pressure ≥140/90) and proteinuria are present in approximately 85 %, 15% have diastolic blood pressure (BP) >90 mm Hg but either or both may be absent in women with severe HELLP syndrome (Sibai, 2004). Some patients are asymptomatic, major complications can occur despite normal blood pressure and proteinuria. These include DIC, abruptio placentae, acute renal failure, pulmonary edema, subcapsular liver hematoma, retinal detachment or stroke. Jaundice and ascites may also be present. Bleeding may occur due to thrombocytopenia. Thrombocytopenia is usually moderate, with counts rarely <20,000/µL. Major hemorrhage is uncommon. Maternal thrombocytopenia reaches a nadir at 24-48 hours postpartum. The maternal mortality rate with HELLP is 1%. The perinatal mortality rate is 11%. Fetal growth restriction is common. Neonates may be at increased risk for thrombocytopenia.

Treatment

Management is like preecclapsia .Delivery is the ultimate cure and should be planned immediately if >34 weeks or can be delayed for 24-48 hours if <34 weeks' gestation to administer corticosteroids if the patient is asymptomatic and the fetal testing is normal. Magnesium sulfate ($MgSO_4$) should be administered intrapartum and postpartum, regardless of blood pressure levels, to prevent seizures (eclampsia). Approximately 6-10 units of platelets is administered at the time of skin incision, and an additional 6 units are administered if oozing is noted during the surgery. Also platelet transfusion is indicated if the platelet count is less than 20,000 cells/uL. If cesarean delivery is planned platelet transfusion, is recommended to achieve platelet count greater than 50,000 cells/uL. Thrombocytopenia and elevated liver function tests worsen postpartum but should start normalizing by the third postpartum day. The use of steroids for HELLP is controversial.

Management of hepatic complications — Marked elevations in serum aminotransferases are not typical of uncomplicated HELLP; when they occur, the possibility of hepatic infarction, subcapsular hematoma, or viral hepatitis should be considered. Marked elevation in serum aminotransferases (usually 1000 to 2000 IU/L or higher) associated with right upper quadrant pain and fever is characteristic of hepatic infarction; this diagnosis can be confirmed by hepatic imaging. These infarcts resolve post partum. These patients may have an underlying procoagulant state, such as the antiphospholipid syndrome. HELLP may be complicated by hepatic rupture with development of a hematoma beneath Glisson's capsule. Histology of the liver adjacent to the rupture shows periportal hemorrhage and fibrin deposition, along with a neutrophilic infiltrate(hepatic preeclampsia). The hematoma may remain enclosed, or rupture, with hemoperitoneum . A hepatic hematoma rarely occurs in the absence of preeclampsia or HELLP .It is characterized by abdominal pain and many have severe thrombocytopenia, shoulder pain, nausea, and vomiting. If hepatic rupture occurs, swelling of the abdomen from hemoperitoneum and shock is seen. The aminotransferases are elevated, and values of 4000 to 5000 IU/L can occasionally be seen. Imaging using CT or MR is more sensitive than ultrasonography for these lesions. The management of a contained hematoma is to support the patient with volume replacement and blood transfusion, as needed, with consideration of percutaneous embolization of the hepatic arteries. It takes months for the hematoma to resolve completely. Surgical intervention is indicated if there is hemodynamic instability, persistent bleeding, increasing pain, or continued expansion of the hematoma. Operative management includes packing, drainage, hepatic artery ligation, and/or resection of affected areas of the liver. For patients with intractable hemorrhage, administration of recombinant factor VIIa and liver transplantation are recommended. Patients who survive have no hepatic sequelae.

Postpartum couse – Decreasing platelet counts continue until 24 to 48 hours after delivery, while serum LDH concentration usually peaks 24 to 48 hours postpartum. An upward trend in platelet count and a downward trend in LDH concentration should be seen by the fourth postpartum day in the absence of complications. Recovery can be delayed in women with DIC, platelet count less than 20,000 cells/uL, renal dysfunction or ascites.

Outcome is generally good; however, serious complications are relatively common. In a series of 437 women with HELLP syndrome at a tertiary care facility, the following complications were observed DIC – 21 %, Abruptio placentae – 16 %, Acute renal failure – 8 %, Pulmonary edema – 6 %, Subcapsular liver hematoma – 1%, Retinal detachment – 1 %. In addition, 55 % of the patients required blood or blood products, and 2 % required laparotomies for intraabdominal bleeding. 1 % died. Other complications include: adult respiratory distress syndrome, sepsis, and stroke. Wound complications secondary to bleeding and hematomas are common in women with thrombocytopenia. Fetal complications include prematurity (70 %), intrauterine growth restriction and abruptio placenta, and depend largely upon the severity of the disease and the gestational stage. The overall perinatal mortality is 7 to 20 %. However, surviving babies do not have an increased risk of liver disease or thrombocytopenia. Although most liver function tests return to normal postpartum , rarely high total bilirubin may be seen in 20 % even till 3 years post partum. HELLP syndrome with or without renal failure does not affect long-term renal function. The rate of recurrence is 2 - 27 %. Recurrent hepatic rupture in a subsequent pregnancy have been reported, suggesting there may be a genetic predisposition to this condition. Women with a history of HELLP syndrome are at high risk for developing preeclampsia in a subsequent pregnancy. The incidence of preeclampsia varies from 20-50 percent in normotensive women to 75 percent in those with underlying hypertension. There is no evidence that any therapy prevents recurrent HELLP syndrome.

2.1.5 Microangiopathies

Microangiopahy is seen in pre eclampsia. Two other important conditions where microangiopathy in pregnancy is seen are Thrombotic thrombocytopenic purpura (TTP) and hemolytic uremic syndrome (HUS) which are characterized by thrombocytopenia, hemolytic anemia, and multiorgan failure. Incidence is 1 in 25,000 births. TTP is known for central nervous system involvement, while HUS predominantly affects the kidneys. Significant overlap exists in the clinical manifestations of TTP and HUS.

Pathogenesis of microangiopathies -Normally the endothelium is smooth and platelets do not adhere to the endothelium. In microangiopathies the endothelium is damaged and there is formation of thrombi. Complement activation plays an important role in endothelial damage.

Role of complement-Complement is a system of serum proteins.The complement cascade is activated through three pathways (i.e., classical, lectin, and alternative pathways) that converge in the generation of C3 convertase. Because the alternative pathway is initiated spontaneously, the alternative C3 convertase (C3bBb) is tightly regulated by plasma and membrane-bound factors, mainly factor H (FH), factor I(FI), membrane cofactor protein (MCP), and decay-accelerating factor (DAF).Complement activation leads to endothelial damage.

Role of platelets-Platelets are nonnucleated cells derived from megakaryocytes in the bone marrow and normally live in the peripheral circulation for as long as 10 days. Platelets play a critical initiating role in the hemostatic system. Primary hemostasis begins when platelets adhere to the site of endothelial disruption, leading to platelet clumping. This is followed by platelet activation, characterized by release of granules containing von Willebrand factor, adenosine 5'-diphosphate (ADP), and serotonin. This attracts other platelets into the platelet plug, which stops the bleeding. Simultaneously, the synthesis of thromboxane A_2 and release of serotonin leads to vasoconstriction to reduce blood loss at the site of vascular injury. The secondary hemostatic phase begins when the coagulation pathway is activated on the surface of the activated platelets to form a secondary thrombus with fibrin. Abnormal intravascular platelet aggregation leads to microthrombi formation, which results in thrombocytopenia, intravascular hemolysis from the breakage of red blood cells through partially occluded vessels, and end organ ischemia.

Genesis of thrombocytopenia-The platelet count in nonpregnant women is 150,000-400,000/µ L. Average platelet count in pregnancy is decreased (213,000/µ L vs 250,000/µ L). Low platelet count is due to hemodilution, increased platelet consumption, and increased platelet aggregation driven by increased levels of thomboxane A_2.Thrombocytopenia can be defined as platelet count less than 150,000/uL or platelet count below the 25 th percentile for pregnant patients (116,000/µ L). In pregnancy mild,moderate and severe thrombocytopenia are defined as platelet count of 100,000-150,000/µL; 50,000-100,000/µ L and <50,000/µ L respectively.

Development of TMA-An acquired or constitutional deficiency in ADAMTS13, a von Willebrand factor (vWF)-processing enzyme, is an important cause of of a peculiar type of TMA. ADAMTS13 levels fall during the last two trimesters of pregnancy, hence TTP is more common at this time. (Fadi Fakhouri, 2010).

Development of HUS-The pathogenesis of pregnancy-associated atypical hemolytic uremic syndrome (P-aHUS) remains obscure and viral illness, retained placental fragments, drugs eg oxytocics, ergot and oral contraceptives have been implicated. The severe deficiency in the von Willebrand factor cleaving protease (ADAMTS13) seen in TTP is rarely present in patients with HUS. P-aHUS may be related to alternative C3 convertase dysregulation. A lack of control of the alternative C3 convertase leads to complement-induced lesions of the endothelial cells. Acquired (anti-FH antibodies) or constitutional (inactivating mutations in FH, FI, or MCP coding genes or activating mutations in factor B and C3 coding genes) with dysregulation of the alternative C3 convertase has been established as a risk factor for the occurrence of aHUS. It is assumed that excessive activation of the alternative C3 convertase leads to complement activation. Pregnancy may trigger the onset or subsequent relapses. Mutations in the SCR19-20 domains of factor H are less frequent in P-aHUS patients compared with non-pregnancy-related aHUS.

2.1.5.1 Hemolytic uremic syndrome(HUS)/Idiopathic post partum failure

It occurs in primipara and is characterized by renal failure, anemia and hypertension. The risk for P-aHUS is highest during a second pregnancy. Onset is within hours to days post partum. Symptoms can begin before delivery, but the onset in most cases is delayed for 48 hours or more after delivery (mean four weeks). HUS may follow a normal pregnancy or be preceded by findings indistinguishable from preeclampsia. HUS with severe renal failure more frequently presents in the postpartum period. Presenting symptoms are often nonspecific , although majority (60%) present with bleeding. Hypertension is seen in 75% of cases. Hemolysis and anemia may be absent at presentation in 50% of cases. DIC is rare.

Labs - Obligate findings include hemolytic anemia (hematocrit < 30% with schistocytes on peripheral smear) and thrombocytopenia under 100,000/µ L (50% of patients will have counts < 20,000/µ L). LDHis usually >600 U/liter. Hemolytic anemia is coomb's negative. There may be hypocomplemententemia, deficiency in prostaglandins or antithrombin levels. HUS is a clinical diagnosis. Tissue biopsy is not required. In problematic cases when renal biopsy is done it shows mesangiolysis and glomerular simplification.

Outcomes- The outcomes are poor. 80-90% survive acute episode. There is a high maternal mortality of 18-44% and fetal loss is seen in 80%. 62% reached ESRD by 1 month. Outcomes do not differ between patients with pregnancy-related and non-pregnancy-related aHUS. Pregnancies in female patients with complement abnormalities are complicated by fetal loss and preeclampsia in 4.8% and 7.7%,respectively. (Fadi Fakhouri,2010) Almost half have residual neurologic or chronic renal failure. Recurrences occur in 50%. Long-term sequelae, such as hypertension and chronic renal failure, are observed in 44% of patients with HUS. The perinatal mortality rate is as high as 30%.

Treatment includes Plasmapheresis. Plasma infusion alone is less effective. Steroids, anti-platelet therapy, Immunoabsorption, splenectomy, IV gamma globulin therapy have been used in different studies. Renal failure is managed by hemodialysis. Antihypertensives are used for control of blood pressure. Platelet transfusions should be avoided. Heparin and fibrinolytic agents and anti thrombin III concentrates may be used. Dilatation and curettage should be considered when the disease occurs very close to delivery.

2.1.5.2 Thrombotic thrombocytopenic purpura

TTP is characterized by the pentad of microangiopathic hemolytic anemia, thrombocytopenia, renal insufficiency, fever, and neurologic abnormalities. TTP usually occurs antepartum , about 12 % in the first trimester, 56 % in the second trimester, and 33 % in the third trimester/postpartum(Egerman RS, 1996), There may be mild renal failure and severe neurological involvement (headache, altered consciousness, seizures, hemiparesis), and fever. Severe thrombocytopenia and hemolytic anemia may be seen. Examination shows petechiae, ecchymoses, and nose and gum bleeding . Rarely hematuria, gastrointestinal bleeding and intracranial bleeding may occur. Bleeding associated with surgery is uncommon unless the platelet counts are lower than 50,000/µ L. Clinically significant spontaneous bleeding is rare unless counts fall below 10,000/µ L.

Treatment

Plasmapheresis is the recommended therapy. Plasmapheresis removes platelet-aggregating substances causing TTP. Treatment is 90% successful with TTP but is less successful with HUS. Steroids are used along with plasmapheresis. However, steroids are less effective than plasmapheresis (25% response rate).Platelet transfusions should be avoided when possible because they can cause a clinical deterioration. Platelet transfusions should be used only for uncontrolled bleeding or intracranial hemorrhage. Other therapies include immunosuppressive agents (vincristine, azathioprine, cyclosporine)and splenectomy for TTP. Premature termination of pregnancy has been associated with relapse. Delivery should be considered only when no response to other therapies occurs. (George JN, 2010)

Differential diagnosis

TTP, HUS and preeclampsia need to be differentiated as prognosis and treatment vary. The distinction between HUS-TTP and severe preeclampsia is often difficult. TTP is characterized by severe thrombocytopenia, hemolytic anemia, neurologic abnormalities (headache, altered consciousness, seizures, hemiparesis), and fever. Renal involvement may occur in 80% of cases of TTP; TTP occurs in 2nd /3rd trimester . von Willebrand factor-cleaving protease (ADAMTS-13) activity <5 percent is seen in 33 to 100 percent of women with TTP.Unlike HELLP the condition may continue or worsen after delivery with TTP. If suspected preeclampsia/HELLP does not improve within 48-72 hours after delivery, consider TTP. TTP like HUS is associated with isolated platelet consumption; thus, although thrombocytopenia is seen, the other findings of DIC are typically absent. A peripheral blood smear can also be useful. The percentage of schistocytes on peripheral smear is higher in TTP (2 to 5 percent).

HUS is characterized by thrombocytopenia, hemolytic anemia, acute renal failure with proteinuria, hematuria, or oliguria/anuria). Neurological manifestations are uncommon. The absence of DIC, onset more than two days after delivery, and/or persistent disease for more than one week are the main findings that characterize HUS. Neurologic involvement may be seen in 50% of cases of HUS. A peripheral blood smear can also be useful. The percentage of schistocytes on peripheral smear is higher in HUS (2 to 5 percent).ADAMTS deficiency is rare in HUS.

History of preceding proteinuria and hypertension favor preeclampsia , preeclampsia-HELLP does not occur before 20 weeks of gestation and most cases are diagnosed in the third trimester. Delivery leads to resolution with preeclampsia, HELLP is associated with thrombocytopenia, and in severe cases, there may be DIC with prolongation of the PT and aPTT, and reductions in the plasma concentrations of factors V and VIII. The percentage of schistocytes on peripheral smear is low (<1%). ADAMTS deficiency is not seen in PIH.

In addition, only a few select laboratories are able to perform complement-associated mutational analysis. Studies of larger heterogeneous populations need to be performed before recommending genetic analysis for patients with pregnancy-associated TTP-HUS. It has not been shown that distinguishing TTP from HUS alters treatment of such patients.

2.1.6 Antepartum and post partum hemorrhage

Significant blood loss due to antepartum or postpartum hemorrhage may cause ischemic injury and lead to obstetric acute renal failure.

Antepartum hemorrhage may be due to placenta praevia or concealed hemorrhage due to abruptio placentae which is usually associated with PIH. Treatment consists of intravascular volume repletion and blood transfusions. If the acute renal failure is due to pre renal intravascular volume depletion and is corrected rapidly the patient may recover without dialysis. However if the insult is prolonged it may lead to acute tubular necrosis for which dialysis is needed.

2.1.7 Puerperal sepsis

It is an important cause of AKI. According to World Health Organization puerperal sepsis is defined as infection of the genital tract occurring at any time between the rupture of membranes or labor and the 42 day post partum in which 2 or more of the following are present: pelvic pains, fever oral temperature 38,5°C or higher on any occasion, abnormal vaginal discharge (example presence of pus), abnormal smell or foul odour of discharge, delayed uterine involution. The causative organisms are gram positive streptococcus pyogenes, staphylococcus aureus, coliforms,Chlamydia and Clostridium tetani. (Momoh ,2010)Causes are prolonged rupture of membranes, obstructed labour, frequent vaginal examinations, anemia, caesarean section etc. .The source of infection may be from the retained products of conception where there may be a history of foul smelling lochia and the retained products can be demonstrated on imaging. High vaginal swab culture may help to identify the causative organism. Other sources may be urinary tract infection or mastitis. Hence a detailed physical examination including the breast examination should be undertaken. Treatment consists of appropriate antibiotics according to the culture sensitivity reports. Surgery to remove the retained products or abscess drainage even hysterectomy in extreme cases may be needed.

2.1.8 Urinary Tract Infections (UTI)

Another important cause of renal failure in pregnancy is UTI. UTIs are the most common renal disease occurring during pregnancy and range from asymptomatic bacteriuria to pyelonephritis. UTIs have been associated with SGA babies, premature labor, IUD, anemia and hypertension in mother. In some cases upper UTI may be associated with renal failure. Pregnant females are at risk for development of UTIs (2-10%), because of anatomic and physiologic changes that occur in normal pregnancy.UTI may be classified as:

2.1.8.1 Asymptomatic bacteriuria

Bacteriuria occurs in 2 to 7 % of pregnancies, particularly in multiparous women, a similar prevalence as seen in nonpregnant women. A clean-voided specimen containing more than 1 lakh organisms per milliliter suggests infection. Bacteriuria often develops in the first month of pregnancy and is frequently associated with a reduction in concentrating ability. 30% of patients develop pyelonephritis if asymptomatic bacteriuria is left untreated. Universal screening is therefore recommended in all pregnant females. Screening for asymptomatic bacteriuria should be performed at 12 to 16 weeks gestation (or the first prenatal visit, if that occurs later). Rescreening is generally not performed in low risk women, but can be considered in women at high risk for infection (eg, presence of urinary tract anomalies, hemoglobin S, or preterm labor). Dipstick has a sensitivity of <50% and routine microscopy and culture are needed. Urinalysis with culture should be performed on a monthly basis after resolution. Treatment with a course of oral antibiotics (Nitrofurantoin 100 mg orally every 12 hours for five to seven days, Ampicillin ,Amoxicillin (500 mg orally every 12 hours for three to seven days), Amoxicillin-clavulanate (500 mg orally every 12 hours for three to seven days),Cephalexin (500 mg orally every 12 hours for three to seven days) and Fosfomycin (3 g orally as a single dose)and sulphonamides are some of the safe regimes. Treatment reduces incidence of pyelonephritis to 3%. Fluoroquinolones should be avoided in pregnancy. The safest course is to avoid using nitrofurantoin in the first trimester if another antibiotic that is safe and effective is available. Sulfonamides should be avoided in the last days before delivery because they can increase the level of unbound bilirubin in the neonate. Trimethoprim (FDA category C) is generally avoided in the first trimester because it is a folic acid antagonist, has caused abnormal embryo development in experimental animals, and some case control studies have reported a possible association with a variety of birth defects. Ceftrioxone should be avoided the day before parturition because it displaces bilirubin and may cause kernicterus. Recurrence occurs in 35%. If bacteriuria is persistent, suppressive therapy (Nitrofurantoin 50-100 mg at night , cephalexin 250-500 mg or amoxycillin) is indicated.

2.1.8.2 Cystitis

Cystitis (3%) is associated with dysuria, urgency and frequency, without systemic signs. It usually occurs in 2nd trimester and is common even in patients with negative urine cultures. Though cystitis recurs in 17% it does not progress to acute pyelonephritis. It should be aggressively treated with oral antibiotic regimens. The symptoms of cystitis and pyuria accompanied by a "sterile" urine culture finding may be due to *Chlamydia trachomatis* urethritis. There may be mucopurulent cervicitis, hence erythromycin therapy is effective.

2.1.8.3 Pyelonephritis-(3%)

Majority (70%) patients with PN have asymptomatic bacteriuria. 50% cases occur in 2 nd trimester. Onset is abrupt with fever, chills, flank pain, anorexia, nausea, vomiting and costovertebral tenderness. The etiologic organisms include *Escherichia coli*, *Klebsiella*, *Enterobacter* and *Proteus* . 10% are due to Gram+ organsisms. 15% patients have concurrent bacteremia. Other complications include hemolysis, sepsis, adult respiratory distress syndrome, hepatic dysfunction and death. Pyelonephritis requires hospitalization and intravenous antibiotics and fluids till fever resolves. Effective regimens include ampicillin plus gentamicin or a third-generation cephalosporin followed by oral administration of antibiotics for 14 days .This leads to complete resolution of infection in 70%. Antibiotics can be further adjusted according to culture sensitivity results. In infections recurring in 2 weeks, 2-3 wks of treatment and suppressive therapy throughout the pregnancy should be given. Post coital cephalexin 250mg or NFT 50 mg may be preventive. Perinephric or cortical abscesses may be seen. Although renal function is well maintained during acute pyelonephritis, some pregnant women develop acute renal failure. Renal biopsy may reveal focal microabscesses and recovery after antimicrobial therapy may be incomplete due to irreversible injury.

2.1.9 Acute Fatty Liver of Pregnancy (AFLP)

It is a rare complication of pregnancy. AFLP is unique to pregnancy. There is no predilection for any geographical area or race. It occurs more commonly in nullipara and primipara than multipara. It was first described in 1940 by Sheehan as an "acute yellow atrophy of the liver". The incidence of AFLP is 1 case per 20,000 births in the UK. Incidence of AFLP from non-UK studies based on hospital case series estimate 1 in 4000 deliveries to 1 in 16000 births. AFLP is associated with AKI in 60%. AFLP occurs in the third trimester or the immediate period after delivery however it can be seen as early as 26 weeks of gestation. (Buytaert,1996) It is due to mutation in enzyme for long chain 3 hydroxy acyl CoA dehydrogenase leading to disordered metabolism of fatty acids by mitochondria in the mother. The most common mutation found in acute fatty liver of pregnancy is the E474Q missense mutation (IJlst L,1997) This gene mutation is recessive; therefore, in non pregnant state, women have normal fatty acid oxidation. However, if the fetus is homozygous for this mutation, it will be unable to oxidize fatty acids. These acids are passed to the mother, who, because of diminished enzyme function, cannot metabolize the additional fatty acids. This results in hepatic strain leading to the development of AFLP, which can be relieved by delivery of the infant. The accumulation of long-chain 3-hydroxyacyl metabolites produced by the fetus or placenta is toxic to the liver and may be the cause of the liver disease. It is characterized by jaundice, hypoalbuminemia, mild renal failure, DIC, PIH, hypoglycemia, pancreatitis and encephalopathy. Laboratory findings may be consistent with disseminated intravascular coagulation (DIC), specifically, prolongation of prothrombin time, low fibrinogen, and low antithrombin levels. This results in a clinical picture similar to DIC; however, in AFLP, the values are abnormal, not due to consumption of the clotting factors but rather to decreased production by the damaged liver. Bilirubin levels are elevated. This elevation is primarily the conjugated form, with levels exceeding 5 mg/dL. This can result in jaundice, which is rarely seen in patients with other forms of pregnancy-related hepatic injury, including preeclampsia. The diagnosis should be suspected in a woman with preeclampsia who has hypoglycemia, hypofibrinogenemia, and a prolonged PTT in the absence of abruptio placentae, high bilirubin, normal/ high transaminases, microvesicular steatosis and rarely liver necrosis. Criteria for diagnosis of AFLP include six or more of the following features in the absence of another explanation: Vomiting, abdominal pain, polydipsia / polyuria, encephalopathy, elevated bilirubin, hypoglycemia, elevated urate, leucocytosis (>11x109/l), ascites or bright liver on ultrasound scan, elevated transaminases (aspartate aminotransferase or alanine aminotransferase >42 IU/l), elevated ammonia, renal impairment, coagulopathy (prothrombin time >14 s or activated partial thromboplastin time >34 s), microvesicular steatosis on liver biopsy. (Ch'ng,2002). The liver biopsy is diagnostic but is not always feasible especially in patients with severe coagulopathy (Bacq, 2006) and it seldom influences acute management. Ultrasound and computed tomography have been used but false negative results are common. Renal biopsy shows Acute tubular necrosis (ATN). Delivery of the fetus, regardless of gestational age, is the only treatment for acute fatty liver of pregnancy (AFLP) once the diagnosis has been made. Treatment includes intravenous fluids, cryoprecipitate, Fresh frozen Plasma and glucose. It reverses with delivery. C section is preferred over vaginal delivery. Liver transplant is the treatment of choice in patients with liver necrosis. There is 20-25% maternal and fetal mortality and the syndrome can recur in subsequent pregnancies with a calculated genetic risk of 25%.The other causes of jaundice during pregnancy include cholestasis, cholelithiasis, viral hepatitis and pre-eclampsia with or without HELLP syndrome. Intrahepatic cholestasis of pregnancy may present during the third trimester but itching is the characteristic symptom and serum bilirubin concentration is rarely higher than 6mg/ dl. Cholelithiasis may occur at any time during pregnancy and is accompanied by pain in the right upper quadrant, and fever, and

USG is usually diagnostic. Acute viral hepatitis in pregnancy presents as a systemic illness with fever, nausea, vomiting, fatigue, and jaundice, however, aminotransferase concentrations are markedly elevated (>500U/liter). The manifestations of pre-eclampsia are usually observed in the second half of pregnancy, whereas the symptoms of HELLP syndrome and AFLP frequently appear in the third trimester. The incidence of HELLP syndrome is much higher (1:5,000). Morbidity of the infant includes increased risk of cardiomyopathy, neuropathy, myopathy, nonketotic hypoglycemia, hepatic failure, and death associated with fatty acid oxidation defects in newborns.

2.1.10 Urinary tract obstruction

Functional hydronephrosis rarely cause renal failure. The diagnosis can be established in some cases by the normalization of renal function in the lateral recumbent position and its recurrence when supine. In some cases, either insertion of a ureteral catheter or delivery of the fetus is required. Rarely, acute urinary tract obstruction in pregnancy is induced by a kidney stone.

2.1.11 Antiphospholipid Syndrome (APS)

It refers to a syndrome characterized by arterial or venous thrombosis or specific pregnancy complications in women with laboratory evidence of antibodies to proteins bound to anionic phospholipids. International consensus conferences have proposed and revised classification criteria for definite APS (Sapporo criteria)(Miyakis 2006). Definite APS is considered present if at least one of the following clinical criteria and at least one of the following laboratory criteria are satisfied.

1. Clinical —(a)Thrombosis — Unequivocal imaging or histologic evidence of thrombosis in any tissue or organ, OR (b) Pregnancy morbidity - Otherwise unexplained death at ≥10 weeks gestation of a morphologically normal fetus, OR One or more premature births before 34 weeks of gestation because of eclampsia, preeclampsia, or placental insufficiency, OR Three or more embryonic (<10 week gestation) pregnancy losses unexplained by maternal or paternal chromosomal abnormalities or maternal anatomic or hormonal causes.
2. Laboratory — The presence of antiphospholipid antibodies (aPL), on two or more occasions at least 12 weeks apart and no more than five years prior to clinical manifestations, as demonstrated by one or more of the following: (a)IgG and/or IgM aCL in moderate or high titer (>40 units GPL or MPL or > 99th percentile for the testing laboratory),(b)Antibodies to ß2-glycoprotein-I (ß2-GP-I) of IgG or IgM isotype at a titer >99th percentile for the testing laboratory when tested according to recommended procedures.(c)Lupus anticoagulant (LA) activity detected according to published guidelines

Clinical manifestations include deep vein thrombosis, thrombocytopenia, livedo reticularis, stroke, superficial thrombophlebitis, pulmonary embolism, fetal loss, transient ischemic attack, and hemolytic anemia. In rare patients, APS results in multiorgan failure because of multiple blood vessel occlusions, a condition referred to as "catastrophic antiphospholipid syndrome" In patients with preeclampsia or the HELLP syndrome, catastrophic APS must be considered, in patients with histories of thrombosis or spontaneous abortions . Thrombotic renal disease occurs in a minority of patients with APS. Glomerular capillaries and other renal vessels, both arteries and veins of all sizes, can be affected. The disease may be silent or produce acute or chronic renal failure with proteinuria. APLS may cause glomerular lesions like membranous nephropathy, minimal change disease or proliferative glomerulonephritis.

Laboratory diagnosis

A history of a biologic false positive serologic test for syphilis (BFPTS) may be a clue to the presence of any type of aPL: aCL, ß2-GP-I antibodies, or an LA. However, because of the nonspecific nature of the BFPTS, the presence of one or more aPL should be confirmed with one of the tests (A)The presence of aPL may be demonstrated directly by: ELISA testing in the case of aCL and antibodies to ß2-GP-I and (B) Clotting assay that demonstrates effects of an aPL on the phospholipid-dependent factors in the coagulation cascade (LA test).The lupus anticoagulant phenomenon refers to the ability of aPL to cause prolongation of in vitro clotting assays such as the activated partial thromboplastin time (aPTT), the dilute Russell viper venom time (dRVVT), the kaolin clotting time or, the prothrombin time. This prolongation is not reversed when the patient's plasma is diluted 1:1 with normal platelet-free plasma.

Treatment includes heparin, oral anticoagulants ie warfarin, antiplatelet drugs eg aspirin and clopidogrel and hydroxyl chloroquin.

2.1.12 Miscellaneous causes

The other miscellaneous causes of acute renal failure in pregnancy include Acute gastroenteritis, infections ,drugs and other causes similar to the varied causes of AKI in non pregnant states.

2.2 Pathology

Pathology of pregnancy related AKI varies with etiology.

2.2.1 Glomerular endotheliosis

It is the typical finding in PIH. Glomeruli look enlarged and the endothelial cells are swollen. This lesion was first described by Spargo. It resolves by the end of post partum period.

2.2.2 Acute tubular necrosis

May be seen in cases of ischemic or toxic insult.

2.2.3 Acute interstitial nephritis

May be commonly due to infection or drug.

2.2.4 Cortical necrosis

It is one of the dreaded histopathological lesions . 50% of all cortical necrosis is pregnancy related. Causes include Abruptio (esp if concealed hemorrhage), septic abortion, placenta previa, prolonged IUD, or amniotic fluid embolism. It is commoner in post partum than antepartum AKI. Renal cortical necrosis may be patchy or total. The triad of anuria, gross hematuria, and flank pain seen in cortical necrosis is unusual in the other causes of renal failure in pregnancy. The diagnosis can be established by ultrasonography which shows a subcapsular hypoechoic band . Renal calcifications on plain film of the abdomen suggest cortical necrosis (6 weeks). CT scanning demonstrates hypoechoic or hypodense areas in renal cortex or may demonstrate cortical tram track calcification by 3 weeks. Angiogram shows abrupt cut off of vascularity which is called pruning. No specific therapy is effective. Many patients develop chronic kidney disease. In our study from Osmania General Hospital, Hyderabad, India over 7 years there were total of 105 patients with Renal cortical necrosis (RCN). The mean age was 28.125 ± 12.40 years. Forty one cases (39.04%) resulted from obstetric complications. The most common histology type of RCN was patchy cortical necrosis in 65 patients (62%). All patients required dialysis and the mean duration of dialysis was 3 ± 1weeks. Thirty three (31.42%) patients progressed to end stage kidney disease while 3 underwent renal transplantation. 10(9.5%) patients succumbed to the acute kidney injury (AKI).(Manisha Sahay)

2.2.5 Vascular changes

May be seen in HUS with glomerular and arteriolar fibrinoid necrosis and thrombi. Glomeruli show mesangiolysis and glomerular simplification.

2.3 Dialysis in pregnancy

Early dialysis is necessary in pregnant women with renal failure and should be considered when the serum creatinine reaches 3.5 mg/dL or the glomerular filtration rate (GFR) is less than 20 mL/min or blood urea nitrogen is more than 100mg/dl. Longer, more frequent dialysis (20 h/wk) is associated with the best fetal outcome. Hemodialysis may therefore be necessary at least 5 days per week. Careful avoidance of hypotension is important. As pregnancy is a procoagulant state the dose of heparin needs to be increased. Peritoneal dialysis with smaller volumes and frequent exchanges is another option. Peritoneal dialysis may be difficult in the third trimester due to increased uterine size. Premature labor and fetal size that is small for the gestational age are typical in women who deliver on dialysis. Nutritional support that allows weight gains of 0.3 to 0.5 kg/wk should be maintained in the second and third trimesters. Although the spontaneous abortion rate is approximately 50% for pregnant women who require dialysis, the fetal survival rate for pregnancies that continue is as high as 71%.

3. References

ACOG practice bulletin. Diagnosis and management of preeclampsia and eclampsia. Number 33, January 2002.ACOG Committee on Practice Bulletins—Obstetrics,Obstet Gynecol. 2002;99(1):159.

American College of Obstetrics and Gynecology (2004)ACOG (American College of Obstetrics and Gynecology) Practice Bulletin: nausea and vomiting of pregnancy. Obstet Gynecol. ;103(4):803.

August P, Mueller FB, Sealey JE, Edersheim TG. (1995) Role of rennin angiotensin system in blood pressure regulation in pregnancy. *Lancet*, 345:896–897.

Ananth Karumanchi S ,Franklin H Epstein (2007)Renal complications in pregnancy In *Comprehensive Clinical Nephrology: edn 3rd Edited by John Feehally, Jurgen Floege, Richard J. Johnson .Mosby Elsevier* .483-504.

Bacq Y. (2006)The liver in pregnancy. In: Schiff ER, Sorrell MF, Schiff L, Maddrey WC, editors. Schiff's Diseases of the liver. 10th ed. Lippincott Williams and Wilkins (LWW); .p. 1281-1304.

Baylis C: (1987) Glomerular filtration and volume regulation in gravid animal models. *Clin Obstet Gynaecol* , 1:789.

Baylis,C, John M Davidson: Renal Physiology in normal pregnancy.(2007) *In Comprehensive Clinical Nephrology: edn 3rd Edited by John Feehally, Jurgen Floege, Richard J. Johnson .Mosby Elsevier*,475-481.

Beaufils MB. Pregnancy. In: Davidson AM, Cameron JS, Grunfeld JP, et al., editors. (2005)*Clinical nephrology*. 3rd ed. New York: Oxford University Press; pp. 1704–28.

Buytaert IM; Elewaut GP; Van Kets HE. (1996) Early occurrence of acute fatty liver in pregnancy. Am J Gastroenterol Mar; 91(3):603-4.

Ch'ng CL, Morgan M, Hainsworth I, et al. (2002)Prospective study of liver dysfunction in pregnancy in Southwest Wales. Gut; 51: 876–80.

Chugh KS. (1987) Etiopathogenesis of acute renal failure in the tropics. *Ann Natl Acad Med Sci (India)*;23:88–99.

Egerman RS, Witlin AG, Friedman SA, Sibai BM. (1996) Thrombotic thrombocytopenic purpura and hemolytic uremic syndrome in pregnancy: review of 11 cases. *Am J Obstet Gynecol.* ;175(4 Pt 1):950-6.

Fadi Fakhouri, Lubka Roumenina,Franc¸ ois Provot,Marion Salle´ e,Sophie Caillard, Lionel Couzi,Marie Essig, David Ribes, Marie-Agne` s Dragon-Durey, Frank Bridoux,Eric Rondeau,and Veronique Fre´ meaux-Bacchi (2010)Pregnancy-Associated Hemolytic Uremic Syndrome Revisited in the Era of Complement Gene Mutations J Am Soc Nephrol 21: 859–867.

George JN (2010) How I treat patients with thrombotic thrombocytopenic purpura: Blood.;116(20):4060.

Hou S. (1998) The kidney in pregnancy. *In: Greenberg A. Primer on Kidney Diseases. 2nd ed. Academic Press;* :388-394.

IJlst L, Oostheim W, Ruiter JP, Wanders RJ (1997). "Molecular basis of long-chain 3-hydroxyacyl-CoA dehydrogenase deficiency: identification of two new mutations". J. Inherit. Metab. Dis. 20 (3): 420–422

Levine, RJ, Lam, C, Qian, C, et al. (2006) Soluble endoglin and other circulating antiangiogenic factors in preeclampsia. N Engl J Med; 355:992.

Lindheimer MD, Katz AI(1991) : The kidney and hypertension in pregnancy.In *The Kidney, edn 4. Edited by Brenner BM, Rector FC. Philadelphia:WB Saunders Co;* :1551–1595.

Levi M (2009) Disseminated intravascular coagulation (DIC) in pregnancy and the peri-partum period. Thromb Res. 2009;123 Suppl 2:S63.

Lucas MJ, Leveno KJ, Cunningham FG (1995) A comparison of magnesium sulfate with phenytoin for the prevention of eclampsia. N Engl J Med. 333(4):201.

Manisha Sahay Cortical necrosis in tropics, accepted for publication, Saudi journal of Kidney disease and transplantation .

Maynard S, Min J, Merchan J, Lim K, Li J, Mondal S, Libermann T, Morgan J, Sellke F, Stillman I, Epstein F, Sukhatme V, Karumanchi S (2003). "Excess placental soluble fms-like tyrosine kinase 1 (sFlt1) may contribute to endothelial dysfunction, hypertension, and proteinuria in preeclampsia". *J Clin Invest* 111 (5): 649–58.

M.A. Momoh, O.J. Ezugworie and H.O. Ezeigwe (2010) Causes and Management of Puerperal Sepsis: The Health Personnel View Point Advances in Biological Research 4 (3): 154-158.

Miyakis S, Lockshin MD, Atsumi T, Branch DW, Brey RL, Cervera R, Derksen RH, DE Groot PG, Koike T, Meroni PL, Reber G, Shoenfeld Y, Tincani A, Vlachoyiannopoulos PG, Krilis SA(2006) International consensus statement on an update of the classification criteria for definite antiphospholipid syndrome (APS).J Thromb Haemost. ;4(2):295.

Naqvi R, Akthar F, Ahmad E, Shaikh R, Ahmed Z, Naqvi A, et al. (1996) Acute renal failure of obstetrical origin during 1994 at one centre. *Ren Fail.* ;18:681–3.

NHBPEP. Report of the National High Blood Pressure Education Program Working Group on High Blood Pressure in Pregnancy. (2000) *Am J Obstet Gynecol.* ;183(1):S1-S22.

Reubinoff BE, Schenker JG. HELLP syndrome--a syndrome of hemolysis, elevated liver enzymes and low platelet count--complicating preeclampsia-eclampsia. Int J Gynaecol Obstet 1991; 36:95.

Schrier RW, Gottschalk C. Kidney diseases in pregnancy. (1997) *In: Diseases of The Kidney. 6th ed. Lippincott Williams & Wilkins.*

Sheehan HL. The pathology of acute yellow atrophy and delayed chloroform poisoning. J Obstet Gynaecol Br Emp. 1940;47:49–62.

Sibai, BM, Villar, MA, Mabie, BC. (1990) Acute renal failure in hypertensive disorders of pregnancy. Pregnancy outcome and remote prognosis in thirty-one consecutive cases. *Am J Obstet Gynecol* ; 162:777.

Sibai, BM, Ramadan, MK. (1993) Acute renal failure in pregnancies complicated by hemolysis, elevated liver enzymes, and low platelets. *Am J Obstet Gynecol* ; 168:1682.

Stone JH. (1998) HELLP syndrome: hemolysis, elevated liver enzymes, and low platelets. JAMA 280:559.

Sibai BM, Taslimi MM, el-Nazer A, et al. (1986) Maternal-perinatal outcome associated with the syndrome of hemolysis, elevated liver enzymes, and low platelets in severe preeclampsia-eclampsia. Am J Obstet Gynecol; 155:501.

Sibai BM. (1990) The HELLP syndrome (hemolysis, elevated liver enzymes, and low platelets): much ado about nothing? Am J Obstet Gynecol; 162:311.

Sibai BM, Ramadan MK, Usta I, Salama M, Mercer BM, Friedman SAAm J Obstet Gynecol. 1993Maternal morbidity and mortality in 442 pregnancies with hemolysis, elevated liver enzymes, and low platelets (HELLP syndrome);169(4):1000.

Sibai BM (2004) Diagnosis, controversies, and management of the syndrome of hemolysis, elevated liver enzymes, and low platelet count. Obstet Gynecol.;103 (5 Pt 1):981.

Venkatesha, S; Toporsian M, Lam C, Hanai J, Mammoto T, Kim YM, Bdolah Y, Lim KH, Yuan HT, Libermann TA, Stillman IE, Roberts D, D'Amore PA, Epstein FH, Sellke FW, Romero R, Sukhatme VP, Letarte M, Karumanchi SA. (2006). "Soluble endoglin contributes to the pathogenesis of preeclampsia". *Nat Med* 12 (6): 642–9.

World Health Organization. 2009. Managing puerperal sepsis. Geneva Switzerland: WHO press.

Zhou, CC, Zhang, Y, Irani, RA, et al. (2008) Angiotensin receptor agonistic autoantibodies induce pre-eclampsia in pregnant mice. *Nat Med* ; 14:855.

Evaluation of Acute Kidney Injury in Intensive Care Unit

Itir Yegenaga
Department of Internal Medicine
University of Kocaeli Medical School, Kocaeli
Turkey

1. Introduction

Acute kidney injury (AKI), impairment of kidney function requires special attention in intensive care unit's (ICU), because if multiorgan failure affect the kidney, it carries a greater risk for worse outcome and furthermore survivors have higher risk then normal population for chronic renal failure. It was reported that they also have higher mortality and morbidity rates compared to normal population (Kellum, 2008 & Shiffle, 2006).

Acute tubular necrosis (ATN) is the primary causes of AKI in hospital and ICU and sepsis, ischemic or toxic insults were reported as the most common reason for ATN. The rates of AKI have been reported in hospitalized patients to be between 3.2%-20% and in ICUs this rate rises up to 22% and even to 67% depending on the population studied and the definition used (Murugan 2011). Based on the administrative data, the incidence of severe AKI (defined requiring dialysis) from 1988 to2002 has increased from 4 to 27 per 100000 population. But fortunately in hospital mortality, has decreased from 41.3 to28 % (p<0.001) (Waikar, 2008). Likewise a progressive 2.8% annual increase in incidence of AKI and progressive 3.8% annual decrease in AKI associated mortality(95%CI:-4.7 to-2.12:p<0.001) was observed from 1996-2005 in a large database in Australia and New Zealand (Pisoni, 2008&Bagshaw, 2007). Despite the fact that mortality might be decreasing in ICU patients with AKI, it is still high and reported to be up to 43-88%. Mortality rate becomes even higher when patients require renal replacement therapy (Kellum, 2008).

Interestingly, it was reported that irreversible AKI requiring chronic dialysis therapy increased from 3.7% in 1984 to 18.2% in 1995 in surviving patients. Even higher number of patients (33-68%) at discharge whose kidney failed to recover and who needed long term dialysis. This changing renal outcome in the survivors of ICU acquired AKI cases might be related to increasing number of older patients, several co morbid conditions, more severe AKI cases than before and in addition, complication of the more aggressive renal replacement therapies currently used (Shiffle, 2006).

Since AKI in critical ill patients have high mortality rate and even if patients survive, they are at risk for End Stage Renal Disease (ESRD) and higher mortality than the normal population, it is important to recognize the clinical picture of AKI and to institute prevention as early as possible. Thus, physician should be alarmed and be ready for early intervention in this particular group of patients. With the introduction of the RIFLE classification for the definition of AKI, the viewpoint of this subject has changed and now it is possible to be aware of patients with high risk for AKI(Bellomo 2004). Nevertheless recently several biomarkers have been introduced to diagnose AKI even before creatinine starts to increase(Waiker, 2008).

In this review, new perspective and favorable improvement of this subject will be discussed; furthermore definition, epidemiology, risk factors, biomarkers of AKI will be evaluated.

2. Definition

Patients in ICU comprise heterogeneous population, and around 30 different definitions were used to describe acute deterioration of renal failure, which both caused difficulties to interpret studies and to discuss the conclusions. Since even small changes in renal function makes prominent differences, it was suggested that re-evaluation of the definition of AKI was mandatory. For the consensus of the definition and improvement of the quality of studies on AKI, Acute Dialysis Quality Initiative (ADQI) group was established. They recommended the term of AKI instead of ARF, since spectrum of AKI is broader and covers different degrees of severity of the disease. In 2002, for a uniform definition of AKI, they described three categories for severity (Risk of ARF, Injury of the kidney, and Failure of kidney function) and two classes for kidney outcome (Loss of kidney function and ESRD), which is called shortly RIFLE criteria(Table1) (Bellomo, 2004). Since AKI is not a stable condition, definition based on changes in function seems to be more suitable. Two measures to reflect kidney function have been recommended for the purpose of definition of AKI; changes in serum creatinine level and urine output. Importantly, these criteria were validated based on ability to distinguish the patients with higher risk for the worst outcome (death and requirement for renal replacement therapy).

The RIFLE criteria have been validated in more then 550,000 patients worldwide. Many studies confirmed that a rise in mortality rates occurred with progressing RIFLE criteria in ICU cases (Murugan, 2011). RIFLE criteria validated in a study on two Turkish tertiary hospital ICU population. This study also showed that increasing mortality rate with increase in severity, difference in mortality rate between stages was statistically significant (χ^2=15.037, $p<0.001$) (Yegenaga, 2010).

Later on in 2007, ADQI group with worldwide collaboration of nephrologists and critical care societies developed Acute Kidney Injury Network (AKIN), which intends to improve worldwide coordination and provokes the development of uniform standards in the AKI area. RIFLE criteria were refined by this group and reported a new AKIN classification, which classified AKI in three stages (stages 1, 2, and 3) according to the degree of damage and outcome categories Loss and ESRD were removed (Mehta, 2007). The purpose of these modifications were to include a small but important group of patients with early and mild AKI who experience a change in renal function that is greater than physiological variation but less than the 50% increase required for the RIFLE criteria. Thus, an absolute increase in serum creatinine levels of at least 0.3mg/dl in 48 hours was recommended to include in stage 1. Patients who required renal replacement therapy (RRT) are classified as stage 3 AKI, regardless of their serum creatinine levels and urine output. Nevertheless there is no common worldwide guideline about the timing to initiate of RRT, using it as criteria to describe stage 3 may cause some misunderstandings. In particular, patients with underlying chronic kidney disease (CKD) may be missed by the original RIFLE criteria but not by AKIN since it counts even smaller changes in serum creatinine level. In addition, 48-hours time

	Serum Creatine Criteria	Urine output criteria
RIFLE class		
Risk	Serum creatine increase to 1.5-fold OR GFR decrease >25% from baseline	<0.5ml/kg/h for 6h
Injury	Serum creatine increase to 2.0-fold OR GFR decrease >50% from baseline	<0.5ml/kg/h for 12h
Failure	Serum creatine increase to 3.0-fold OR GFR decrease >75% from baseline OR serum creatine ≥354μmol/l (≥4mg/dl)with an acute increase of at least 44μmol/l (0.5mg/dl)	Anuria for 12h
AKIN Stage		
1	Serum creatine increase ≥ 26.5 μmol/l (0.3mg/dl) OR increase to 1.5-2.0-fold from baseline	<0.5ml/kg/h for 6h
2	Serum creatine increase ≥ 2.0-3.0 fold from baseline	<0.5ml/kg/h for 12h
3	Serum creatine increase >3.0-fold from baseline OR serum creatine ≥354μmol/l (≥4.0mg/dl) with an acute increase of at least 44μmol/l (0.5mg/dl) OR need for RRT	<0.3ml/kg/h for 24h OR anuria for 12h OR need for RRT

Table 1. Two definitions of AKI

interval for the diagnosis of AKI was introduced to ensure that the process is acute. Unlike RIFLE, in AKIN criteria there has been an attempt to resolve some easily reversible causes of azotemia (for example, volume depletion and urinary obstruction). AKIN criteria declare that diagnosis based on the urine criterion alone will require exclusion of urinary tract obstructions and other easily reversible causes of decreased urine output.

Determination of baseline renal function: Since AKI was defined as rapid decline in renal function from baseline levels, it is important how to measure baseline renal function. The baseline serum creatinine level has been recommended for use as a marker to reflect the renal function. The baseline serum creatinine value has been estimated in various ways, such as the serum creatinine level on hospital admission, the minimum creatinine level during the hospital stay, the serum creatinine value estimated from the MDRD calculation (assuming estimated GFR=75ml/min/1,73m^2) or the lowest value among these (Ricci,

2011). The choice of estimation technique used to obtain the baseline creatinine value has a marked effect on the prevalence of AKI, severity of disease, and mortality risk associated with various stages of AKI. When premorbid renal function is not known ADQI group has recommended back- estimation of the baseline serum creatinine level value using the MDRD formula. In a study, involving 4,863 hospitalized patents, investigators studied the performance of these three potential surrogates for the baseline serum creatinine level and they concluded that all three surrogates resulted in bidirectional misclassification of AKI. Although the use of serum creatinine level at admission found to be more specific in this study, this parameter had the lowest sensitivity (38.9%) for diagnosis of AKI (Siew, 2010).

Subgroup analysis of data from the Beginning and Ending Supportive Therapy for the Kidney (BEST) study also compared observed baseline serum creatinine levels with MDRD back estimated values to determine the RIFLE class. They found that MDRD back estimated serum creatinine value performed reasonably well for the determination of the RIFLE categories when premorbid renal function was near normal, but should be cautiously used in patients with suspected CKD (Bagshaw, 2009).

As a conclusion investigators should make every effort to find out true baseline creatinine level before using any estimated values. An appropriate baseline serum creatinine value should express normal renal function of patients, such as outpatients serum creatinine level measured within the past year (prefereably in the past 3 months). When an outpatient serum creatinine level is not available, serum creatinine level on admission to hospital or ICU could be used as a second choice. However, use of admission serum creatinine level is specific but insensitive, and may underestimate the incidence of AKI.

Which classification is better RIFLE or AKIN? Based on the studies to compare these two classifications; AKIN did not seem to show any improvement in the sensitivity and predictive ability of the definition and classification of AKI. Acute Physiology Score (SAPS)3 database in 2009 re-evaluated and compared the performance of the RIFLE and AKIN criteria (Joannidis, 2009). They concluded that RIFLE seems to be more sensitive for diagnosing AKI and to have a greater ability then AKIN criteria to predict the mortality. These data confirm that neither classification offers clear advantage over the other; and both systems still have some limitations. Similarly Bagshaw et al. compared AKIN classification and RIFLE criteria in 120,123 critically ill patients during the first 24 hours after admission to the ICU (Bagshaw, 2008). They concluded that AKIN classification did not improve the sensitivity and predictive ability of RIFLE criteria for the definition and classification of AKI in the first 24 hours in ICU. Based on these large database studies there is no evidence about superiority of any of these classifications. Both criteria can be used for the evaluation of critically ill patients, as long as the clinician is aware of the limitations mentioned above.

3. Etiology and risk factors for AKI

Early detection of AKI in ICU is crucial to perform early intervention and prevent further complications, thus it may be lifesaving to determine the risk factors for the impairment of the renal function.

The Program to Improve Care in Acute Renal Disease (PICARD) is prospective observational extensive cohort study, which was done in USA from 1999 to 2001 (Mehta,

2004). This study revealed that, etiology of AKI was ATN (acute tubular necrosis) in 50% of cases with no specific determined cause. The next most common etiologies included nephrotoxin administration (26%), cardiac disease (20%) including myocardial infarction, cardiogenic shock, and congestive heart failure, ATN from hypotension (12%), sepsis (19%), unresolved prerenal factors (16%) and liver disease (11%). They found that predictors of mortality using proportional hazards Cox regression at the day of diagnosis of ARF were age, BUN, liver failure. At the day of consultation; age, Log urine output, creatinine (<2mg/dl), BUN, liver failure, ARDS (acute respiratory distress syndrome) and platelet count were related to mortality. When the day renal replacement therapy started, the predictive factors for survival were found as age, platelet count, liver failure, sepsis or septic shock. Oliguria, sepsis, respiratory failure, and hepatic failure would be consistently associated with mortality in AKI (Chertow, 2006).

The largest cohort with most participant of AKI to date was the Beginning and Ending Supportive Therapy for Kidney (BEST) study (Uchino, 2005). Out of 29.269 critically ill patients, there were 1.738 (5.7%) patients with AKI. The most common cause of AKI was septic shock (47.5 %), followed by major surgery (34%), cardiogenic shock (27%), hypovolemia (26%) and nephrotoxin administration (19%). In-hospital mortality varied from 50.5% to 76.8% between centers. A multivariate logistic regression model to identify independent correlates of in-hospital mortality yielded several previously identified risk factors, including delayed diagnosis of AKI, age, sepsis, and known disease severity score that included BUN and urine output, which are consistent with the previous studies.

Based on the previous reports; most common and complicated cause of AKI in ICU was found as sepsis and its prevalence have been reported to be 9-40% (Brivet, 1996 & Liano, 1998 & Bellomo,2008). Therefore, we prospectively evaluated 257 patients with sepsis or systemic inflammatory response syndrome who were admitted to the surgical and medical ICU during 12 months in 2001 to determine the risk factors for acute renal failure (ARF) development (Yegenaga, 2004). In this study, ARF was defined as serum creatinine level >2 mg/dL, based on this definition out of 257, twentynine (11%) patients were diagnosed as ARF. Mortality rate was 72% in patient with sepsis and ARF and in those with sepsis without ARF this rate was found as low as to 24 %. Multivariate logistic regression analysis of data showed that older age (OR:1.1, CI:1.03-1.13) serum bilirubin >1.5 (OR:9.7, CI:1.65-60.3), higher baseline serum creatinine level (OR:1.02,CI:1.007-1.04), and higher central venous pressure (CVP) (OR:1.5,CI:1.26-1.80) were predictive for the development of ARF (Yegenaga, 2004). It was mandatory to evaluate fluid status of these patients, since it was found that CVP is an independent risk factor for the development of AKI (Van Biesen & Yegenaga, 2004). And subgroup analysis of these patients revealed that higher colloid fluid loading for the first 3 days (2037±1681vs 1116±1220, p<0.03) and lower diuresis (1347±649vs1849±916mL, p=0.005) was associated with poor outcomes and in addition interestingly the fraction of inspired oxygen (FiO2) needed to be increased significantly on the second day of sepsis in the ARF group but remained unchanged in non ARF group. These patients developed ARF despite further fluid loading and in addition, respiratory function deteriorated. Against the classical knowledge; this study brought up the idea that in critically ill patient fluid loading should be performed in cautious. It is more likely that in dehydrated patients fluid loading can prevent ARF development but in critical ill patients with sepsis it might bring more risk for ARF and also to increase the mortality rate (Payen, 2008).

A similar study was designed previously for the Turkish ICU population of two tertiary hospitals, and RIFLE criteria were used for the definition of AKI (Yegenaga, 2010). In this Turkish ICU population, AKI incidence was 56,8% including Risk of RIFLE, and mortality rate was 65% in AKI and and it was found 35% in non AKI group. In this study it was observed that mortality rate was correlated well with the severity of RIFLE criteria; in the risk group 56%, in injury 68%, and in failure it was found as 72%. Multivariate logistic regression revealed that unlike the previous study age and serum bilirubin level were not significant anymore, but SOFA score (OR: 1.49, CI:1.085-2.205, $p=0.045$), baseline serum creatinine level (OR: 1.87,CI:1.391-2.520, $p<0.001$), and every 1 liter of extra positive fluid balance (OR: 1.56, CI:1.029-2.373, $p=0.036$) were independent risk factors for AKI. This study also brought up the importance of fluid overload in critically ill patients with sepsis; despite more vasopressor use and more fluid resuscitation, kidney damage starts very early and that is difficult to reverse. Previously in this particular population fluid loading was known as early intervention, but based on the observation in this and in some other recent reports fluid therapy should be performed cautiously. It is claimed that fluid overload may increase intra-abdominal pressure, leading to abdominal compartment syndrome, which has been recently recognized as an important cause of AKI in critically ill patients (Schrier, 2004). Furthermore fluid overload has been demonstrated to cause other organ failure in addition to kidney in ICU patients (Malbraina, 2005); for example impairment of cardiac function, worsens the lung injury (Essen, 2002).

4. Biomarkers

The reduction in glomerular filtration rate (GFR) is the main abnormality which is responsible for the clinical picture of AKI. Since serum creatinine level (SCr) is negatively correlated with GFR value, SCr level has been used worldwide as a marker to estimate renal function for years. But it is understood now that creatinine may not be appropriate marker for couple of reasons to measure the GFR in AKI. Addition to tubular secretion; there are some factors which effect serum creatinine concentration for example; age, sex, muscle mass, metabolism of creatinine, and volume status. Therefore the measurement of SCr level only has very limited utility to evaluate total kidney function. It was understood that serum creatinine value is neither perfectly sensitive nor specific as a biomarker to determine GFR value. However Cystatin C was reported recently as the best alternative to SCr as an endogenous GFR marker and also it is able to predict AKI 1-2 days earlier than SCr. Cystatin C is a low molecular weight protein produced by all nucleated cells that is freely filtered by the glomerulus and then reabsorbed and metabolized by the proximal tubule (Herget-Rosenthal, 2005). Serum levels of Cystatin C are dependent not only on clearance but also on production rate and acute changes in volume of distribution. Higher dose of corticosteroid and hyperthyroidism may increase serum Cystatin C level and it may be decreased by hypothyroidism.

However, tubular cell injury may precede but not always lead to a reduction of GFR. The relationship between functional and structural changes in the kidney is inconsistent. For instance, in sepsis, changes in kidney function might be severe but in contrast histological findings may not be clear. The earliest sign of ischemic or nephrotoxic AKI may not be decreasing in GFR level, therefore in this particular condition biomarkers should be able to identify tubular injury even before GFR falls and increasing in serum SCr level. Furthermore early identification of kidney injury will be critical for future developments in treatment or prevention of AKI (Cruz, 2010).

Several more biomarkers of AKI have been introduced recently, Neutrophil Gelatinase-Associated Lipocaline (NGAL) also known as Lipocalin-2 or siderocalin is one of the best studied biomarker of AKI to date. And it is rapidly up-regulated in the blood and in urine post-AKI. It was reported that; even though Cystatin C seems to be a better marker for AKI then SCr, Urine NGAL is superior to Cystatin C for earlier detection of AKI. In fact, cystatin C is mainly a marker of clearance, and its serum concentration may increase only after the GFR begins to decrease. Unlikely, NGAL which is rapidly induced in kidney tubule cells in response to ischemic injury, and its appearance in urine and serum is independent of the GFR but is highly predictive of a subsequent decline in GFR (Mishra, 2003).

Another promising biomarker is KIM-1, a type-1 transmembrane glycoprotein that is highly expressed in proximal tubule cells after ischemic and nephrotoxic injury. In a study with patient undergoing cardiac surgery, urine KIM-1 levels peaked 12 hours after injury in AKI and predicted the need for dialysis or mortality in hospitalised patients. KIM-1 seems to be more specific to ischemic and nephrotoxic kidney injury than NGAL and it is not significantly affected by chronic kidney disease or urinary tract infection (Liangos, 2007).

A pro-inflamatory cytokine IL-18 was also reported to be up-regulated and easily detected in the urine of animals with ischemic AKI. In a study, urine IL-18 levels were found markedly increased in patient with AKI but not in the patients with urinary tract infection, chronic kidney disease, nephritic syndrome, and prerenal failure. Urinary IL-18 showed sensitivty > 90% and specifity>95% for the diagnosis of AKI (Parikh, 2008). Both urine IL-18 and NGAL were found as sequential predictive biomarkers of AKI in children undergoing cardiac surgery. The patients in whom AKI developed 2-3 days after surgery, urine NGAL peaked at 25 fold within 2 hours and declined 6 hours after surgery, whereas urine IL-18 levels peaked 12 hours after surgery (Parikh, 2006).

5. Conclusion

Since AKI increases mortality rate and significantly worsens patients' outcome, it is important to determine the patient with risk for AKI in ICU. The consensus has been achieved for the definition of AKI. This definition focuses on the association of hospital mortality, instead of renal failure requiring dialysis or clinical syndrome defined by pathology. Every patient who is admitted to the ICU should be evaluated and categorized based on the creatinine level. Furthermore, close follow-up of renal function is crucial. Recently introduced biomarkers can be used for early diagnosis of AKI even before SCr level starts to increase. During treatment of these patients intensivist should be alert against fluid overload which is described as an independent risk factor to develop AKI.

6. References

Kellum JA. Acute kidney injury. Crit Care Med 2008;36 (Suppl 4): S141-145.

Schiffl H. Renal recovery from acute tubular necrosis requiring renal replacement therapy: a prospective study in critically ill patients. Nephrol Dial Transplant 2006 21:1248-1252

Murugan R & Kellum JA. Acute kidney injury: What is the prognosis? Nat Rev Nephrol 2011, 7:209-2178

Waiker SS, Liu KD & Chertow GM. Diagnosis, epidemiology and outcome of acute kidney injury. Clin J Am Soc Nephrol 2008, 3:844-861

Bagshaw SM, George C & Bellomo R, ANZICS Database management committee, Changes in the incidence and outcome for early acute kidney inkury in a cohort of Australian intensive care units. Crit Care 2007,113):R68

Pisoni R, Wille KM & Tolwani AJ. The epidemiology of severe acute kidney injury: from BEST to PICARD, in acute kidney injury: New concepts. Nephron Clin Practice 2008, 109:c188-191

Bellomo R, Ronco C, Kellum JA, Mehta RL & Palevski P, and the ADQI workgroup. Acute renal failure - definition, outcome measures, animal models, fluid therapy and information technology needs: the Second International Consensus Conference of the Acute Dialysis Quality Initiative (ADQI) Group. Crit Care 2004;8;R204-212.

Yegenaga I, Tuglular S, Ari E, Etiler N, Baykara N, Torlak S, Acar S, Akbas T, Toker K & Solak ZM. Evaluation of sepsis/systemic inflammatory response syndrome, acute kidney injury, and RIFLE criteria in two tertiary hospital intensive care units in Turkey. Nephron Clin Pract 2010;115:c276-282.

Mehta RL, Kellum JA, Shah SV, Molitoris BA, Ronco C, Warnock DG& Levin A.; Acute Kidney Injury Network. Acute Kidney Injury Network: report of an initiative to improve outcomes in acute kidney injury. Crit Care 2007;11:R31.

Ricci Z, Cruz DN & Ronco C. Classification and staging of acute kidney injury; beyond the RIFLE and AKIN criteria. Nat Rev Nephrol 2011, 7:201-208.

Siew ED, Matheny ME, Ikizler TA, Lewis JB, Miller RA, Waitman LR, Go AS, Parikh C & Peterson JF.Commonly used surrogates for baseline renal function affect the classification and prognosis of acute kidney injury.Kidney Int 2010, 77:536-542

Bagshaw SM, Uchino S, Cruz D, Bellomo R, Morimatsu H, Morgera S, Schetz M, Tan I, Bouman C, Macedo E, Gibney N, Tolwani A, Oudeman-van Straaten HM, Ronco C & Kellum JA.A comparison of observetion versus estimated baseline creatinine for determination of RIFLE class in patients with acute kidney injury. Nephrol Dial Translant 2009, 24:2739-2744

Joannidis M, Metnis B, Bauer P, Schusterschitz N, Moreno R, Druml W & Metnitz PGH. Acute kidney injury in critically ill patients classified by AKIN versus RIFLE usin the SAPS 3 database. Intensive Care Med 2009, 35:1692-1702

Bagshaw SM, George C & Bellomo R; ANZICS Database Management Committe. A comparison of the RIFLE and AKIN criteria for acute kidney injury in critically ill patients. Nephrol Dial Transplant 2008;23:1569-1574

Mehta RL, Pascual MT, Soroko S, Savage BR, Himmelfarb J, Ikizler TA, Paganini EP & Chertow GM: Spectrum of acute renal failure in the intensive care unit: The PICARD experience. Kidney Int 2004, 66:1613-1621

Chertow GM, Soroko SH, Paganini EP, Cho KC, Himmelfarb J, Ikizler TA & Mehta RL: Mortality after acute rena failure: models for prpgnostic stratification and risk adjustment. Kidney Int 2006,70:1120-1126

Uchino S, Kellum JA, Bellomo R, Doig GS, Morimatsu H, Morgera S, Schetz M, Tan I, Bouman C, Macedo E, Gibney N, Tolwani A & Ronco C. Beginning and Ending Supportive Therapy for the Kidney (BEST Kidney) Investigators. Acute renal failure in critically ill patients. A Multicenter Study. JAMA 2005, 295:7: 813-818

Brivet FG, Kleinknecht DJ, Loirat P & Landais PJ. Acute renal failure in intensive care units—causes, outcome, and prognostic factors of hospital mortality; a prospective, multicenter study. French Study Group on Acute Renal Failure. Crit Care Med 1996;24:192-198.

Liano F, Junco E, Pascual J, Madero R & Verde E. The spectrum of acute renal failure in the intensive care unit compared with that seen in other settings. The Madrid Acute Renal Failure Study Group. Kidney Int Suppl 1998;66:S16-24

Bellomo R, Wan L, Langenberg C & May C. Septic acute kidney injury: new concepts. Nephron Exp Nephrol 2008;109:e95-100.

Yegenaga I, Hoste E, Van Biesen W, Vanholder R, Benoit D, Kantarci G, Dhondt A, Colardyn F & Lameire N. Clinical characteristics of patients developing ARF due to sepsis/systemic inflammatory response syndrome: results of a prospective study. Am J Kidney Dis 2004;43:817-824.

Van Biesen W, Yegenaga I, Vanholder R, Verbeke F, Hoste E, Colardyn F & Lameire N. Relationship between fluid status and its management on acute renal failure (ARF) in intensive care unit (ICU) patients with sepsis: A prospective analysis. J Nephrol 2005, 18:54-60

Payen D, de Pont AC, Sakr Y, Spies C, Reinhart K & Vincent JL. Sepsis Occurrence in Acutly Ill Patients (SOAP) Investigators. A positive fluid balance is associated with a worse outcome in patients with acute renal failure. Crit Care 2008,12(3):R74.

Schrier RW & Wang W. Acute renal failure and sepsis. N Eng J Med 2004, 51:2:159-169

Malbraina ML, Deeren D & De Potter TJ. Intra-abdominal hypertension in the critically ill: it is time to pay attention. Curr Opin Crit Care 2005, 11:156-171.

Esson ML & Schrier RW. Diagnosis and treatment of acute tubular necrosis. Ann Intern Med 2002, 137:744-752.

Herget-Rosenthal S, Pietruck F, Volbracht L, Philipp T & Kribben A. Serum Cystatin C: A superior marker of rapidlt reduced glomerular filtration after uninephrectomy in kidney donors compared to creatinine. Clin Nephrol 2005, 64:41-46

Cruz DN, Ronco C & Katz N. Neutrophil gelatinase-associated lipocalin: A promiising biomarker for detecting cardiac surgery-associated acute kidney injury. L Thorac Cardiovasc Surg 2010, 139:1101-6

Mishra J, Ma Q, Prada A, Mitsnefes M, Zahedi K, Yang J, Barasch J & Devarajan P. Identification of neutrophil gelatinase assotiated lipocalin as a novel early urinary biomarker for ischemic renal injury. J Am Soc Nephrol 2003,14:2534-43

Liangos O,Perianayagam MC, Vaidya VS, Han WK, Wald R, Tighiouart H, MacKinnon RW, Li L, Balakrishnan VS, Pereira BJ, Bonventre JV &. Jaber BL. Urinary N-acetyl-beta-(D) glucosaminidase activity and kidney injury molecule-1 level are associated with adverse outcomes in acute renal failure. J Am Soc Nephrol 2007:18:904-912

Parikh CR & Devarajan P New biomarkers of acute kidney injury. Crit Care Med 2008, 364):S159-S16

Parikh CR, Mishra J,Thiesse-Philbrook H, Dursun B, Ma Q, Kelly C, Dent C, Devarajan P& Edelstein CL. Urinary IL-18 is an early predictive biomarker of acute kidney injury after cardiac surgery. Kidney Int 2006,70:199-203

9

Vancomycin-Induced Nephrotoxicity

Ahmad Bilal*[1,2], Omar Abu-Romeh*[1,2], Talla A. Rousan[2] and Kai Lau[1,2,3]
[1]*Section of Nephrology*
[2]*Department of Medicine*
[3]*VA Medical Center*
University of Oklahoma Health Sciences Center
University of Oklahoma Medical Center and VA Medical Center
Oklahoma City, OK
USA

1. Introduction

Nephrotoxicity associated with vancomycin administration has been a topic of debate for over five decades (Tables 1 & 2). Vancomycin is a glycopeptide antibiotic excreted by the kidney and has been used extensively, especially for methicillin-resistant staphylococcus aureus (MRSA) and for many strains of pathogenic staphylococcus epidermis. The nephrotoxic potential of vancomycin is neither fully appreciated nor well characterized. Previously, most reports of acute kidney injury (AKI) associated with vancomycin had blamed the acute renal failure (ARF) on early, relatively impure formulations of vancomycin (impurities popularly known as Mississippi mud). This conventional belief and the ensuing ambiguity if not controversy in the literature about its nephrotoxic potential have led to common notion that it is rather innocuous. Its popularity as an inexpensive and effective anti-staph medication and its widespread use had contributed to the increased incidence of AKI. But the impurity theory no longer holds because the modern purified preparations are devoid of additives.

The incidence of vancomycin (Van)-induced AKI (Van-AKI) has been on the rise due to (1) the staphylococcal epidemic, (2) the increasing incidence of health-care associated pneumonia (HCAP) and osteomyelitis (due to mounting use of prosthetic hard-wares and more ready diagnosis by routine MRI and CT scans), and (3) wider acceptance and practice of protracted vancomycin administration as outpatient or in nursing homes, where unfortunately physician involvement and toxicity monitoring are inherently less vigorous.

This issue is further compounded by the poor recognition and/or delayed diagnosis due to (1) the outdated notion that vancomycin is relatively benign and safe (Sorrel et al 1985, Kalil et al 2010), (2) the lack of modern guidelines in drug and creatinine monitoring, (3) the recent Infectious Disease (ID) recommendation to target trough levels of 15-20 mg/L in treating MRSA with potentially higher minimal inhibitory concentration (MIC) than the typical sensitivity range of <1 mg/L, (4) the prevailing assumption of renal tolerance based on absolute serum creatinine levels below certain rather arbitrary threshold, instead of using changes in serum creatinine or changes in estimated creatinine clearance from baseline, and

---

* Both authors contributed equally to the work in this Chapter)

Authors & Publication years	Aim of study	Key Results and Conclusions
Farber et al 1983	Retrospective study of toxicity of preparations of Vancomycin from 1974 to 1981	Possibility of additive toxicity between vancomycin and aminoglycosides should be considered
Sorrell et al 1985	A prospective study of adverse reactions of vancomycin therapy	Vanomycin is a safe drug with minimal side effects as long as levels are kept below 10 mg/L
Bailie et al 1988	Literature review of vanomcyin induced nephrotoxicity and ototoxicity.	Area under the curve (AUC) is more important in determining the toxicity of vancomycin as compared to magnitude of peak concentration.
Goetz et al 1993	Prospective study to compare toxicity of vancomycin and aminoglycosdies in combination and alone.	Combination of vancomycin and aminoglycosides is more nephrotoxic than individual agents alone
Vance-Bryan et al 1994	Comparative assessment of vancomycin toxicity in young and elderly hospitalized patients	Risk of nephrotoxicity in elderly is greater than young and independent of aminoglycoside administration
Ingram et al 2008	To identify risk factors of nephrotoxicity with continuous vancomycin infusion in outpatient setting	Serum steady-state vancomycin levels >28 mg/L markedly increase the risk of nephrotoxicity
Pritchard et al 2008	Relationship between increasing vancomycin trough concentrations and incidence of nephrotoxicity	Increasing trough vancomycin levels >14 mg/L and length of therapy increase the risk of nephrotoxicity
Lodise et al 2008	To determine nephrotoxic potential of vancomycin based on dosage and compare to linezolid	Vancomycin > 4 g/day are associated with 3-fold increased rates of nephrotoxicity vs. < 4 g/day; both doses associated with higher risks than linezolid
Pertel et al 2009	To determine efficacy and safety of daptomycin vs vancomycin against cellulitis	Daptomycin is superior to vancomycin in treating cellulitis and has with minimal side effect profile
Kalil et al 2010	Linezolid vs vancomycin or teicoplanin for nosocomial pneumonia	Vancomycin and teicoplanin are not associated with more renal dysfunction as compared to linezolid.
Colomo et al 2010	Impact of administration of vancomycin or linezolid to critically ill patients	Vancomycin should be used with caution in critically ill patients with acute renal failure

Table 1. Literature on Vancomycin-induced Nephrotoxicity: Large Epidemiologic Surveys and Drug Toxicity & Efficacy Monitoring Studies

(4) the failure to appreciate AKI causes accumulation of the renally excreted vancomycin, excess of which in turn inflicts further damage to the kidney, setting up a vicious cycle. Indeed, the literature is replete with observational studies (Table 1) and case reports (Table 2) which in the overall aggregate provide a large body of evidence in support of the contention that vancomycin could be nephrotoxic. Although published studies monitoring

Authors and publication dates	No. of patients	Highest serum vancomycin levels (mg/L)	Other Unexcluded Confounding or Contributing Factors to ARF
Duton and Elmes (1959)	4	Not given	Pre-existing renal disease in all 4; given 6-13 g over 2-5 days & as boluses in 30 min
Farber et al (1983)	12	39 - 65	Use of aminoglycosides, pre-existing renal disease
Odio et al (1984)	4	Not given	Concurrent aminoglycosides, 3 patients had pre-existing renal disease
Frimat et al (1995)	1	50	None
Sokol et al (2004)	1	Not given	Bacteremia, concomitant nephrotoxins (piperacillin/tazobactam, amikacin)
Barraclough et al (2007)	1	66	None
Ladino et al (2008)	5	42 - 86	Sepsis in 1, Bacteremia in 1, and acute allergic interstitial nephritis in 1
Psevdos et al (2009)	2	38.6 - 60.5	HIV
Shah-Khan et al (2011)	1	64.7	Sepsis secondary to Serratia marcescense
Bilal, Abu-Romeh, Rousan & Lau (2011) [current study]	6	38 - 110; Mean ± SE (70 ± 10)	None

Table 2. Case reports describing Vancomycin-induced Nephrotoxicity

adverse events in large cohorts usually succeeded in identifying a substantial and statistically significant incidence of renal complications (Bailie et al., (1988); Colomo et al., (2010); Farber et al., (1983); Goetz et al., (1993); Hidayat et al., (2006); Ingram et al., (2008); Lodise et al., (2008); Pritchard et al., (2008); Rybak et al., (1990); Vance-Bryan et al., (1994)), due to the inherently retrospective and epidemiologic nature, most if not all such large-group analyses were unable to capture sufficient key details in the affected individual patients to unequivocally establish a cause-and-effect relationship. There are also growing numbers of case reports, albeit is less than two dozen spanning over 50 years, which attributed the AKI to vancomycin (Barraclough et al., (2007); Dangerfield et al., (1960); Dutton & Elmes et al., (1959); Frimat et al., (1995); Ladino et al., (2008); Odio et al., (1984); Psevdos et al., (2009); Shah-Khan et al., (2011); Sokol et al., (2004)). But as will be reviewed in detail below, they often failed to definitely exclude other potential causes of acute renal failure (ARF), including sepsis, allergic interstitial nephritis, urinary tract obstruction, hemodynamic derangements, other concomitant nephrotoxic agents, radio-contrast dyes, ischemia, volume depletion, and other intrinsic renal insults.

2. Objectives

We have three objectives in writing this chapter. One, we shall draw upon the evidence from a thorough review of the published literature and from the detailed analyses of our own experience to argue for the existence of Van-AKI. Two, based on the insights deduced from these two sources, we will describe and characterize the typical picture of Van-AKI, the renal functional profile in the evolution of the ARF and the recovery. We will also outline the lessons that could be learned for safer but equally effective administration of vancomycin. Three, we will recommend some simple practical guidelines designed to prevent and/or ameliorate the emergence of Van-AKI.

3. Methods

Objective 1: To better document and more firmly establish the existence of Van-AKI

We approached this objective in two ways. First, we performed a systematic search and a careful review of the existing literature (Tables 1 & 2) using Pub-Med, Web of Science, Medline (OVID), Journal Citation Reports (ISI), Cochrane Database of Systematic Reviews, and Current Contents. Secondary references cited from these primary sources were also considered and reviewed with a focus on the published evidence in support of or against the entity of vancomycin nephrotoxicity. Search terms included acute renal failure (ARF), AKI, acute tubular necrosis, nephrotoxicity, renal insufficiency, renal failure, elevated creatinine, decline or deterioration in renal function or glomerular filtration rate or creatinine clearance, all cross-referenced with vancomycin. All studies with sufficient details on methods that are amendable to critical reviews were considered and only those with conclusions supported by the presented data or results were then included in Tables 1 & 2.

Second, we carefully and objectively analyzed the data from 101 consecutive patients evaluated for ARF (from among a total of 153 cases referred for renal consultation in the course of the month of services (Table 3). The renal consultative service was provided to adult patients admitted to the Hospitals of the University of Oklahoma Health Sciences Center (OUHSC) with a 450-bed capacity for acute or tertiary care. After excluding pre-renal and post-renal causes for ARF using the traditional or conventional clinical criteria and renal ultrasound, we found intra-renal insults in 78 patients from among the 101 with ARF (Table 4). Additional diagnostic studies and analyses of the clinical presentation and subsequent course allowed us to assign an etiologic factor accounting for the intra-renal ARF (Table 5). We have identified 6 patients with ARF with clinical and laboratory data and subsequent recovery course that unequivocally support the causal role of vancomycin in the AKI.

1. Inter- or concurrent issues in patients with known end-stage renal diseases (N=41).	
2. Issues unrelated to acute kidney injury (AKI), acute renal failure (ARF) or chronic kidney diseases (N=11).	
electrolytes disorders	n=4
transplantation issues	n=2
fluid management	n=4
drug overdose	n=1
3. AKI or ARF (N=101).	

Table 3. Indications for Renal Consultations (analysis of the 153 cases seen over a month)

In analyzing the potential etiologies of their AKI, we have vigorously ruled out sepsis, bacteremia, urinary tract obstruction, volume depletion, and any conceivable concomitant nephrotoxic antibiotics or intra-renal or intrinsic insults so that we could convincingly pin down vancomycin as the principal culprit. Based on serial drug levels, daily and cumulative administered doses, the temporal relationship between drug administration and changing renal function, the profile of renal failure, and the course of recovery upon stopping vancomycin, we believe other confounding variables could be excluded with a high degree of certainty. As opposed to the previous era when vancomycin was typically and invariably administered to patients along with an aminoglycoside or amphotericin B (typically for overt or presumed sepsis, bacteremia, or neutropenic fever), the recent practice of treating HCAP with triple antibiotics consisting of vancomycin but no other known nephrotoxins has provided a unique opportunity to witness and document AKI in the absence of other nephrotoxic insults. The absence of bacteremia or sepsis also helps eliminate a key confounding variable that previously precluded isolation of vancomycin as the culprit. Similarly, with the heightened detection and increased diagnosis of osteomyelitis by CT or MRI, more and more patients have been treated with long-term antibiotic regimen composed of vancomycin but not aminoglycoside. Since these patients are relatively asymptomatic and generally free of bacteremia on pre-treatment blood cultures, their subsequent development of AKI could reasonably be attributed to the adverse effects of antibiotics like vancomycin. Thus these two groups of patients (vancomycin-treated HCAP or osteomyelitis of undefined pathogens) have unwittingly provided a wonderful chance for clinicians to document the diagnosis of Van-AKI, an entity which had previously been questioned and debated because of the presence of other potential but unexcluded nephrotoxic insults.

A. Post-renal or obstructive nephropathy (N=4 or 4% of all AKI).
B. Pre-renal (N=19 or 19% of all AKI)
volume depletion, n=8;
hemodynamic issues, n=11; (atrial fibrillation, bleeding, myocardial ischemia, or hypotension).
C. Intra-renal insults (N=78 or 77% of all AKI).

Table 4. Acute Kidney Injury (AKI) *or Acute Renal Failure (ARF) (N=101)*

Objective 2: To describe and characterize the clinical and renal function profile for a typical Van-AKI, using lessons and insights from the reviewed literature and our own experience

To this end, we examined and tested the validity of the various independent risk factors proposed from the literature, namely serum vancomycin levels, total dose administered, and the duration of administration in our group of 6 patients. We attempted to generate insights from our own experience and that of the literature by doing the following statistical analyses. We first grouped their demographic data and clinical characteristics including hematologic data. We abstracted and tabulated the various parameters and indices of vancomycin therapy and longitudinal renal function, for each patient and also the entire group, using 100/serum creatinine as the estimate of creatinine clearance (CrCl) (Table 6). We analyzed their serial serum creatinine (and the associated CrCl) by calculating group means (and variance as standard errors), throughout the entire course of their AKI (Figure 7), starting from their initial baseline, to the days just before serum vancomycin reached its peak, through the days of peak vancomycin levels, then the days of peak serum creatinine,

		Number	% of Intra-renal Insults
(1)	Sepsis or septic shock	(45)	(58%)
(2)	Unknown or multifactorial	(11)	(14%)
(3)	Allergic interstitial nephritis	(7)	(9%)
(4)	Radio-contrast dye	(3)	(4%)
(5)	Rhabdomyolysis	(2)	(3%)
(6)	Nephrotoxic antibiotics	(10)	(13%)
	(a) Colistin	(1)	(1.3%)
	(b) Amphotericin B	(1)	(1.3%)
	(c) Vancomycin	(4 solo)	(5%)
		(4 major)	(5%)

Table 5. For Intra-renal insults (N = 78 or 77% of the 101 cases of Acute Kidney Injury)

the days of nadir vancomycin levels, and finally to the days of nadir serum creatinine at maximal recovery 60 days after the initiation of vancomycin. We also plotted serial vancomycin levels against the renal functional profile to evaluate and define the temporal relationships between drug levels and kidney function during the evolution of and recovery from AKI (Fig 7).

Objective 3: To generate and provide simple practical guidelines and recommendations to minimize vancomycin nephrotoxicity

Inferences from the analyses performed for Objective 2 will provide the basis for us to formulate the proposed guidelines designed to prevent and /or ameliorate the emergence of Van-AKI. These will be elaborated as a narrative in the Results section and presented in a tabulated format (Table 7) in the final Conclusion and Recommendations.

4. Findings

Results for objective 1: Evidence for the existence of Van-AKI

Towards objective 1, the findings of our current studies reported here belong to two sections. In the first section (A), we have performed and will present a comprehensive, systematic, and an up-to-date literature review to draw on all described indirect and circumstantial evidence cited to support the concept and the existence of Van-AKI. In the second section (B), we shall describe the 6 patients we personally saw and helped manage who were consulted for acute renal failure and in whom we found compelling evidence for the diagnosis of Van-AKI. We will detail their presentation and the clinical course of their ARF. We shall provide serial laboratory findings to document the causality of vancomycin, including their recovery course following the discontinuation of the offending agent.

(A) Evidence for Van-AKI based on literature review

The literature has provided two independent sources of indirect evidence in support of the issue of Van-AKI. The first body of evidence (1) (Table 1) comes from several epidemiologic surveys and drug toxicity monitoring studies performed in sizable patient cohorts taking vancomycin, which suggested an association between the drug and acute elevation of serum creatinine (Farber et al. (1983), Sorrell et al. (1985), Bailie et al. (1988), Rybak et al. (1990), Goetz et al. (1993), Vance-Bryan et al. (1994), Hidayat et al. (2006), Lodise et al, (2008), Pritchard et al. (2008), Ingram et al. (2008), Pertel et al. (2009), Kalil et al. (2010), Rodriguez Colomo et al. (2010). The second body of evidence (2) (Table 2) is based on the growing number of case reports describing the association between acute nephrotoxicity and vancomycin (Dutton & Elmes et al.(1959), Dangerfield et al. (1960), Odio et al. (1984), Frimat et al. (1995), Sokol et al. (2004), Barraclough et al. (2007), Ladino et al. (2008), Psevdos et al. (2009)).

(A) (1): Epidemiologic and drug toxicity monitoring studies

These studies have collectively provided four lines of evidence implicating vancomycin in the pathophysiology of AKI: (a) Correlation between acute rise in serum creatinine and high serum vancomycin levels (Rybak et al 1990, Hidayat et al 2006, Ingram et al 2008, Lodise et al 2008, Pritchard et al 2008); (b) Increased incidence of acute renal failure (or potentiation of nephrotoxicity) when vancomycin was also administered concurrent with aminoglycosides (Farber et al 1983, Rybak et al 1990, Goetz et al 1993); (c) Increased incidence of AKI with prolonged duration of vancomycin therapy (Hidayat et al, 2006, Pitchard et al 2008); (d) Increased incidence of AKI with vancomycin compared to linezolid in comparable cohorts with similar patient characteristics (Lodise et al 2008, Colomo et al, 2010). The studies providing these four lines of evidence will be presented in the same order.

a. ARF was more often associated with a higher steady-state or trough serum vancomycin levels and linked to higher daily doses.

Rybak et al reported in 1990 that higher serum trough vancomycin levels were associated with the development of elevated serum creatinine (Rybak et al., 1990). In the ensuing two decades, this observation was not only confirmed but also extended by the studies of Hidayat et al (2006), Ingram et al (2008), and Lodise et al (2008).

Since the new millennium, the widespread use of vancomycin has led to the expected emergence of strains of methicillin resistant staphylococcus aureus (MRSA) that have only intermediate sensitivity to vancomycin, based on higher than the classical minimum inhibitory concentration (MIC) of 1 mg/L. Accordingly, the Infectious Disease (ID) guidelines have recommended higher trough concentrations like between 15-20 mg/L (Rybak et al., 2009) in order to maximize the chances of eradicating such infections. One unintended consequence was the apparent rise in the incidence of AKI by following such guidelines too rigidly but without closer vigilance of the level of renal function.

Thus, in a prospective study on the efficacy and toxicity of vancomycin during treatment of these relatively resistant MRSA strains by targeting and achieving the higher trough level of 15-20 mg/L, Hidayat et al. (2006) not only noted a higher mortality rate and a poorer end-of-treatment response, but also the development of nephrotoxicity in the subset of patients with demonstrably higher trough levels.

In 2008, Ingram et al. performed a retrospective cohort study of 102 adults to identify risk factors for nephrotoxicity during continuous outpatient vancomycin administration between 2004 and 2007. The incidence of nephrotoxicity, defined as ≥ 50% increase in baseline serum creatinine, was about 15.7%. Based on their analyses, a steady-state serum vancomycin concentration of ≥ 28 mg/L was thought to be an independent risk factor for developing nephrotoxicity.

Since the published new ID guidelines to keep trough level between 15-20 mg/L for resistant strains of MRSA, a good number of clinicians have increased the dose to >4 g/day to achieve the recommended required trough levels. This approach has afforded an opportunity for Lodise et al. (2008) to conduct a retrospective cohort study to describe the impact of ≥ 4 g/day of vancomycin on renal function. They found a 3-fold greater incidence of nephrotoxicity in patients receiving >4 g vancomycin/day (34.6 %) versus those receiving <4 g /day (10.9%). In the same review, these investigators also found a much lower incidence of renal failure in similar patients who received only linezolid (6.7%) as opposed to either > 4 or < 4 g /day of vancomycin (*P*=0.001).

Pritchard et al. (2008) conducted a retrospective analysis of ~ 3,000 courses of vancomycin given between 2003 and 2007. The aim of their study was to determine the relationship between vancomycin trough concentrations and nephrotoxicity. They noted that trough levels >14 mg/L was an independent risk factor for renal injury among others to be elaborated below.

In contrast, when serum trough vancomycin levels were prospectively limited to the lower range of 5 to 10 mg/L and if peak levels were kept ~ 28 mg/L, in 1985, Sorrel et al found no AKI with vancomycin (when used alone in two patients) and < 8% incidence of AKI even if combined with an aminoglycoside among the 54 patients studied. Taken together, these findings indicate that vancomycin must be considered nephrotoxic, especially at high serum levels, although it was found to be relatively safe at low trough or steady-state levels.

Parenthetically, Bailie et al. (1988) had reviewed the utility of peak serum levels as an indicator of vancomycin induced nephrotoxicity and ototoxicity. They determined that peak vancomycin concentration per se may be relatively minor in producing and predicting nephrotoxicity as opposed to the total area under the serum concentration-time curve (AUC).

b. Increased incidence of AKI when vancomycin was concurrently administered with an aminoglycoside.

At least three to four studies have found the synergistic nephrotoxic potential between vancomycin and aminoglycosides. In a retrospective study, Farber et al in 1983 found that more patients who received both vancomycin and gentamicin (12 of 34) had suffered from nephrotoxicity as compared to those getting vancomycin alone (3 of 60) with a p value of <0.001. In the studies by Sorrel et al (1985), AKI was found in 4 of 54 vancomycin-treated patients, but all 4 had also received aminoglycosides. In contrast, no AKI was found in the two on vancomycin alone.

These findings, however, were not uniformly observed (Downs et al. in 1989, Cimino et al. in 1987, Mellor et al. in 1985), perhaps due to intrinsic differences in their patient characteristics, definitions of acute renal failure, and the divergence in their study methods. In contrast, in 1990 Rybak et al. confirmed that the combination of aminoglycosides and vancomycin was more nephrotoxic than either drug alone.

The prospective studies by Goetz & Sayer published in 1993 provided corroboration for the additive nephrotoxic potential between vancomycin and aminoglycosides. The incidence of nephrotoxicity was 19% in patients receiving vancomycin alone, 12% in patients receiving an aminoglycoside alone and 24% in patients receiving combined vancomycin and an aminoglycoside.

c. Increased incidence of AKI with prolonged vancomycin administration.

Several studies have led to the conclusion that prolonged therapy with vancomycin was a risk factor for AKI (Goetz & Sayer 1993, Hidayat et al 2006, Pritchard et al 2008). Besides showing the synergism between aminoglycosides and vancomycin in causing AKI, Goetz & Sayer observed that a duration of >21 days posed greater risk for renal toxicity. In the prospective studies by Hidayat et al on targeting higher trough vancomycin levels for MRSA strains with high MIC, they not only confirmed the previous association between high trough levels and nephrotoxicity, but also a link between prolonged treatment and AKI.

The retrospective review by Pritchard et al in 2008 also identified the duration of vancomycin administration as an independent risk factor. In their studies of ~ 3,000 courses of vancomycin given between 2003 and 2007, they observed that therapy over 7 days was associated with AKI. They also suggested baseline serum creatinine > 1.7 mg/dl as another independent risk factor. It is however unclear if this association merely reflects a heightened sensitivity of the clinicians to AKI, an enhanced detection of renal failure with an already elevated baseline creatinine, and/or intrinsically greater susceptibility of chronically diseased kidneys to new and acute insults.

d. Increased incidence of AKI or slower recovery from pre-existing ARF if treated with vancomycin versus linezolid.

In the retrospective review by Lodise et al (2008) on the impact of ≥ 4 g/day of vancomycin, they also found a significantly lower incidence of renal failure in patients on linezolid (6.7% vs. 34.6% in patients on > 4 g /day or 10.9 % in those on < 4 g /day) (P=0.001). In the treatment of nosocomial pneumonia, Kalil et al (2010) performed a meta-analysis to test the hypothesis of the superiority of linezolid over vancomycin. But they found no significant difference in either vancomycin efficacy or risks of renal dysfunctions, although the study was not powered to compare the nephrotoxic potential between the two drugs.

Rodriguez Colomo et al. (2010) conducted a retrospective, multicenter observational study in patients in intensive care unit with pre-existing renal failure. They found that those patients treated with linezolid had a better renal recovery than those treated with vancomycin, implying either continued nephrotoxic susceptibility or superimposed injury with vancomycin in these cohorts.

In brief, despite the mounting body of indirect evidence summarized above suggesting a role of vancomycin in AKI, firm and unambiguous proofs for a cause-and-effect linkage remain elusive. Virtually all of the studies cited and reviewed above did not offer sufficient details on those individual patients with presumed Van-AKI to allow independent and objective confirmation of a causal and unequivocal relationship. Inherent in the nature of these large-cohort surveys and drug toxicity monitoring studies, despite showing statistical significance among different cohorts, none of the other known and potential etiologic factors for the ARF could be readily evaluated in individual affected patients, let alone vigorously excluded. For instance, the evolution of their serial renal function and the subsequent clinical course after cessation of vancomycin were either not provided or extractable from those individuals afflicted with AKI. A larger prospective study with sufficient clinical details is therefore needed to objectively eliminate all other confounding variables and to prove the implied cause-and-effect relationship.

(A) (2): Evidence for Van-AKI based on published case reports

Between 1956 and 1986, 57 cases of ARF were described in the course of vancomycin administration and had been attributed to vancomycin. However, over a half of them were reported within the first 6 years of vancomycin use, when impurities were considered to be the most likely culprit (Bailie & Neal 1988)

Although they spanned out over 5 decades in the medical literature, there have been but fewer than two dozen well documented cases of ARF which can be confidently and objectively attributed to vancomycin (Dutton & Elmes et al (1959), Dangerfield et al (1960), Odio et al (1984), Frimat et al (1995), Sokol et al (2004), Barraclough et al (2007), Ladino et al (2008), Psevdos et al (2009), Shah-Khan et al (2011)) (Table 2).

A very early case series was described by Dutton & Elmes (1959) who reported that 4 out of 9 vancomycin-treated patients developed renal failure (Table 2). The authors did not measure vancomycin or report drug levels. Unfortunately, all 4 affected patients had suffered from pre-existing renal diseases. Most remarkably, they had all received relatively high doses of vancomycin (between 6-13 grams over 2-5 days). One described method of administration involved rather rapid direct injection in 20 ml saline over only 5 minutes. In retrospect, the high dose and the bolus injection might have resulted in excessive blood and renal tissue concentrations and contributed to the high rates of acute nephrotoxicity, as clearly demonstrated by the dosage comparison studies of Lodise et al (2008).

Dangerfield et al (1960) described nephrotoxicity in 11 out of 85 patients in their series. They defined nephrotoxicity as an otherwise unexplained elevation in serum creatinine ≥ 0.5mg/dl. Eight of these patients had no pre-existing renal disease. Follow up demonstrated a return to baseline renal function in 3-4 weeks. No serum vancomycin concentrations were reported. More importantly, no details on these 11 patients were provided for an objective review or an independent confirmation that no other factors could have contributed to the ARF. Since patients with serious infections requiring vancomycin therapy could have concurrent sepsis, hemodynamic derangements, volume depletion and/or dehydration, it remains unclear if the well known etiologies for AKI had been systematically and definitively excluded, especially if the criterion for ARF was a simply fixed serum creatinine elevation of 0.5 mg/dl irrespective of the starting baseline levels. The actual drop in glomerular filtration rate (GFR) is relatively minor (~ 10 ml/min or ~ 10 %) if serum creatinine rose from a baseline of 2 to 2.5 mg/dl, which could be easily explained by many pre-renal factors. In contrast, a rise in serum creatinine from a baseline of 1 to 1.5 mg/dl could easily reflect ~33 ml/min or ~33 % drop in GFR. Thus at the very best, these generalized descriptions offer no stronger evidence for Van-AKI than that inferred from large efficacy and toxicity studies reviewed and commented above [(A) (1); Table 1].

Each of the report by Frimat et al (1995) and by Barraclough et al (2007) described a case in which they found no alternative explanations for the ARF except vancomycin (Table 2). In the former report, the patient received 39 grams of vancomycin over 17 days, with a peak drug level of 50 mg/L. The patient needed 2 sessions of hemodialysis before the renal function very slowly recovered over > 2 months. In the latter report, the patient had a peak vancomycin level of 66 mg/L and had no other plausible explanation for ARF. Kidney function recovered to baseline in 5-6 weeks. In our opinion, these 2 cases demonstrated rather convincingly the causal relationship between vancomycin and the associated ARF, very similar to our 6 patients to be described below (see Fig 1-6 and Table 6).

In 2008 Ladino et al. presented a case series of 5 patients believed to be Van-AKI. Vancomycin levels were reported to be between 42-86 mg/L and renal function recovered in 3-4 weeks after stopping vancomycin. These authors believed that they had ruled out other causes of ARF. However, in three of the five, there were equally viable etiologic explanations. Thus, one patient had full-blown sepsis, another had bacteremia, and the third had evidence for acute interstitial nephritis (AIN), making it difficult to accept vancomycin as the principal or sole culprit.

In 2011 a case of renal biopsy-proven acute tubular necrosis (ATN) was reported. The authors attributed the ARF to 5 g of intravenous vancomycin given in < 24 h to a 103-kg young man with chills, high fever, tachycardia and catheter infected with Serratia (Shah-Khan et al (2011)). He appeared to be septic from a PICC line and exit site infection although peripheral blood culture was negative and there was no frank hypotension. Serum creatinine rose from 0.97 to 4.26 mg/dl in a day and required three hemodialysis treatments for several days of severe oliguria, a serum vancomycin of 64.7 mg/L on day 4, and a sustained elevation of creatinine > 9 mg/dl from days 4 to 9. Although urine output rose to 1-2.5 liters a day since day 5, serum creatinine remained elevated at 1.24 mg/dl even by day 30. The AKI in this man confirmed the observation and caution by Lodise et al (2008) that >4 g of vancomycin /day posed extra nephrotoxic risks. The rapidity of his functional recovery, albeit incomplete, might be related to the single day of brief exposure to vancomycin although excessive in total quantity.

The difficulty of identifying in 5 decades even 2 dozen cases of definite or probable Van-AKI serve to explain the uncertainty and continued controversy regarding the nephrotoxicity of vancomycin. Although there have been many other reports of vancomycin-associated nephrotoxicity, most of them turned out to have been very poorly documented. In most of them, some other renal insults could be easily identified to explain their ARF if only the clinical details were more meticulously, comprehensively, and/or objectively analyzed. In general, often overlooked and/or frequently missed were the concomitant aminoglycosides or nephrotoxic medications, coexisting sepsis or bacteremia, hypotension, hemodynamic factors, pre-existing renal diseases, radio-contrast dye insults, and/or allergic interstitial nephritis. In all objectivity, these factors proved to be the more reasonable and probable etiologies for the ARF without necessarily invoking vancomycin.

To offer more vigorous evidence for Van-AKI, we will describe in the following section B our 6 patients. We shall provide sufficient details to demonstrate the causal role of vancomycin, having carefully considered and then excluded most if not all described confounding factors or other potential etiologies. In all six patients, we shall also provide complete information about their entire clinical course showing the temporal evolution of the AKI (in an individual set of three figures per patient as well as a separate case report for each). High-lighted will be the initial renal dysfunctions and the subsequent recovery upon cessation of vancomycin, against the temporal profile of the rising and falling serial vancomycin levels (Figs 1-6).

Results for objective 1:

(B) Evidence for VAN-AKI derived from 6 cases observed at OUHSC

Of the 101 cases referred for acute renal failure (ARF) (Table 4), 78 (77%) were attributable to intra-renal causes (Table 5), as opposed to pre-renal factors like hemodynamic etiologies or volume depletion (19 or 19%) , or post-renal causes like obstructive nephropathy (4 or 4%). Among the 78 patients with AKI due to intra-renal etiologies (Table 5), 45 (or 58%) could be attributed to sepsis or septic shock, 11 (or 14%) to multiple or unidentifiable factors, 7 (or 9%) to allergic interstitial nephritis, 3 (or 4%) to radio-contrast dye insults, 2 (or 2.6 %) to rhabdomyolysis, and 10 (or 13%) to nephrotoxic antibiotics. Of the 10 patients with antibiotic-induced AKI, one was linked to colistin, another to amphotericin B, 4 solely caused by vancomycin and 4 principally due to vancomycin. We shall focus on 6 of these 8 (4 solely due to vancomycin and two others with vancomycin as the uncontested primary etiology). Demographic details and clinical characteristics at baseline for the entire group are tabulated in Table 6A. The usual pre-renal and obstructive etiologies were excluded by conventional clinical and laboratory studies. None exhibited signs of hypotension, sepsis or bacteremia despite mild leukocytosis. There were no physical, hematologic or urinary evidence to suggest allergic interstitial nephritis. Although two patients had received radio-contrast dye injection, these were temporally unrelated to the AKI.

These 6 cases will also be individually presented in narrative form, along with an accompanying 3-part figure per patient. Three of them were treated for MRSA or Health Care Associated Pneumonia (HCAP) (Cases 1, 4, 5) and three for osteomyelitis from proven or presumed MRSA (Cases 2, 3, 6) (Table 6A). The individual figure serves to illustrate the changes in serum creatinine (A), changes in 100/serum creatinine, as an estimate of CrCl (B), and changes in the levels of serum vancomycin (C) as a function of time from the first day of vancomycin therapy through day 80 since the initiation or the last day of follow-up whichever was longer (Fig 1-6). Thus individually and collectively these 6 cases offer the strongest support for the concept and diagnosis of Van-AKI, especially in the context of the previously reviewed literature.

Case I:

A 48-year-old white man was admitted to the general internal medicine ward with delirium tremens, diverticulitis, and community acquired pneumonia. He had a past medical history significant for rheumatic fever, rheumatic heart disease, history of infective endocarditis 6 years earlier with septic emboli. There was also a history of diverticulitis and alcoholism. His heart rate was 125 beats/minute and his blood pressure was 143/85 mmHg. The patient was agitated and hallucinating, but otherwise physical examination was unremarkable. Initially white blood cell count was 11.1 K/mm^3 and hemoglobin of 12.4 g/dL. Blood chemistries were significant for Na of 130 mEq/L, K of 2.6 mEq/L, and Cl of 85 mEq/L. His serum creatinine was 0.93 mg/dl. He had elevated liver enzymes and bilirubin (aspartate aminotransferase 306 units/L, alanine aminotransferase126 units/L, total alkaline phosphatase 203 units/L, and total bilirubin 2.7 mg/dl), which all eventually resolved in the course of general and specific therapy during his hospitalization. Serum alcohol level was < 10 mg/dl. Chest X ray revealed perihilar right lower lobe and left lower lobe pneumonia as well as right middle and left lingular pneumonia. Computed tomography (CT) scan of the abdomen and pelvis with intravenous and oral contrast showed findings consistent with sigmoid diverticulitis. Blood and urine cultures were negative.

The patient was given lorazepam as needed for alcohol withdrawal symptoms. Regarding his antibiotic regimen, he was initially started on moxifloxacin 400 mg intravenous once daily; the antibiotic regimen was changed on day 3 to vancomycin, piperacillin/tazobactam, and ciprofloxacin given his poor clinical response. Later on day 5, levofloxacin substituted ciprofloxacin for the same reason. Vancomycin was initially started at a dose of 1 g intravenously q12 h (from hospital days 3 through 5). The dose was increased to 1 g intravenously q8 h on day 6 because of a low vancomycin trough level of < 5 mg/L. The dose was further increased on day 7 when trough level was 8 mg/L.

On hospital day 10, vancomycin trough level was found to be 68 mg/L. Vancomycin was therefore discontinued. Creatinine level ranged between 0.57 and 0.93 mg/dl during the first 9 hospital days, but it increased to 2.34 mg/dl on day 10 and continued to rise to a peak of 4.69 mg/dl on day 15 (Fig 1A). Urinalysis done on day 10 of hospital stay was normal with no urinary sediment. Renal ultrasound was unremarkable. Serum creatinine started to decline after that and reached 1.07 mg/dl on day 33 (two days prior to his discharge). Random vancomycin levels were checked periodically after stopping the drug. Level declined to 5 mg/L on day 20. The patient improved clinically throughout his hospital stay with resolution of his pneumonia and improvement of the diverticulitis. He was discharged with follow up in the general medicine clinic after completing his course of antibiotics.

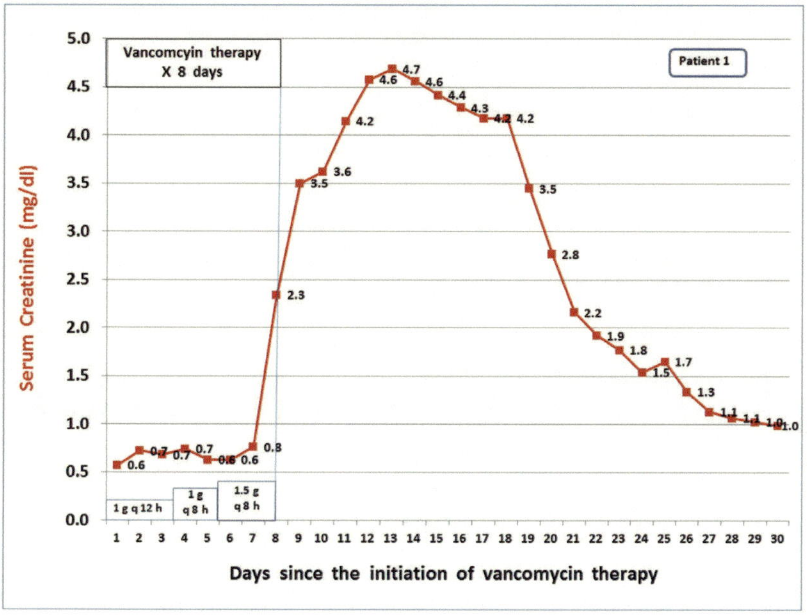

Fig. 1. A

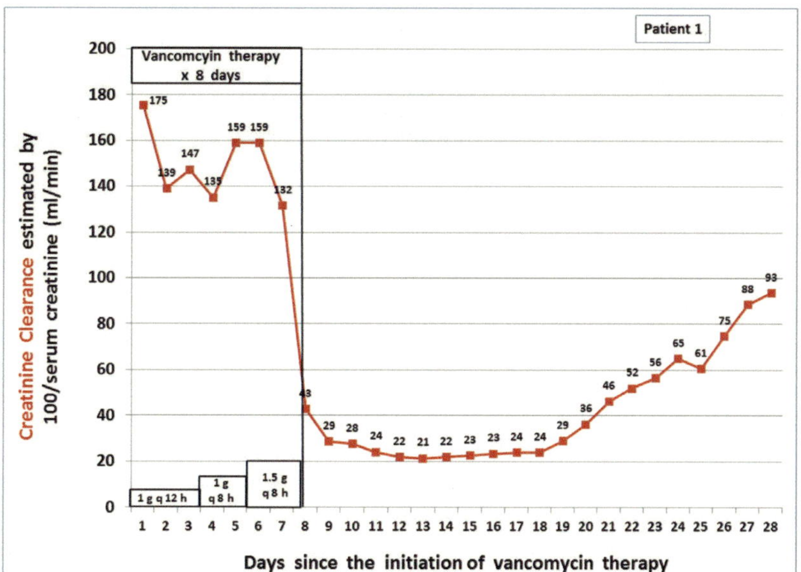

Fig. 1. B

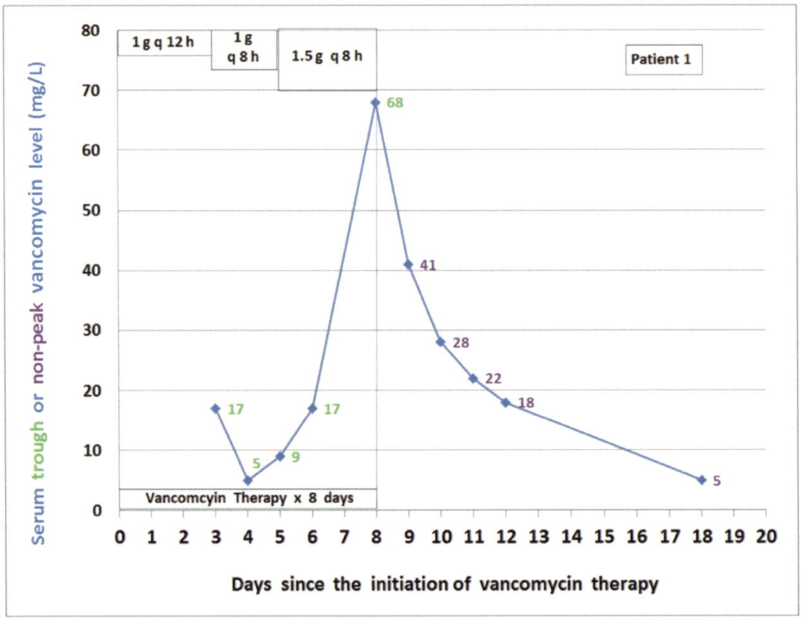

Fig. 1. C

We believed his acute kidney injury (AKI) was secondary to direct vancomycin nephrotoxicity based on the temporal relationship between the continually escalating dosage and documented excessive trough vancomycin levels on the one hand and the worsening kidney function on the other hand. Although he had received IV contrast on day 1, his serum creatinine did not rise until day 8. All pre-renal hemodynamic factors and post-renal causes were excluded, as were the absence of other intrinsic nephrotoxins. His recovery upon stoppage of vancomycin gave additional credence to our formulation. Although he had pneumonia, at no times did he have bacteremia or any signs of sepsis or hypotension. There were also no signs of allergic interstitial nephritis by serial exam, blood or urine eosinophilia. The patient was on multiple medications when he developed his AKI, including vancomycin, levofloxacin, piperacillin/tazobactam, ondansetron, enoxaparin, lorazepam, morphine sulfate, ompeprazole, sucralfate, and thiamine. But all these medications (except for vancomycin and enoxaparin, the latter replaced by unfractionated heparin) were continued during his subsequent renal recovery, arguing against any possible pathogenic role in the AKI.

Case 2:

This was a 53-year-old man with recurrent and recalcitrant osteomyelitis admitted for acute renal failure. He was known to suffer from diabetes mellitus, hypertension, chronic hepatitis C infection, alcohol abuse, and cocaine dependence. The patient sustained a right ankle fracture secondary to a fall and status post intramedullary nailing for fusion of right tibiotalar and subtalar joints. The patient's course was complicated by two episodes of right ankle osteomyelitis post surgery; the first episode happened about four months after the surgery which was treated with intravenous vancomycin and piperacillin/tazobactam in addition to the removal of 2 screws from the right foot. The second episode took place five months thereafter. At that time he underwent removal of the remaining screws and nail and was started on intravenous vancomycin at 1 g every 12 h with an intended duration of treatment for eight weeks.

On a regular out-patient follow up towards the end of antibiotic therapy, the patient was found to have a creatinine of 6.9 mg/dl from a baseline of 1.1 mg/dl (Fig 2A). On admission, he did not have any significant complaints. Outpatient medications included amlodipine, clonidine, glipizide, hydrochlorothiazide, lisinopril, hydrocodone, insulin, omeprazole, tramadol, and naproxen. Lisinopril dose had been constant for at least two years prior to admission. The patient admitted to taking two tablets of naproxen 500 mg daily for about seven months previously for pain relief.

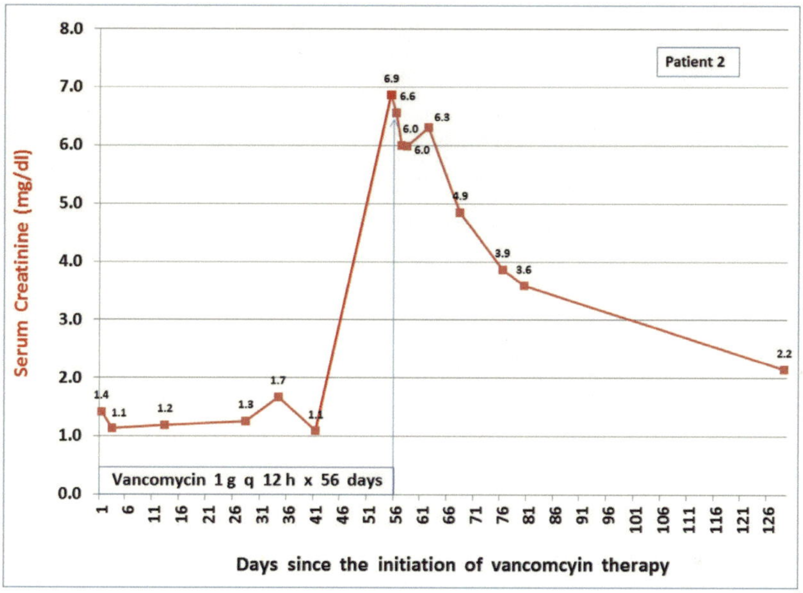

Fig. 2. A

Examination was significant for right ankle pitting edema and for a sinus tract over the lateral malleolus draining serous fluid. Initial laboratory revealed a white blood cell count of 7.3 K/mm^3 and hemoglobin of 10.0 g/dl. Chemistry was significant for BUN of 63 mg/dl, bicarbonate of 16 mEq/L, and creatinine 6.87 mg/dl. Previously, his serum trough vancomycin levels ranged between 11.5 mg/L and 20.9 mg/L since the initiating the antibiotics, with a level of 11.5 mg/L measured two weeks prior to admission (Fig 2C). On admission, random vancomycin level was however found to be 67 mg/L. Urine was positive for eosinophils. Urine creatinine was 87.6 mg/dl and urine protein 37 mg/dl, yielding a ratio of 0.42. Renal ultrasound revealed horseshoe kidneys with dimensions of 11.3 x 5.3 x 5.1 cm and 11.1 x 5.1 x 4.7 cm respectively for the right and left kidneys.

On day 1, vancomycin was discontinued along with stopping lisinopril and naproxen. Creatinine started to trend down reaching 2.15 mg/dl about 10 weeks later (Fig 2A). Since all medications except vancomycin had previously been taken without producing any renal toxicity, the temporal relationship between the high vancomycin level and elevated creatinine strongly suggests Vancomycin-AKI. His subsequent clinical course of a slow but steady recovery upon cessation of vancomycin lends further support to this formulation.

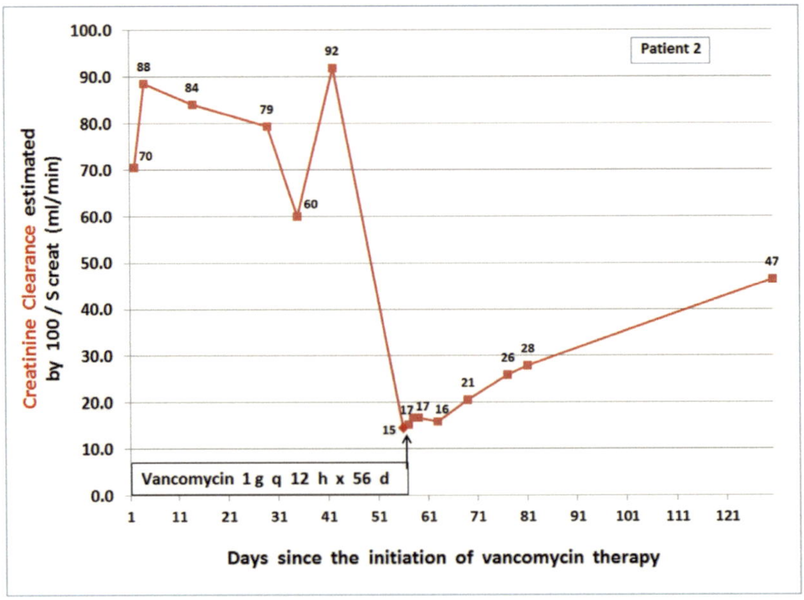

Fig. 2. B

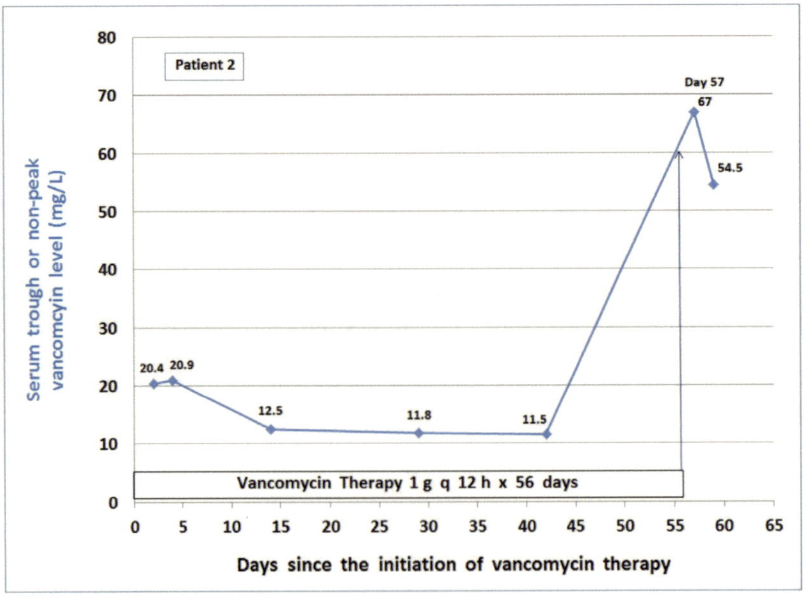

Fig. 2. C

We found no other stigmata of allergic interstitial nephritis (to either vancomycin) or other potential offending agents. Similar to the other patients, all pre-renal and post-renal factors had been carefully considered and excluded, including the absence of other known intra-renal insults in our patient.

Case 3:

This patient was a 56 year old man admitted for chronic open draining wound on right foot. He had a history of diabetes mellitus of unknown duration, although he was not taking any medications for diabetes. He reported chronic drainage from his right foot with worsening pain. Otherwise, the review of system was negative, notably for the absence of fever, chills, vomiting, diarrhea, dyspnea, and chest pain. He denied taking any NSAID or recent hospitalizations.

On admission he was normotensive and afebrile. He had no orthostatic hypotension. The big toe on his right foot had a large ulcer with purulent drainage and surrounding cellulitis. Nuclear scan confirmed osteomyelitis. Blood cultures and wound cultures were negative. His serum creatinine was 0.9 mg/dl on admission. He was treated with 1 g vancomycin q 12 h. On hospital day 3 his creatinine was 2.56 mg/dl and rose to a peak of 7.4 on hospital day 12, falling down to 4.85 at the time of discharge (Fig 3A).

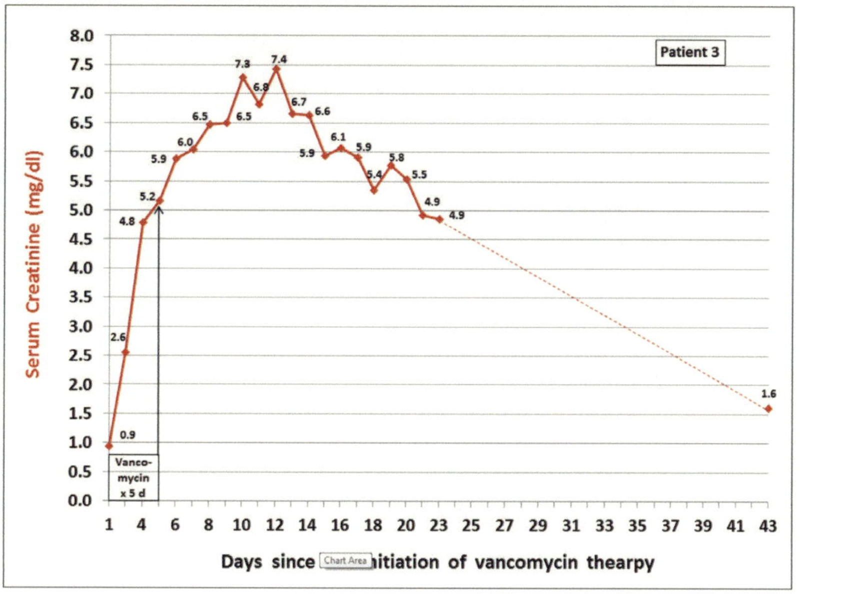

Fig. 3. A

Throughout his hospital stay, he was normotensive and received no other potential nephrotoxic insults including radio-contrast dyes. Due to persistent though mild leukocytosis and a low grade fever, he had undergone above knee amputation on his right side on hospital day 9. This was also prompted by the consideration that he had failed medical treatment and the wound was deemed to have very poor chance of healing based on vascular studies and transcutaneous oxygen tension gradients. He had received 2 g of vancomycin daily for the first 5 hospital days and given his extremely high serum trough or random vancomycin levels (Fig 3C) and the temporal relationship with the acute rise in serum creatinine, his AKI was best explained by vancomycin. In addition, all other etiologic factors, both pre-renal and post-renal causes, had been vigorously excluded. Three weeks after discharge, his amputation wound was healing well and his serum creatinine fell to 1.6 mg/dl, towards his normal baseline although still significantly elevated considering the loss of his right leg (Fig 3 A).

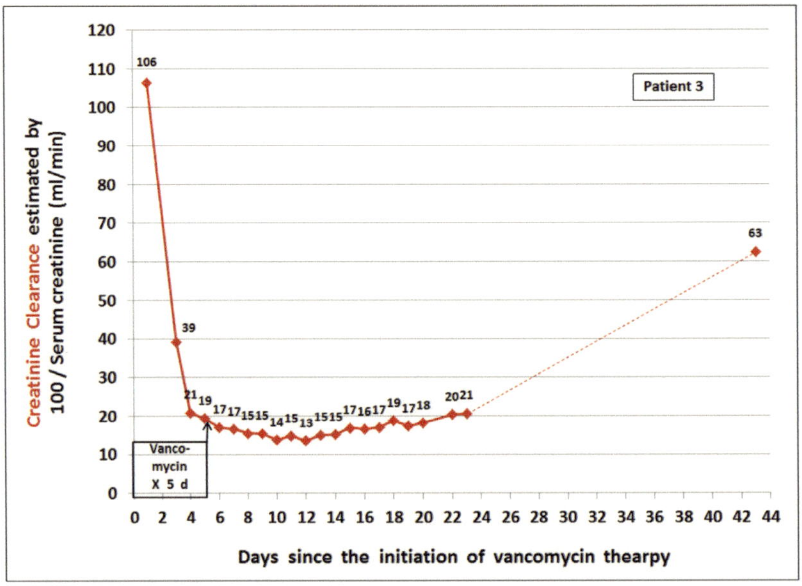

Fig. 3. B

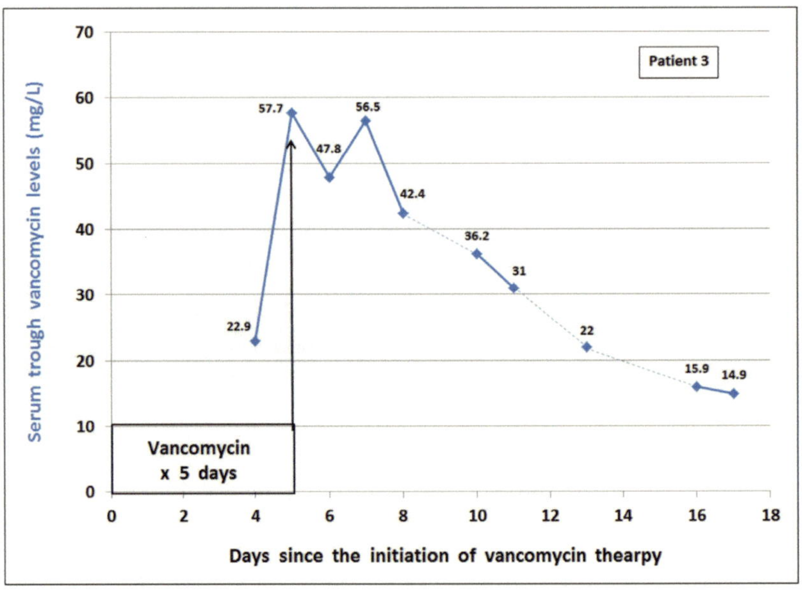

Fig. 3. C

Case 4:

This patient was a 33 year old man with a past medical history of Hirschsprung disease as a child admitted to the trauma service of our Medical Center after an alleged assault. He was intubated at the scene and subsequently treated for multiple facial fractures, right orbital fractures and intracranial hemorrhage. His hospital course was significant for having developed left lower lobe pneumonia attributed to MRSA cultured from the tracheal aspirate on the fourth hospital day. This was treated initially with vancomycin 1.5 g every 8 h. After 3 doses, trough vancomycin level was 10 mg/L. Thus vancomycin was increased to 2 g every 8 h, a regimen which was continued for the ensuing 10 days. His vancomycin trough levels on days 4, 5 and 9 of administration were respectively 15, 17 and 20 mg/L (Fig 4C).

His serum creatinine was 1.3 mg/dl on admission. After repletion of his extracellular fluid volume, it dropped to 0.6 and stayed in that range for a week (Fig 4A). On days 9 to 10 of vancomycin therapy, his serum creatinine began to climb slightly to 0.9 mg/dl. It rose to 1.2 on day 11 and to 2.8 mg/dl on day 12 of vancomycin administration. It peaked and plateaued at 3.5 to 3.6 mg/dl two weeks after the initiation of vancomycin (Fig 4A). Of note, his serum trough vancomycin level was found to be 110 mg/L eight hours after the last dose of vancomycin. Although there was a peripheral eosinophilia of 12.5% with a peak absolute count of 1,400 ten days after the last dose of vancomycin, his serum creatinine level then was already trending down, arguing against an allergic interstitial nephritis. There was no significant granulocytosis despite an intermittent low-grade fever and mild leukocytosis. All blood cultures drawn throughout his hospital course were negative. Hemophilus influenza grew out from his tracheal aspirate on hospital day 9 and treated for 9 days withpiperacillin/ tazobactam. The patient was hemodynamically stable throughout his hospital stay and he made a slow but steady and significant physical recovery to be able to transfer to a full rehabilitation center on hospital day 36. At that time his serum creatinine had also returned to 0.84 mg/dl, very close to his normal baseline.

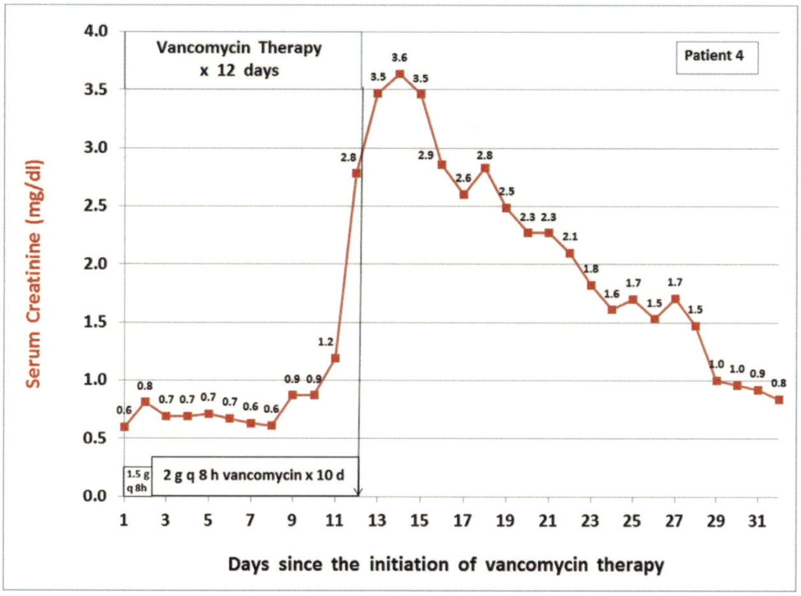

Fig. 4. A

Although he had received IV contrast on day 1, his serum creatinine had remained in the normal range and stable over the first 2 weeks of his hospitalization. All known nephrotoxic insults, pre-renal and post-renal factors were excluded as potential explanation for his AKI.

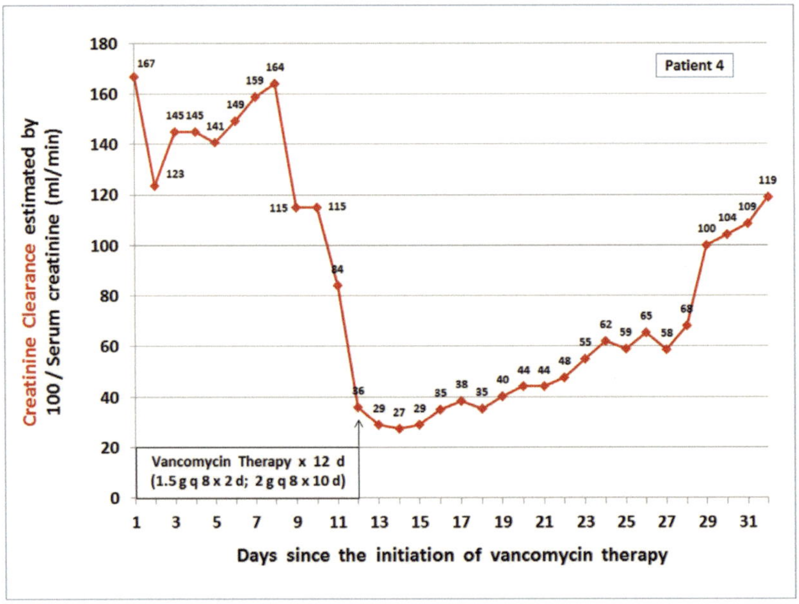

Fig. 4. B

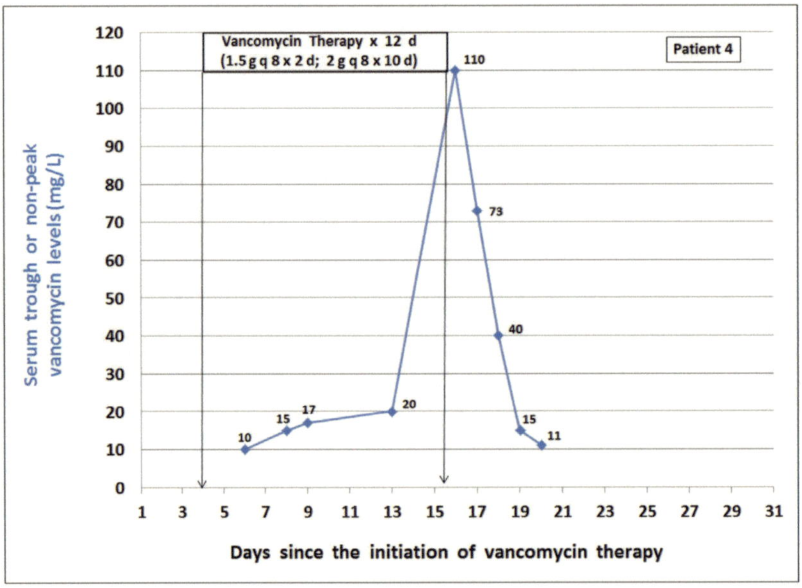

Fig. 4. C

Thus we believe his clinical course and renal function profile were best explained by acute vancomycin nephrotoxicity. His kidney recovery 3 weeks after stopping vancomycin was also consistent with the typical picture of improved serum creatinine over this time frame as in classical Van-AkI shown here and in the few documented cases published in the literature.

Case 5:

This man was a 75 year old resident of a skilled nursing facility admitted to our medical center because of altered mental status. He had a history of dementia and old cerebrovascular accidents and his outside medications included no nephrotoxic medications.

On examination, he appeared to be confused and disoriented, responsive only to painful stimuli. His blood pressure was 126/70 mm Hg. His pulse rate was 67. Temperature was 36.1 C and his respiratory rate was 18. On room air, his pulse oxygen saturation was 95%. He had coarse crackles in left lower lobe with decreased air entry. No other sources of infection were found on physical examination.

The white blood cell count was 11.3 K/mm^3. A chest X ray showed left lower lobe consolidation and a small pleural effusion. A CT scan of the head revealedno acute intracranial process. His serum creatinine was 2.42 mg/dl (versus a baseline of 1.5mg/dl). He was thought to be volume depleted. After receiving intravenous fluids, his serum creatinine returned to normal and on day 5, it was 1.11 mg/dl. In the mean time he was given vancomycin 1g q12 h and piperacillin/tazobactam 2.25 g q 6 h (adjusted dose for his renal function) for the treatment of his HCAP. On day 5 of his admission, he was discharged back to nursing home to complete a 2 week course of HCAP treatment.

Six days later, he was re-admitted to the hospital, again with altered mental status and decreased oral intake. His serum creatinine was elevated to 3.45 mg/dl (Fig 5 A). He was hemodynamically stable with blood pressure of 147/96 mm Hg and a pulse rate of 89. White blood cell count was 8.4 K/mm^3. Serum Na was 153 mEq/L and K was 3.8 mEq/L. BUN was 15 mg/dl. The urine fractional excretion of Na (FENa) was 13.8%, suggestive of intrinsic or intra-renal disease. Despite intravenous fluids, his serum creatinine continued to rise during the first few days (Fig 5A).

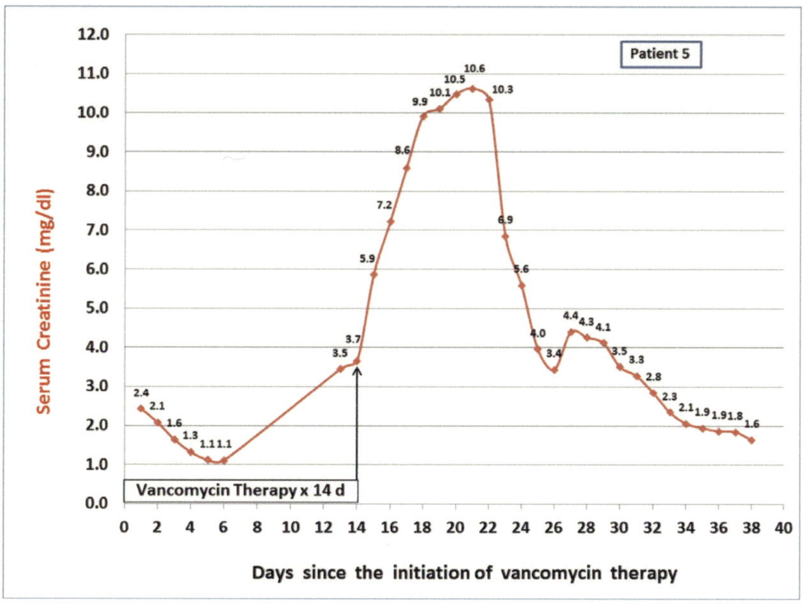

Fig. 5. A

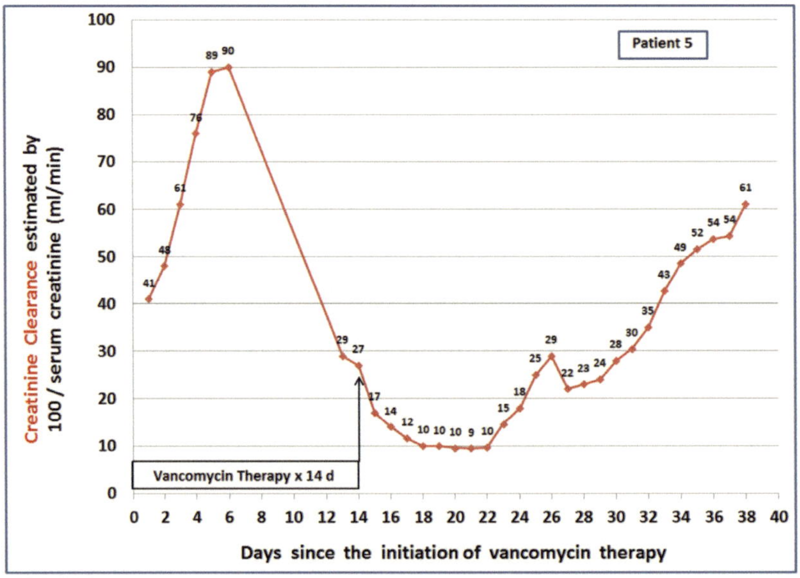

Fig. 5. B

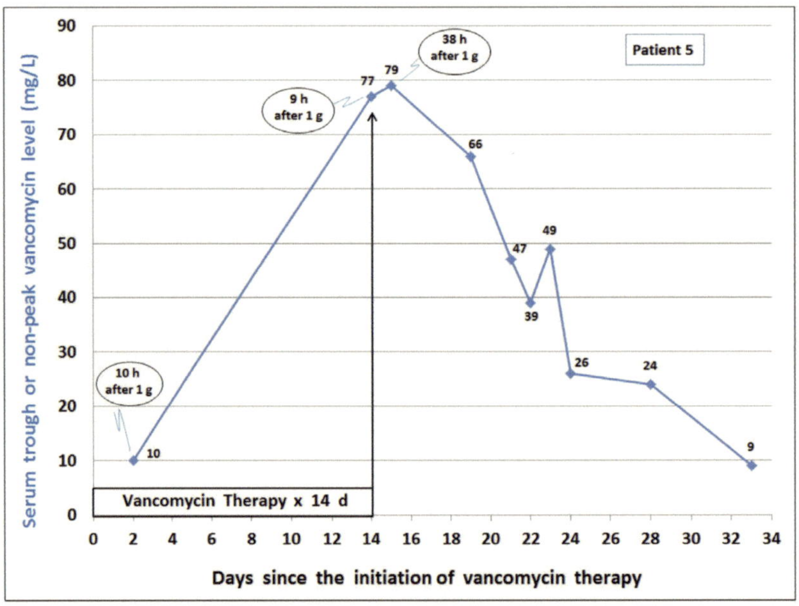

Fig. 5. C

In the nursing home his vancomycin level was not monitored. On re-admission, the vancomycin level (77 mg/L) was found to be in toxic range. Vancomycin was thus discontinued. 5 days later serum creatinine was 6.6mg/dl and it continued to climb to a peak level of 10.3 mg/dl on hospital day 7 (Fig 5A).

Patient appeared clinically stable and euvolemic. A kidney ultrasound did not show any obstruction. Of note other causes of acute renal failure were ruled out. He did not have acute interstitial nephritis as there was no rash, peripheral eosinophilia or eosinophiluria. He showed no signs of sepsis and his blood cultures remained negative. He did not receive any nephrotoxic agents or radio-contrast dyes. His antibiotics were switched to ciprofloxacin 400 mg IV q 24 h and cefepime 1g q12 h.

On days 7 and 9 of his second hospitalization, he underwent two sessions of hemodialysis to help manage his oliguria and to help remove the cumulated vancomycin. After the hemodialysis his serum creatinine and serum vancomycin levels both trended down. As vancomycin disappeared from his system, his kidney function improved significantly. Although he required furosemide drip to help manage his oliguria, he became relatively polyuric in the recovery phase of his AKI. Four weeks after discontinuation of vancomycin, his serum creatinine was 1.64 mg/dl close to though still higher than his best baseline value. But he was vastly improved and able to be discharged. At that time vancomycin level was 9 mg/L.

Case 6:

This patient was a 65 year old man hospitalized for hand osteomyelitis. He had a significant and complicated past and ongoing medical history due to uncontrolled type 2 diabetes mellitus, hypertension, hyperlipidemia, atrial fibrillation, previous stroke, degenerative joint disease of his left hip and knee, status-post knee replacement, gastro-esophageal reflux disease, diabetic neuropathy, and a chronic but recently resolved MRSA diabetic left foot ulcer.

His present illness related to his left thumb pain that was initially treated with local steroid injections by his outside doctor. Subsequently, he had a draining ulcer at the first metacarpal joint of his left hand. Four days prior to his transfer from a local hospital to our medical center, MRI showed first metacarpal osteomyelitis and tendonitis. He was started on vancomycin, initially at a dose of 1.5 g every 18 hours three days before the transfer. On the 2nd hospital day with us, gram stain and culture from the left thumb wound showed MRSA. MRSA was also confirmed by intra-operative bone biopsy culture on the 3rd hospital day. Vancomycin was continued targeting 24-h trough levels ≥ 15 mg/L.

The patient was discharged on the 5th hospital day to complete a prolonged course of vancomycin at a dose of 1.5 g daily at the recommendation of ID consultants. Blood for vancomycin levels and basic metabolic profile was drawn and checked by home health nurse once weekly. After two weeks, his vancomycin dose was increased to 2.0 g daily. Four more weeks later, it was further raised to 2.5 g daily to keep level >15 mg/L (Fig 6C). Three weeks after the last dose increase, although the 24-h trough levels finally reached 17-19 mg/L (Fig 6C), his serum creatinine had also risen from 1.3 to 2.3 mg/dl (Fig 6 A). This represented a further hike from initial baseline of 0.8 at the start of vancomycin therapy.

Meloxicam, an NSAID, and lisinopril, which he had taken for years, were temporarily stopped, along with holding his vancomycin for 3 days. When his serum creatinine appeared to stop rising and seemed to stabilize at ~ 2.1 mg/dl, vancomycin was resumed albeit at a reduced dose of 1 g daily. This was however stopped completely due to the persistent elevation of his serum creatinine at 2 mg/dl (Fig 6A). By having excluded obstruction with renal ultrasound, pre-renal or hemodynamic factors, bacteremic or septic etiologies and other intra-renal insults, we believe his subacute decline in renal function (Fig

6B), at least in retrospect, was best explained by the protracted vancomycin exposure with unmeasured peak levels which could have inflicted steady but sustained chronic damage.

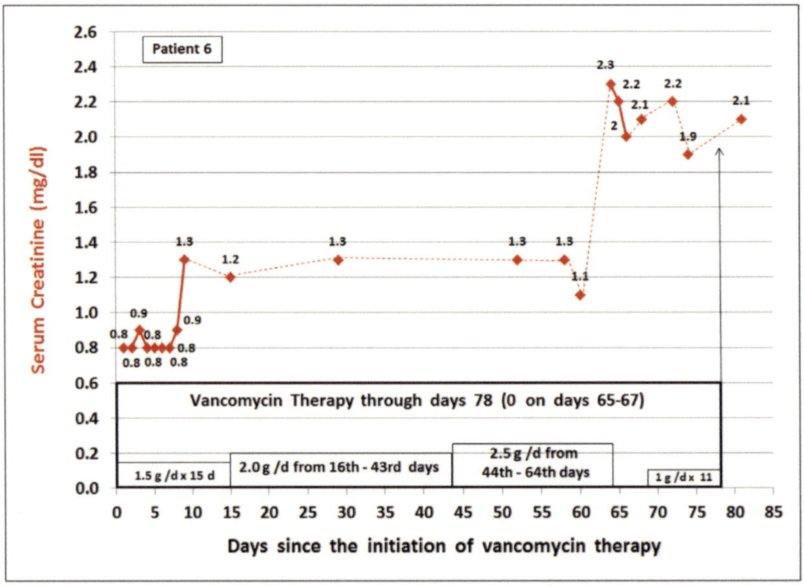

Fig. 6. A

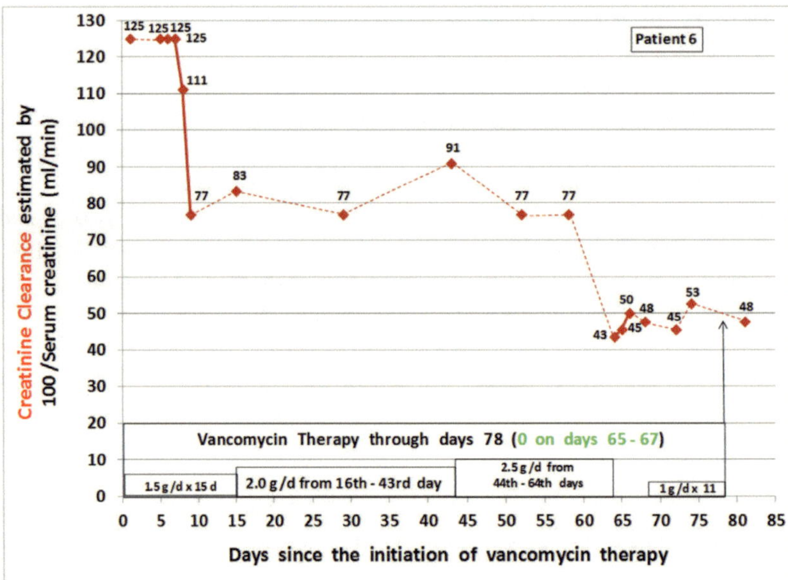

Fig. 6. B

The most informative was the marked drop in his creatinine clearance 2 weeks into vancomycin therapy (from ~ 125 to ~ 80 ml/min) (Fig 6B), which had easily escaped clinical

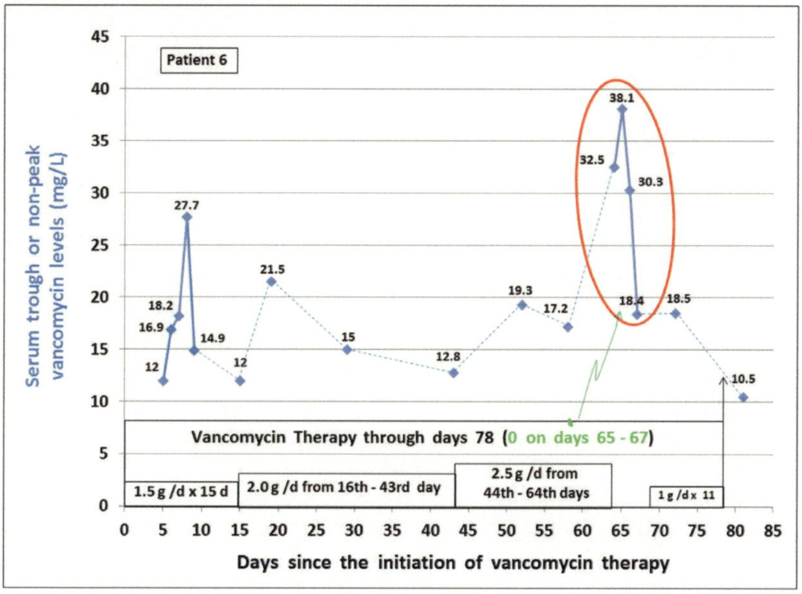

Fig. 6. C

detection by most physicians if evaluated simply based on examining the absolute values at one point in time or judged by the modest rise in creatinine from ~ 0.8 to 1.3 mg/dl (Fig 6A), the latter typically attributed to pre-renal or volume-related issues. Only when serum creatinine exceeded the rather arbitrary upper limit of normal of 1.2 mg/dl and only when it remained elevated was the concern of AKI raised in this patient. This issue of renal failure had finally become unequivocal and unmistakable when the entire course was reviewed longitudinally. After 10 weeks of vancomycin exposure, there was a 3-fold elevation in his serum creatinine (0.8 to 2.2 mg/dl) (Fig 6A), or more dramatically though more meaningfully in clinical nephrology, a corresponding 60 % decrease in creatinine clearance (from 125 to 50 ml/min).

Results on objective 2:

Lessons learned and insights deduced from the published literature and our case experience

To generate a typical profile of patients suffering from Van-AKI, we attempted to generalize from the group of our six patients on whom we have a complete set of clinical and laboratory data. When the serial renal function data and vancomycin levels for all 6 patients were plotted as group means on the same figure as a function of the time of vancomycin treatment, a clinical profile of Van-AKI and its recovery become apparent (Fig 7). Table 6 summarizes the group data as mean ± SE on their demographic and hematologic data (Table 6A), serial renal function through the 60th and last day of follow-up (Table 6B), vancomycin dosages (cumulative and average daily dose), duration of treatment, and serial vancomycin levels (Table 6 C). The following statistical statements could thus be made, providingsome insights and lessons on the issue of Van-AKI.

1. For our cohort of 6 patients, the mean duration of vancomycin administration was 28.2 ± 12.7 [SE] days (Table 6 C). Our group of patients, with more delayed diagnosis and

more severe renal failure, certainly confirmed the general impression from both prospective and retrospective studies that the chronicity of administration beyond 7 to 21 days posed independent risks for nephrotoxicity (Goetz & Sayer, 1993; Hidayat et al, 2006; Pritchard et al, 2008). The cumulative dose was 59.3 ± 23.6 g, yielding an average daily dose of 2.4 ± 0.6 g/day (Table 6 C). Since mean body weight (BW) was 85.5 ± 2.8 kg (Table 6A), the average dose was 28 mg/kg BW per day. The last dose given averaged 1.33 ± 0.17g (Table 6 C), equivalent to 15.5 mg /kg body weight. In retrospect if not prospectively, this dose should be considered excessive and probably unnecessary because at the time of this last dose, both serum creatinine (4-6 fold of baseline) and vancomycin level (30 to 70 mg/L) for that day were known to have been significantly elevated (Table 6 B & C and Fig 7). We believe this last dose could have been much reduced or simply skipped (had greater restraints been exercised and more circumspection applied), considering the fore-knowledge of a significantly elevated serum creatinine (mean being 4.1 mg/dl, Fig 7) and high vancomycin levels of 65-70mg/L (Fig 7Fig 7). Existing literature suggests that both pre-existing renal insufficiency (as denoted by serum creatinine >1.7 mg/dl) (Pritchard et al, 2008) and elevated steady state serum vancomycin levels > 28 mg/ (Ingram et al, 2008) or elevated trough levels >14 mg/L (Rybak et al 1990) are independent risk factors for ARF during vancomycin therapy (Hidayat et al, 2006; Pritchard et al, 2008; Lodise et al, 2008).

2. Peak vancomycin levels (group mean 70 ± 10 mg/L), which we defined here as the individual patient's highest value at any time during therapy and irrespective of when it was last given, was observed 26.2 ± 11.1 days after the first dose and 9.5 ± 4.9 hours after the last dose (Fig 7, Table 6 C). Some patients received their last dose, despite in retrospect already exhibiting a very high peak vancomycin level a few hours earlier (Table 6 C). At the point when vancomycin was discontinued, drug level was 65.1 ± 12.5 mg/L (Table 6 C). We would therefore propose that vancomycin orders be written daily (if not every 12 h), similar to coumadin orders in the titration phase of trying to achieve certain target levels or attaining a steady-state concentration, instead of one generic scheduled order for several days at a time. Needless to say, in retrospect, both the peak vancomycin levels for individual patients and the level on the day of stopping vancomycin (65.1 mg/L; Fig 7) were substantially higher than the recommended steady-state cut-off level of 28 mg/L (Ingram et al, 2008) or the trough cut-off level of 14 mg/L (Pitchard et al, 2008).
3. On the day of peak vancomycin level (day 26.2 of therapy), average serum creatinine had already risen to 4.1 ± 0.78 mg/dl (Δ= 3.14 ± 0.67 mg/dl, p<0.005 vs. baseline; Table 6 B) and the corresponding creatinine clearance (CrCl) had fallen to 29.5 ± 5.5 ml/min, (Δ = - 84.7 ± 11.2 ml/min, p<0.001 vs. baseline; Table 6 B).
4. Prior to the actual peak serum vancomycin levels documented on day 26, an earlier serum vancomycin had also been obtained, on ~ day 22 (± 10) or ~ 4.2 ± 2 days earlier. This "pre-peak" vancomycin level (30 ± 9.8 mg/L) was already significantly elevated (Table 6 C & Fig 7). On that day, serum creatinine (1.85 ± 0.48 mg/dl) was numerically higher than baseline (Δ= 0.89 ± 0.4, n.s.). This corresponded to an estimated CrCl of 79.2 ± 21.1 ml/min, or a drop of 35 ± 14 ml/min from baseline, though just shy of significance (p=0.06) (Table 6 B). It is noteworthy that in retrospect, three independent forewarning signs for nephrotoxicity had already emerged on this 22nd day of therapy: (a) duration of administration > the 3rd week previously suggested as a risk factor

(Goetz & Sayer, 1993); (b) mean serum creatinine > the 1.7 mg/dl postulated as a risk thresh-hold (Pritchard et al, 2008); and (c) mean steady state vancomycin levels > 28 mg/L as a risk threshold (Ingram et al, 2008).

5. Indeed, over these interim 4.2 days, serum creatinine had increased further from 1.85 to 4.1mg/dl (Δ = 2.24 ± 0.74 mg/dl, $p < 0.04$; Table 6 B and fig 7). There was also an additional loss of CrCl of 49.7 ± 19.3 ml/min, $p < 0.05$; Table 6 B and Fig 7).
6. Serum creatinine peaked on the average 28.8 ± 9.9 days into vancomycin treatment, which occurred ~ 2 to 3 days after serum vancomycin level had reached its peak. Over this interval, there was a further increase in serum creatinine, climbing from 4.1 to 5.93 ± 1.23 mg/dl (Δ= 1.83 ± 0.73 mg/dl, $p<0.05$; Table 6 B), associated with a further drop in CrCl from the 29.5 to 21.7 ± 5.1 ml/min (Δ= - 7.9 ± 3.0 ml/min, $p<0.05$; Table 6 B).
7. Estimated CrCl fell from the mean baseline of 114.2 ± 15.3 to a nadir value of 21.7 ± 5.1 ml/min, $p < 0.005$ (Fig 7; Table 6 B). This was accompanied by a significant and marked increase in serum creatinine from the baseline of 0.96 ± 0.13 mg/dl to 5.93 mg/dl, a 6-fold increase (Δ = 4.97 ± 1.12 mg/dl, $p < 0.01$). Accordingly, there was a total loss of CrCl of 92.6 ± 13.6 ml/min, $p<0.005$ at the time of the worst (or peak) serum creatinine. Serum creatinine peaked 28.8 days after initiating vancomycin therapy, which was temporally 2.9 ± 1.4 days after the last dose. It is noteworthy that although vancomycin level reached the highest value 9.5 ± 4.9 hours after the last dose, serum creatinine did not reach its peak until 68.7 ± 32.4 hours after the last dose, indicating a delay of ~ 60 hours between reaching peak drug level and the full impact of functional impairment.
8. After vancomycin was stopped, serum creatinine returned towards the baseline, falling to a nadir value of 1.57 ± 0.22 mg/dl ($p<0.02$ vs. peak creatinine of 5.93 mg/dl, Δ = 4.36 ± 1.21 mg/dl; Table 6 B). This was associated with an estimated CrCl of 72.3 ± 12.4 ml/min at the point of maximal functional recovery (Δ = 50.7 ± 13 ml/min, $p < 0.01$ compared to the lowest value at the worst time of the ARF; Table 6 B). The maximal functional improvement was noted 30.8 ± 10.4 days after the last dose, or 59.0 ± 15.7 days after the first dose of vancomycin (Table 6 C).
9. Despite 2 months since vancomycin had been initiated and 1 month after the last dose of vancomycin, once AKI had developed, the functional recovery was unfortunately incomplete even at the time of maximal improvement in the serum creatinine. In the short-term follow-up of ~ 31 days after the last dose or after the onset of ARF, there remained a residual elevation of serum creatinine (Δ = 0.61 ± 0.2 mg/dl, $p< 0.04$), associated with what appeared to be an irreversible decline of CrCl of 41.9 ± 12.9 ml/min, $p < 0.03$ (Table 6 B & Fig 7). Compared to the baseline CrCl of 114.2 ml/min, this represented a 37 % residual loss of renal function. It is possible that with longer period of follow up further return of renal function may ensue.
10. Vancomycin level was ordered and monitored in the recovery period based on decisions by the individual clinicians without any discernible or uniform pattern. In this cohort of 6 patients, the lowest drug level (17.5 ± 7.5 mg/L) was observed 8.0 ± 2.5 days after the last dose (Table 6 C). It is noteworthy that this concentration of vancomycin, 8 days after stopping vancomycin, still fell into if not exceeded most recommended therapeutic ranges.
11. Compared to the duration of vancomycin administration of 28.2 days, the average recovery time for maximal return of renal function was 3.2 ± 1.7 fold longer, indicating significant clinical morbidities (and associated financial burdens) posed by a preventable medication complication.

Results on objective 3:

Practical guidelines for the safe and effective long-term vancomycin administration

The financial and health burden for managing ARF due to Van-AKI is currently unknown and clearly cannot be determined by our retrospective studies, especially with such a small series and observed over such a short time window. Furthermore, we have no good information on the true incidence of Van-AKI. However, it suffices to note that for our first 5 patients, it took between 20 and 70 days of inpatient care and management (a mean of 35 ± 9.6 days after the diagnosis of ARF) before regaining partial renal function for discharge to outpatient follow-up. The clinical impact of Van-AKI was also substantial to affected patients since we found significant residual losses of renal function ~ 37 % (by CrCl) even 31 days after diagnosing ARF or after stopping the drug, using the lowest serum creatinine in the recovery. For these two and other additional reasons, the prevention and amelioration of Van-AKI should be a top priority. Drawing upon our own experience and analyses plus that published in the literature, we would like to turn the lessons and insights (from results on Objective II) into the following guidelines.

1. We propose that vancomycin be viewed as nephrotoxic till proven otherwise, just like aminoglycosides, cis-platinum, amphotericin B, and radio-contrast dyes. If there are no compelling indications, as was the case for 4 of our 6 patients (cases 1, 2, 3, and 5; Table 6 A), vancomycin should not be used, in deference to other safer suitable alternatives (see suggestions under Discussion).
2. If it must be used, the index of suspicion for Van-AKI should be high because even the slightest degree of renal injury (generally undetected by the meager increase in serum creatinine from its normal baseline) will impair excretion, predispose to drug accumulation and excess levels, which in turn inflicts more tissue damage and further compromises elimination, setting up a viscous cycle. Such a rapid buildup of vancomycin with steeply rising serum creatinine was amply illustrated by our patients 4 and 6, the former precipitously over 48 h and the latter in 13 days, but both were mediated by the same mechanism. There had been case reports of similarly steep functional decline caused by sharply increasing vancomycin levels (Shah-Khan et al, 2011).
3. Drug levels and serial renal function should be closely monitored continually throughout treatment, daily the first week, preferably thrice weekly but no fewer than twice weekly thereafter. For example, three of our 6 patients did not have drug levels and/or creatinine measured for 8-21 days immediately prior to their ARF and/or development of excessive vancomycin levels (cases 2, 5 and 6). In at least six subsets of patients who are particularly vulnerable to AKI, these preventive measures should be mandatory.

a. Those treated in the outpatient setting, nursing homes, or long-term care facilities where physician involvement and supervision are inherently minimal, indirect, and less than immediate, like our patients 2, 5 and 6. Lab results must be received, reviewed and acted upon in a timely fashion (within 23 h if dosed daily or within 11 h if dosed every 12 h) by professionals trained to monitor for nephrotoxicity and supervised by physicians experienced in this issue. Timely dose adjustments or stoppage must be feasible and reliable to prevent AKI.

b. Critically ill and complicated patients, like those in the ICU, who are at increased risks for ARF due to other potential nephrotoxic insults or hemodynamic instability (Colomo et al (2010)).

c. Patients infected by MRSA requiring a high vancomycin MIC and therefore high trough levels of ~ 15-20 mg/L and urgent attainment of such high levels by rapid escalation. Only daily vancomycin and daily creatinine level would allow achievement of such target levels without undue risks for unrecognized renal toxicity (also see point # 4 below).
d. Protracted infusion (>2 weeks).
e. Pre-existing CKD.
f. ARF or those with fluctuating serum creatinine.

Pre-emptive renal consultation at the earliest signs of potential nephrotoxicity may prevent costly AKI and y hospitalization.

4. Scheduled vancomycin dosing should be discouraged, and if necessary, written no longer than every 2 to 3 consecutive days because of the known narrow therapeutic window of vancomycin. The duration should be further limited to one day at a time in three particularly susceptible patient cohorts.
a. Elevated serum creatinine, whether before or during vancomycin therapy (e.g. cases 3, 4 and 6), since vancomycin excretion is already impaired,
b. Those in the early non-steady state of initiating therapy (e.g. cases 3 and 5), and
c. Those requiring rapid dose escalations to meet certain target levels (cases 1, 4, and 6).

In cases 1, 4, and 6, for instance, toxic trough vancomycin levels were created and found because of the rapid escalation without attaining a relative steady state at each incremental step. Our experience amply confirmed the virtually identical experience reported in the one case by Barraclough et al in 2007. We would support and re-emphasize their caution regarding the need not only to monitor very tightly and frequently during rapid dose escalation but also ordering one dose at a time.

By routinely refraining from a multi-day scheduled order, physicians could use the latest serum creatinine and vancomycin data to adjust the next dose to avoid further damage which otherwise could easily happen with a standing order. The danger of the latter approach was statistically and pictorially shown in our six patients by the delayed stoppage despite theoretically prior knowledge of vancomycin levels of 70 mg/L and creatinine elevation to 4-fold of the baseline 2 days earlier (Fig 7, Tables 6 B & C). The rationale and justification are identical to writing daily coumadin orders in similar non-steady states like dose titration or escalation. The trade off for the inconvenience and extra though manageable work load would be a far lower incidence of AKI [(and perhaps fewer cases of chronic kidney disease (CKD)] and reduced health care expenses.

5. Based on inferences from our statistical analyses, we recommend three simple practicable thresholds for drastic dose reduction or complete stoppage of vancomycin.
a. A doubling of baseline serum creatinine,
b. A serum creatinine ≥ 1.5 mg/dl for any adult patients,
c. 10- to 12-h trough levels ≥ 20-25 mg/L (Table 6 C, Fig 7) (Ingram et al, 2008).

We urge serious considerations for an immediate stoppage if any 2 of these 3 criteria are present, at least temporarily withholding vancomycin until additional tests show stable or improved renal function and significant decline in vancomycin levels.

6. We would re-emphasize the observation from classical renal physiology that serum creatinine is a very insensitive index of renal function in terms of detecting early decline in GFR. It is also grossly inaccurate in quantifying the loss of renal function, especially when the absolute values are below 1.5 mg/dl or when the changes occur between 0.5 and 2 mg/dl. Sole reliance on the increases of serum creatinine or the absolute values as

indicator of ARF will delay detection and recognition of AKI. Decline in GFR is not linearly related to the rise in serum creatinine. An initial small rise in serum creatinine from a perfectly normal baseline actually represents a marked fall in GFR whereas a marked rise in advanced CKD represents only modest drops. Thus, even small increments from the normal should raise concerns of AKI, especially in the early phase. The 500 ml of IV fluids typically used to deliver the vancomycin q 12 h could easily mask a genuine increase in serum creatinine, making detection of AKI in the early phase even harder unless the index of suspicion is high.

The emaciated 40-kg patient described by Barraclough et al (2007) illustrated this point well because his baseline serum creatinine was only 0.3 mg/dl. Although it went up precipitously to 0.5 mg/dl by day 4 day (already 40% loss of GFR) and then to 1.4 mg/dl (already 79 % loss of GFR) by day 8 day of therapy and with a vancomycin level 66 mg/L, the standing order of 1 g twice daily was not reduced until day 9, when creatinine finally peaked at 1.9 mg/dl (84% loss of GFR).

We thus recommend using the reciprocal (times a convenient constant like 100) as a simple, reliable and accurate estimate of CrCl and its changes reflect *relative changes* in GFR for a given patient. This approach will enhance the sensitivity and detection of early kidney injury, at a time when timely and appropriate dosage reduction or cessation should be made to prevent further nephrotoxicity.

The contrast between using serum creatinine and using 100/serum creatinine is best illustrated in 4 of our patients (cases 1, 3, 4, and 6). Two of them (cases 1 & 3) lost 62 to 76 % of their CrCl or GFR in 1 day (from 132 to 43 ml/min in case 1 and from 106 to 39 ml/min in case 3) if renal function is evaluated by using CrCl (Fig 1 B and Fig 3 B). In contrast, superficially there appeared to be quite "minimal" or "manageable" loss by serum creatinine over the same one day [(0.8 to 2.3 mg/dl in case 1 (Fig 1A) and 0.9 to 2.6 mg/dl in case 3 (Fig 3A)]. Similarly, case 4 lost 62 % of the GFR in 2 days when judged by CrCl (Fig 4 B), contrary to the "modest" rise in serum creatinine from 0.9 to 2.6 mg/dl (Fig 4 A). Likewise, patient # 6 suffered 36% loss of CrCl in 2 days (Fig 6B) as the corresponding serum creatinine went up by a "meager" delta of 0.5 mg/dl (from 0.8 to 1.3; Fig 6A) over the same 2 days.

We therefore recommend quantifying relative GFR loss by the decrements in CrCl, as estimated by 100 /serum creatinine. Specifically, we suggest that 20-30 % drop in GFR estimated by this serum creatinine reciprocal method would provide a better and earlier warning signal for possible nephrotoxicity than the thresholds of doubling of serum creatinine or values ≥ 1.5 mg/dl. As recommended later, a renal consult can be requested to assist with such a less conventional approach of evaluating GFR.

7. As shown in our patients individually and collectively, the current practice of ordering and measuring "random" vancomycin levels, without regard to the timing of the last administered dose, will continue to confuse and confound us. Random levels are essentially un-interpretable, often misleading and unreliable, generally inaccurate as an index of the area under the curve (AUC) relating drug concentration against time, and at times simply useless if not dangerous. For instance, to the best of our knowledge there is no published "normal" range to define what to expect for levels between 4 to 8 hours post-dosing. Such grey-zone times create unnecessary ambiguity and obligate extrapolation and speculation. In addition, there is a general tendency (and thus a common problem) for busy clinicians working as a team to assume a high value or "toxic levels" as "peak" previously ordered by a colleague without always checking

details of the last administration or verifying this assumption. Thus frequently if not invariably, high or "toxic" values are simply attributed to sampling within a few hours of the infusion when in fact they may actually be a 10-12 h trough level. A high peak value (if indeed verified to be peak) may not necessarily require dose reduction or discontinuation although even this assumption may not be correct or safe. But a true trough but high level should mandate immediate consideration of stopping vancomycin (or at least until nephrotoxicity is excluded). Reconstruction of the timing of a "random" level relative to the last infused dose is tedious, time-consuming and prohibitive. They render making sound clinical decisions on proper dosage adjustments very difficult.

On scientific ground, we would discourage if not deplore the practice of "random" vancomycin levels. It condones uncertainties and fosters the culture and attitude of making and accepting subjective arbitrary interpretations. We would therefore endorse getting only a true trough level like 10-12 h (after the last dose if given at q 12 h frequency), or 24- or 48-h troughs (if dosed at 24 to 48 h frequency for whatever reasons).

Parenthetically, though with undefined clinical impact, the AUC per unit time is smaller (thus the nephrotoxic risk lower) if dosed once q 12 h versus dosing q 24 or q 48 h even when the trough levels are identical, say, at 15 mg/L for all three regimens. This is because AUC (or the total drug exposure by time and concentration) has been shown to play a role in Van-AKI (Bailie et al 1988). We would therefore favor and recommend the q 12 h (or at the longest, < q 24 h) dosing schedule over the q 48 h regimen and accordingly suggest measuring the 12-h trough levels unless logistically impossible. If q 24-h dosing is necessary, experience has shown comparable safety compared to q 12 h dosing if the 24-h rough levels were kept below 10 mg/L (Cohen, Dadashev et al. 2002).

8. We propose changing our default mode of ordering vancomycin "*to give* the *next dose only if the trough level falls below the therapeutic target*", as opposed to the current default mode of "*keep giving to sustain the trough level above the target range*". In practice, presently most physicians would re-dose even if the trough level was as high as 20-25 mg/L (or even 30), for fear that if we withhold, the level might drop precipitously below the therapeutic range regardless of the prevailing serum creatinine. Consequently, the actual trough levels are always substantially if not markedly higher than 20-25 mg/L.

Our recommendation of a conservative dosing is based on two considerations. First, by definition all levels prior to the trough would have exceeded 15-20 mg/L, which were shown to pose greater risks for nephrotoxicity (Hidayat et al (2006); Pritchard et al (2008); our series of six patients). Second, there is no published evidence that trough levels of 10-15 mg/L, for example, are necessarily associated with poorer clinical cure or response than levels of 15-20 mg/L if the MIC against a "sensitive" MRSA is supposed to be < 1 mg/L or at the worst < 2 mg/L (Hermsen, Hanson et al. 2010; Chan, Pham et al. 2011).

9. Although the initial loading dose of vancomycin (typically 15 mg/kg) is the same regardless of the level of renal function, the maintenance dose must be reduced in pre-existing renal insufficiency, newly developed ARF, and/or deteriorating function. This basic safety principle was forgotten or ignored in virtually all the reported cases including our 6 patients. We recommend using the nomogram (15 mg x GFR in ml/min) for daily maintenance dose (in mg per day) first suggested by Moellering et al (1981) for renal impairment. This rough guideline has stood the test of time and provides a good though crude first approximation, allowing us to make later and continual adjustments based on subsequent trough levels.

In practice, if serum creatinine is relatively stable, GFR can be estimated by the equation of Cockcroft-Gault for CrCl (in ml/min) [= (140 - age in years) x (lean body mass in kg) / (serum creatinine in mg/dl x 72)] (Cockcroft and Gault (1976)). For instance, the maintenance dose will be ~ 1.5 g /d (=15 mg/d x 100) for a CrCl of 100 ml/min. Likewise, it will be ~ 450 mg/d (=15 mg/d x 30) for a CrCl of 30 ml/min. We should note that even with a steady state creatinine, this equation is known to over-estimate CrCl in the (a) elderly, (b) emaciated, (c) edematous, (d) obese, and (e) paralysis or amputees. An even smaller dose must be considered in these situations.

For patients with changing serum creatinine, it is advisable not only to measure creatinine and vancomycin more frequently due to the non-steady state, but also obtain renal consultation. These patients are at increased risks created by the predictable positive feedback loop between falling GFR (as denoted by steadily rising serum creatinine) and increasing kidney vancomycin exposure (as reflected by rising vancomycin levels). For patients functionally anuric or anephric, 2 mg/kg/d is a reasonable initial dose. In these patients and those with established end-stage renal disease or dialysis dependency, nephrology should be consulted even though they fall outside of the scope of cohorts to be considered in this Chapter (Van-AKI).

10. Although unproven by randomized controlled trial, there are theoretical reasons and some anecdotal evidence to support the consideration of prompt and significant removal of vancomycin by hemodialysis in patients with Van-AKI and burdened with sustained toxic levels and severe renal failure. We would therefore recommend earliest possible referral to nephrology for assistance and support for such a therapeutic option.

Though without personal or literature data to address this issue, we would submit that it is an unresolved theory as to the scientific basis and/or the clinical superiority of targeting trough vancomycin levels between 15 and 20 mg/L for those MRSA with MIC > 1 but < 2 mg/L (Hermsen, Hanson et al. 2010; Chan, Pham et al. 2011).

We would urge exercising circumspection in accepting this recommendation and showing discretion and flexibility in applying the same if the goal is to achieve the bacterial killing without renal toxicity.

5. Discussion

For nearly half a century, vancomycin has been used successfully to treat infections caused by gram positive bacteria, notably MRSA, from various sources and in various organs. The issue of Van-AKI has been controversial due to the difficulty in establishing a cause-and-effect relationship between vancomycin and the alleged ARF. This is true among the affected patients reported in large epidemiologic surveys or drug toxicity monitoring studies because they generally provide little details on individual patients for an objective review or independent determination (Table 1). Similarly, among the two dozen or so reported cases of Van-AKI (Table 2), fewer than 10 had unequivocally excluded the usual confounding variables like sepsis, bacteremia, hemodynamic factors and concurrent nephrotoxins. Many also failed to provide serial vancomycin levels to show the temporal evolution with the ARF. Thus, to date, the existence of Van-AKI has been intensely debated and at times categorically dismissed.

Our first objective was to more firmly establish this clinical entity by performing a vigorous and comprehensive review of the existing literature and by reporting our own experience. We have obtained and presented three lines of evidence to argue for the entity of Van-AKI. First, the drug toxicity monitoring studies in the aggregate have offered a substantial body of indirect evidence to support the existence of Van-AKI, mainly based on the close correlations between increased blood levels and/or increased dosage on the one hand and increased incidence on the other hand (Rybak et al, 2009) (Table 1). Typically, there was observed a very low incidence of Van-AKI with low trough vancomycin levels like < 10 mg/L (Sorrel et al, 1985), but increased incidence with higher trough levels like >14 (Pritchard et al, 2008) or >15-20 mg/L (Hidayat et al, 2006), or with a high steady-state level > 28 mg/L (Ingram et al, 2008), and a 3-fold higher incidence when daily dose >4 g (Lodise et al, 2008).

Additional support was provided by the observations of synergism in nephrotoxicity between vancomycin and aminoglycoside (Farber et al, 1983; Sorrel et al, 1985; Rybak et al, 1990; Goetz & Sayer, 1993), the increased risks of Van-AKI with prolonged administration (Goetz & Sayer, 1993; Hidayat et al, 2006; Pritchard et al 2008), and the enhanced risks of nephrotoxicity (Lodise et al, 2008) or poorer renal outcome with vancomycin (Rodriguez Colomo et al, 2010) compared to linezolid in treating similar patient cohorts.

The second line of evidence was obtained from the 2 dozen cases of ARF associated with vancomycin administration (Table 2). Many were somewhat equivocal in terms of a clear cut etiology for the ARF, especially when no vancomycin levels were given and/or other common etiologies had been or could be vigorously excluded. There however remained about half a dozen well documented and unambiguous cases of Van-AKI, as evidenced by toxic drug levels and the absence of any other contributing factors or confounding variables for the ARF (Frimat et al, 1995; Barraclough et al, 2007; Ladino et al, 2008 [2 of 5 convincing cases]; Shah-Khan et al, 2011; Table 2).

The third and perhaps the strongest line of evidence is derived from our own experience, which includes 6 cases we have encountered and treated in the course of a month of renal consultation. There are probably two reasons for the relative ease with which these 6 patients with Van-AKI were discovered. One is the changing microbiology and characteristics of modern era patients and our obligated responses to these changes and adoption of current dosing practices. Two is the unique patient cohorts treated with vancomycin nowadays compared to the invariably septic or bacteremic patients with shock and pancytopenia in earlier decades. We shall elaborate on these two points.

First, there has been an apparent increase in the incidence of AKI during vancomycin therapy, largely due to three factors. One, the incidence of infections by documented MRSA and MRSE is growing rapidly. Two, there is an exponential increase in the use of vancomycin not only for sensitive and documented pathogens, but also for HCAP and osteomyelitis (especially in diabetics) in whom MRSA must be considered and/or covered, typically by vancomycin. After all, it is inexpensive, time-honored, tried, true, and proven to be effective against MSRA, the most prevalent and the deadliest bacteria. Three due to the widespread use (if not abuse) of vancomycin, there is a steady emergence of organisms sensitive only to rather high MIC, leading to the ID recommendation of trough levels > 15-20 mg/L (Rybak, Lomaestro et al. 2009). These three factors have combined to contribute to a significant upsurge of Van-AKI in our view.

Second, as opposed to the older cases where sepsis, bacteremia, hemodynamic instability, concurrently administered aminoglycosides, amphotericin B or contrast dyes could not be definitely excluded as etiologic factors for the ARF, none of these risk factors could have contributed to the AKI in our 6 patients (3 with HCAP and 3 with osteomyelitis, and none bacteremic or hypotensive) (Table 6 A). By providing and correlating serial vancomycin levels before, during, and after the ARF with the corresponding changes in renal function during the evolution phase and recovery period of the AKI, we believe we have vigorously documented the existence of Van-AKI in these six patients in whom we have complete access to and full review of all their clinical and laboratory data (Fig 1-7).

Collectively, we believe these three independent lines of evidence firmly establish the fact that vancomycin is unquestionably nephrotoxic, no different than aminoglycoside, cisplatinum, and radio-contrast dyes. The degree of renal failure was severe enough to initiate dialysis in one patient though he got less than one week of vancomycin. The other five patients had various degrees of residual renal impairment even a month after the last dose (Table 6 B, Fig 7). We therefore submit that the issue is no longer whether Van-AKI exists, but how to prevent or ameliorate it. To generate some practical guidelines towards this goal (our third objective), we took an intermediate step by pursuing the next objective.

Our second objective was to statistically analyze our 6 patients to generate a clinical pattern and to define a typical profile of Van-AKI, with the intent to abstract some insights and derive some lessons which can eventually help us formulate preventive strategies. Generally speaking, we note that Van-AKI is a real and common complication of vancomycin treatment, especially during rapid dose escalation and/or prolonged infusion of fixed doses without frequent monitoring of drug levels and serum creatinine. Van-AKI could be costly both financially and clinically since significant irreversible functional loss can ensue (Table 6 B, Fig 7). In the detailed analysis of our 6 cases, we found that, in retrospect if not prospectively, most cases of Van-AKI could have been prevented or ameliorated if only the returned results on levels and serum creatinine were carefully examined and interpreted within the clinical context and if only timely and appropriate corrective responses were made.

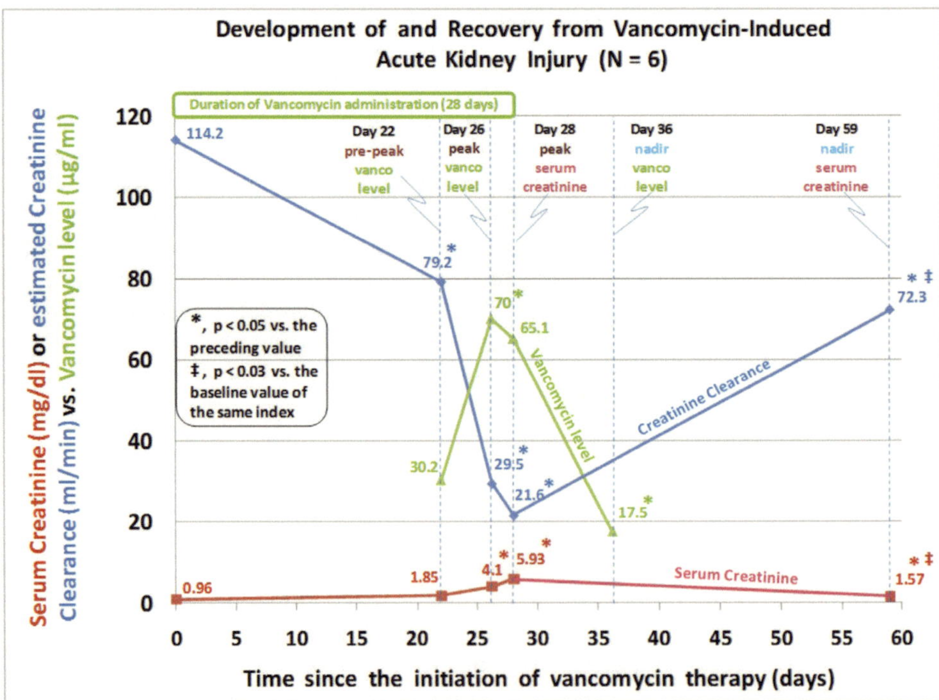

Fig. 7. Renal functional profile and changes in serum Vancomycin levels as averages of the 6 patients with AKI plotted against time since the initiation of vancomycin.

Characteristics (N= 6 patients)	(Mean ± SE)	(Units)
Gender Male : Female	6 : 0	
Age (years)	55.7 ± 6.0	years
Body weights	85.5 ± 2.8	kg
Pre-existing chronic kidney disease	N=2 (33 %)	%
Hypertension	N=3 (50 %)	%
Diabetes mellitus	N=3 (50 %)	%
Congestive heart failure or coronary disease	0	%
History of liver disease or hepatic dysfunction	N=2 (33 %)	%
Signs of volume depletion	N=1 (16 %)	%
Positive blood or urine cultures	0	%
Exposure to radio-contrast agents (but both temporally unrelated to ARF)	N=2 (33 %)	%
Indication for vancomycin: - Pneumonia	N=3 (50%)	(1 MRSA)
Osteomyelitis	N=3 (50%)	(1 MRSA)
Hypotension (SBP <95 x >4 h) or signs of shock	0	%
Fever (temperature > 38 degrees C or 100.5 F)	N=2 (33%)	%
Baseline WBC	10.6 ± 1.9	v
Baseline absolute neutrophils	8.6 ± 1.8	K/mm3
Baseline absolute eosinophils	74 ± 32	per mm3
Urine eosinophils	0	%
Ultrasound evidence for obstructive uropathy	0	%
Overall assessment of the pathogenic role of vancomycin in the AKI	85 ± 1	%

Table 6. A. Demographics and baseline clinical characteristics (N= 6)

We therefore attempted to identify independent common risk factors resulting in Van-AKI. In this pursuit, we have confirmed but extended the three previously reported risk factors for Van-AKI (a) High blood vancomycin levels (Rybak et al, 1990; Hidayat et al, 2006; Pritchard et al, 2008; Ingram et al, 2008; Lodise et al, 2008). In all 6 of our patients, the clinical intent was to dose to achieve a target trough level >12-20 mg/L, but during the execution, toxic levels had developed. (b) Prolonged duration of administration (Goetz & Sayer, 1993; Hidayat et al, 2006; Pritchard et al 2008). Two of our patients (#2 & # 6) had received vancomycin for 56 and 78 days, primarily in the outpatient setting where the monitoring mechanism and dose adjustment and response time were suboptimal. (c) Rapid dose escalation without achieving steady state (Barraclough et al, 2007). Three of our patients (#1, #4, and #6) suffered as a result of the desire to achieve the higher 15-20 mg/L target levels because of the apparent failure to await a steady state between dosage increments. In other two patients (# 3 & # 5), the intent to attain therapeutic levels within the first few days of administration resulted in excessive levels also due to non-steady state kinetics.

In our opinion, therefore, the most important but recurrent lesson to learn from all these cases and the literature would be meticulous avoidance of excess vancomycin levels since low levels were rarely reported to induce Van-AKI. Toxic levels typically develop during the non-steady state of either the initial days of a fixed dose schedule or the early phase of rapid dose escalation. While we have no data to base any proposed recommendation, it is fair to state that the ID recommendation of targeting 15-20 mg/L represents the consensus opinion of a panel of experienced experts in this field. The primary goal of combating infections is of course complete bacterial eradication. Viewed from this perspective, it is understandable and reasonable that the default mode of ordering vancomycin is to *keep giving to sustain trough levels >15-20 mg/L*. In practice though, the empirically observed trough levels would almost always exceed 15-20 mg/L, sometimes even up to 25-30, due to lack of foolproof dosing formula and due to invariably changing renal functions. Thus these drug levels seemed to be constantly at the threshold of flirting with nephrotoxicity. This could occur not only at the time of the documented trough levels but also most certainly during all the preceding hours when levels (though typically not measured) could be expected to be significantly if not markedly elevated.

Renal Function by serum creatinine or Creatinine Clearance estimated by 100/serum creatinine (absolute values or changes)				
	Units	Mean	SE	P VALUES
Baseline serum creatinine	(mg/dl)	0.96	0.13	
Creatinine Clearance (CrCl)	(ml/min)	114	15	
Serum creatinine on the day just before vancomycin level reached the peak (day of "pre-peak" vancomycin)	(mg/dl)	1.85	0.48	n.s. vs. baseline
CrCl on the day of "pre-peak" vancomycin	(ml/min)	79.2	21.1	
Rise in serum creatinine on the day of "pre-peak" vancomycin vs. baseline	(mg/dl)	0.89	0.40	n.s. vs. baseline
Drop in Crcl on the day of "pre-peak" vancomycin	(ml/min)	- 35	14	$p = 0.06$
Serum creatinine on the day of peak vancomycin	(mg/dl)	4.10	0.78	
CrCl on the day of peak vancomycin	(ml/min)	29.5	5.5	
Rise in serum creatinine from baseline to the day of peak vancomycin	(mg/dl)	3.14	0.67	$p < 0.005$
Fall in CrCl from baseline to the day of peak vancomycin	(ml/min)	- 84.7	11.2	$p < 0.001$
Rise in serum creatinine from the day of "pre-peak" vancomycin to the day of peak vancomycin	(mg/dl)	2.24	0.74	$p < 0.04$
Drop in CrCl from "pre-peak" to peak vancomycin	(ml/min)	- 49.7	19.3	$p < 0.05$
Peak serum creatinine	(mg/dl)	5.93	1.23	
Increase in serum creatinine vs. baseline	(mg/dl)	4.97	1.12	$p < 0.01$
CrCl at peak serum creatinine (worst CrCl)	(ml/min)	21.6	5.1	
Fall in CrCl at peak serum creatinine (worst decline)	(ml/min)	- 92.6	13.6	$p < 0.005$
Interval between the first dose and peak serum creatinine	(days)	28.8	9.9	
Further rise in serum creatinine from the day of peak vancomycin level to the day of peak creatinine level	(mg/dl)	1.83	0.73	$p < 0.05$
Further fall in CrCl from the day of peak vancomycin level to the day of peak creatinine level	(ml/min)	- 7.9	3.0	$p < 0.05$
Nadir serum creatinine during recovery	(mg/dl)	1.57	0.22	
CrCl at the time of nadir serum creatinine (maximal recovery)	(ml/min)	72.3	12.4	
Time from the first dose to nadir serum creatinine (recovery time)	(days)	59	15.7	
Drop in serum creatinine between peak & nadir values	(mg/dl)	4.36	1.21	$p < 0.02$
Best CrCl recovery (maximal CrCl - worst CrCl)	(ml/min)	50.7	13	$p < 0.01$
Irreversible increase in serum creatinine vs. baseline	(mg/dl)	0.61	0.2	$p < 0.04$
Residual decline in CrCl despite maximal recovery	(ml/min)	- 41.9	12.9	$p < 0.03$

Table 6. B. Summary of Serial Renal Function data during the Evolution of AKI & during its Recovery (N=6) (Mean ± SE)

On the other hand, to pursue the other equally important goal of prevention of Van-AKI, a more appropriate default mode of ordering vancomycin, we propose, would be to *infuse only if trough levels fall below certain target ranges,* as long as the attained trough levels are sufficiently high to achieve bacterial killing. We submit that these two goals are not mutually exclusive but in fact achievable in the same patient at the same time. At least two retrospective studies could be cited to support this notion. In the treatment of deep-seated MRSA infections, a retrospective cohort study failed to find any difference in clinical outcome between those with measurably high (>15-20 mg/L) and those with demonstrably lower trough levels (Hermsen, Hanson et al. 2010). In another retrospective study on vancomycin in the treatment of MRSA ventilator-associated pneumonia, the authors did not find any significant difference in survival or clinical cure in patients with trough level < 15 mg/L and those with trough levels > 15 mg/L (Chan, Pham et al. 2011).

Vancomycin Dosages and Serum Levels vs. the time course of changing serum creatinine	Units	Mean	S.E.
Cumulative dose	**gram**	**59.3**	**23.6**
Duration of vancomycin treatment	**days**	**28.2**	**12.7**
Average daily dose	**g/day**	**2.4**	**0.6**
Cumulative dose per unit body weight	**mg/kg**	**679**	**260**
Average daily dose per unit body weight	**mg/kg/day**	**28**	**8**
Vancomycin level on the day just before peak level ("pre-peak" day)	**mg/L**	**30.2**	**9.8**
Time from the first dose to the day of "pre-peak" vancomycin level	**days**	**22**	**10**
Time from the day of "pre-peak" level to the day of peak vancomycin	**days**	**4.2**	**2.0**
Peak vancomycin levels (defined as the highest value for a given patient during the entire course irrespective of when it was given)	**mg/L**	**70.0**	**9.8**
Time from the first dose to the day of peak vancomycin level	**days**	**26.2**	**11.1**
Time lag from the last dose to the appearance of peak vancomycin	**hours**	**9.5**	**4.9**
Vancomycin levels just before discontinuation	**mg/L**	**65.1**	**12.5**
Time when the last vancomycin dose given since the day of initiation	**days**	**28.2**	**12.7**
Amount of vancomycin given in the last dose	**g**	**1.3**	**0.2**
Nadir vancomycin level measured and recorded during recovery	**mg/L**	**17.5**	**7.5**
Time from the last dose to nadir vancomycin level in recovery	**days**	**8.0**	**2.5**
Time from the first dose to the day of peak serum creatinine	**days**	**27.2**	**10.7**
Interval between the last dose and the appearance of peak serum creatinine	**hours**	**68.7**	**32.4**
Time from the last dose to nadir serum creatinine (days to nadir)	**days**	**30.8**	**10.4**
Recovery time as a ratio of vancomycin exposure time	**ratio**	**3.2**	**1.7**

Table 6. C. Summary of Vancomcyin dosage and serum levels during the course of AKI and its recovery (N=6)

Additionally, in the treatment of MRSA bacteremia, it has been shown that high trough vancomycin levels of 15 to 20 mg/L per se might not be a good determinant or predictor for therapeutic success, at least not in those with pneumonia or MRSA endocarditis (Walraven, North et al. 2011). Therefore, until prospective randomized control studies comparing certain trough vancomycin level ranges are done to provide hard evidence to prove the importance of trough levels in excess of >15-20 mg/L, we propose physicians exercise appropriate caution, some circumspection, and some discretion in individual patients and base final dosing decisions on the entire clinical contexts, including the prevailing renal function.

Statistical analyses of our group data have yielded some new perhaps noteworthy insights. One, in 4 of our 6 patients (#1, #2, # 3, and # 5), the indication for vancomycin was not compelling, at least in retrospect, since only two had documented MRSA. Thus similar to some of the reported cases, in 2/3 of our patients, Van-AKI could have been avoided. Two, the failure to closely monitor drug levels or renal function had definitely contributed to the unexpectedly toxic levels and to Van-AKI in 3 of our patients (#2, #5, and # 6). In them, levels had not been checked for 8 to 21 days. Two of them (#2 and # 6) were under a designed 10-weeks treatment plan as an outpatient.

Three, there was no appropriate response to the discovery of excessive vancomycin levels (e. g. 30 mg/L) on day 22 of therapy despite a doubling of serum creatinine from the normal baseline (1.85 vs. 0.96 mg/dl) (Tables 6 B and C). Four days had been allowed to elapse, letting the steady climb of vancomycin level to its highest value on day 26, when little to nothing was done to reduce or withhold the dose during this interim. The same concern could be stated for the last dose given on day 28 since it should have been stopped or drastically reduced, as opposed to the 1.3 g dose actually used despite a vancomycin level of 70 mg/L and a serum creatinine of 4.1 mg/dl already noted 1-2 days earlier.

Four, when this highest level of 70 mg/L was finally reported on day 26 of therapy, at a time when serum creatinine (4.1 mg/dl) was already increased 4 fold, there was a 1-2 day time delay before the drug was stopped (Fig 7). Five, there was no evidence for any systematic dose adjustments for the known renal impairment in 3 of our 6 patients (#3, # 4, and # 6), either because of the absence of renal consultation or the lack of familiarity with the nomogram by Moellering et al (1981) [(15 x GFR in ml/min) for daily maintenance dose (in mg per day)]. This general equation has been found to be quite useful as it provides the first though crude approximation for dosages as a function of the residual renal function, permitting later finer adjustments based on subsequent trough levels. In practice, if serum creatinine is relatively stable, GFR can be estimated by using the equation of Cockcroft-Gault for CrCl (in ml/min) [= (140 - age in years) x (lean body mass in kg) / (serum creatinine in mg/dl x 72)] (Cockcroft and Gault, 1976).

The common basic issue among what appeared to have been judgment or logistic errors is either the lack of adequate monitoring or the lack of appropriate timely responses to typically already known warning signals for Van-AKI. Perhaps one additional source of problem or lesson to learn is the ordering, trusting, using and interpreting "random" vancomycin levels, here crudely defined any non-peak or non-trough levels, obtained at times totally without regard to the last administered dose. Such "random" levels are basically un-decipherable, generally misleading and unreliable, typically inaccurate as a surrogate of the AUC relating drug levels vs. time, and often simply useless if not hazardous. There is no published "normal" range statistically derived to define what one can expect for levels 4 to 8 hours post-dosing. This vacuum of information leaves plenty of doubts and much room for inaccurate extrapolations and erroneous speculations, making sound clinical decisions on proper dosage adjustments impossible.

We believe the practice of "random" levels should be abandoned, replaced by true 10-12 h trough levels. It should be noted that the AUC per unit time is smaller (thus nephrotoxic risk lower) if dosed once q 12 h vs. q 24 or q 48 h for identical trough levels for all three schedules. If a q 24-h dosing must be used, published experience would recommend aiming at 24-h trough levels below 10 mg/L to achieve similar safety margins as q 12 h dosing without sacrificing efficacy (Cohen, Dadashev et al. 2002).

The cornerstone to avoiding Van-AKI is abstinence, if not absolutely indicated as for 4 of our 6 patients, and if suitable safer alternatives are available. Despite the vast and positive overall clinical experience with vancomycin as an anti-MRSA antibiotic, several newer, less nephrotoxic or non-nephrotoxic alternatives have emerged, some even proven in clinical trials to confer comparable efficacy in certain bacterial infections. A few of these studies merit our comments and considerations as alternative agents because they demonstrate non-inferiority or comparable efficacy to that of vancomycin, at least for certain organ infections.

Thus, in MRSA ventilator-associated pneumonia, linezolid has been found in one retrospective study to produce similar survival rates but a trend towards higher cure rates than vancomycin (Chan, Pham et al. 2011). Clinical and microbiological outcomes in the treatment of nosocomial pneumonia were also found in one prospective randomized control trial to be comparable between linezolid and vancomycin (Rubinstein, Cammarata et al. 2001).

In patients with SA bacteremia and endocarditis, daptomycin has been shown to produce similar clinical responses as standard vancomycin therapy (Fowler, Boucher et al. 2006) and the reported success rates favored daptomycin over vancomycin among those patients infected with MRSA.

In skin and soft tissue infections, a prospective single-blinded multicenter study reported similar efficacy between daptomycin and vancomycin (Pertel et al, 2009). Similarly, teicoplanin (Van Laethem et al. 1988) and telavancin (Wilson et al. 2009) have been found to yield comparable cure rates as vancomycin for skin and soft tissue infections. It should be noted that teicoplanin is a glycopeptide with similar spectrum of anti-bacterial activities as vancomycin but with one third lower nephrotoxic risks, based on a recent Cochrane review of 24 studies involving 2,400 patients (Cavalcanti, Goncalves et al. 2010).

Finally, two 5th generation cephalosporin prodrugs (ceftaroline fosamil and ceftobiprole medocaril) have been found to possess anti-MRSA activities. Ceftaroline has been shown to produce similar clinical cure rates as vancomycin in complicated skin and skin structure infections (Iizawa, Nagai et al. 2004; Ge, Biek et al. 2008), whereas ceftobiprole was found to show similar efficacy as vancomycin in suspected gram positive infections, diabetic foot and mixed bacterial complicated skin and skin structure infectons (Noel, Bush et al. 2008 a; Noel, Strauss et al. 2008; Noel, Strauss et al. 2008 b).

In summary, several newer antibiotics have been shown to provide a potential equally effective but less nephrotoxic alternative to vancomycin for deep-seated MRSA infections. It is beyond the scope and our goal to comment on the advisability of deploying such alternatives other than updating their availabilities.

Our third and final objective was to use the lessons and insights from the literature and our case series to generate and recommend some simple practical guidelines targeted to the prevention and amelioration of Van-AKI. We will present these recommendations in a summary form in Table 7 below (Section VII).

6. Conclusions and recommendations

In conclusion, the era of vancomycin administration has spanned over half a century. Due to the widespread use of antibiotics whether indicated or not, there has been a growing emergence of microorganisms increasingly resistant to the existing antibiotics. MRSA has dictated the greater reliance on vancomycin. This in turn breeds the development of strains relatively insensitive to vancomycin, forces physicians to target higher drug levels and

1. Vancomycin is nephrotoxic and should be used only if truly indicated and in the absence of other safer suitable alternatives.
2. Close surveillance for Van-AKI must be performed throughout treatment by measuring drug levels and serial serum creatinine, once daily the first week, thrice weekly the second week, and no fewer than twice weekly thereafter. These preventive measures should be mandatory and in some cases done daily for the following cohorts at increased risks for AKI. (a) Those treated in the outpatient setting, nursing homes, or long-term care facilities; (b) Critically ill and complicated patients; (c) Patients needing high trough levels of ~15-20 mg/L and/or rapid dose escalation; (d) Protracted duration > 2 weeks; (e) Pre-existing CKD; (f) ARF or unstable/fluctuating serum creatinine.
3. Scheduled vancomycin dosing should be abandoned, and if absolutely necessary, written for less than 2 - 3 days at a time (like titrating Coumadin dosage in anticoagulation). To take advantage of the latest creatinine and vancomycin levels, daily orders should be written for (a) pre-existing elevated serum creatinine or changing levels, (b) the first week of initiating therapy due to the inherent non-steady state, and (c) rapid dose escalation.
4. Vancomycin should be stopped or drastically cut if any of the following thresholds emerges: (a) Doubling of normal baseline serum creatinine, (b) A serum creatinine ≥ 1.5 mg/dl for adults, (c) 10- to 12-h trough levels > 20-25 mg/L. Vancomycin must be stopped immediately if (a) or (b) plus (c) are present. A better safeguard will be a standard protocol by which the ordering MD &/or the RN executing the order is required to review, register, and document the latest trough level and the latest serum creatinine *before* administering the vancomycin (similar to blood sugar documentation before giving the next dose of insulin).
5. Since serum creatinine is an insensitive and inaccurate index of GFR, its reciprocal x 100 (100/serum creatinine) should be used to better estimate CrCl (and GFR). For a given patient, the decrement in CrCl will yield a more accurate measure of relative GFR losses and if this exceeds 20-30 %, nephrotoxicity should be considered and vancomycin stopped or reduced.
6. Ordering "random" serum vancomycin levels should be discouraged because they are un-interpretable (without published data to extrapolate to or correlate with the AUC). Reconstruction of the timing of a "random" level relative to the last dose is tedious, time-consuming and prohibitive. Since they tend to confuse and mislead in clinical decisions on proper dosage adjustments, only true 10-12 h trough levels (or in some special necessary cases 24- or 48-h) should be obtained.
7. For safety reasons, the default mode should be to *"give* the *next dose only if the trough level falls below the therapeutic target"*, as opposed to *"keep giving to sustain the trough level above the target range"*.
8. After an initial loading dose (identical regardless of renal function), the daily maintenance dose must be reduced in CKD and/or ARF, using the published nomogram (15 x CrCl in ml/min) (in mg per day). If serum creatinine is stable, CrCl (in ml/min) can be estimated by the Cockcroft-Gault formula [(140 - age in years) x (lean body mass in kg) / (serum creatinine in mg/dl x 72). A smaller dose than calculated must be given in: (a) elderly, (b) emaciated, (c) edematous, (d) obese, and (e) paralysis or amputees because the formula will over-estimate CrCl in these conditions.

9.	Since it is unproven that achieving trough levels of 15-20 mg/L is necessarily and unequivocally associated with superior clinical response than 10-15 mg/L (Hermsen, Hanson et al. 2010, Chan, Pham et al. 2011), a balance must be struck for a given patient between the efficacy in combating infection and the avoidance of Van-AkI in the actual dosing to achieve certain recommended target ranges.
10.	For patients with ARF, rapidly rising serum creatinine, and/or sustained vancomycin levels in the toxic range (>45 mg/L), renal consultation should be considered to assist with dosage adjustment and perhaps removal by hemodialysis, possibly to ameliorate nephrotoxicity and accelerate recovery.

Table 7. Recommendations for the Prevention of Vancomycin-induced Nephrotoxicity

consequently increasing the incidence of Van-AKI. The growing incidence of diagnosed diabetic foot ulcers and osteomyelitis and the mounting incidence of HCAP have further escalated the prescriptions of vancomycin, contributing to the increasing appearance of Van-AKI. Though unproven, it appears from personal and anecdotal experience of the senior author over the last 4 decades that the incidence of vancomycin-induced nephrotoxicity has been under-recognized, under-diagnosed, and under-reported.

Although vancomycin levels are typically monitored (albeit without any systematic or rational pattern) the primary goal is to ensure a relative drug excess and therefore adequacy of bacterial killing, not to prevent nephrotoxicity. Generally, renal safety almost appears to be an afterthought, only considered when serum creatinine is found to be very high or vancomycin level is in the blatantly toxic range. This is because to date Van-AKI as a real clinical entity of major concern has remained a debatable issue and eluded the attention of the most physicians except the ID experts and nephrologists. We believe and hope this chapter has firmly and fully established this as a serious and significant predictable adverse consequence of vancomycin administration, especially during dosage escalation, during prolonged therapy, used at rather high doses, and/or given without any following tight and close safety precautions.

There have been few if any published specific and pragmatic guidelines aimed at preventing and/or ameliorating AKI. Until large and prospective studies have been conducted to generate better alternatives, we would recommend the following interim and tentative guidelines.

7. References

Bailie, G. R. and D. Neal (1988). "Vancomycin ototoxicity and nephrotoxicity. A review." *Med Toxicol Adverse Drug Exp* 3(5): 376-386.

Baker, R. J. and C. D. Pusey (2004). "The changing profile of acute tubulointerstitial nephritis." *Nephrol Dial Transplant* 19(1): 8-11.

Barraclough, K., M. Harris, et al. (2007). "An unusual case of acute kidney injury due to vancomycin lessons learnt from reliance on eGFR." *Nephrol Dial Transplant* 22(8): 2391-2394.

Cavalcanti, A. B., A. R. Goncalves, et al. (2010). "Teicoplanin versus vancomycin for proven or suspected infection." *Cochrane Database Syst Rev*(6): CD007022.

Chan, J. D., T. N. Pham, et al. (2011). "Clinical Outcomes of Linezolid vs Vancomycin in Methicillin-Resistant Staphylococcus aures Ventilator-Associated Pneumonia: Retrospective Analysis." *J Intensive Care Med.*

Cimino, M.A., C. Rotstein, et al. (1987). "Relationship of serum antibiotic concentrations to nephrotoxicity in cancer patients receiving concurrent aminoglycoside and vancomycin therapy." *Am J Med* 83: 1091-1097.

Cockcroft, D.W.,M.H. Gault (1976). "Prediction of creatinine clearance from serum creatinine." *Nephron* 16:31-35.

Cohen, E., A. Dadashev, et al. (2002). "Once-daily versus twice-daily intravenous administration of vancomycin for infections in hospitalized patients." *J Antimicrob Chemother* 49(1): 155-160.

Dangerfield, H. C. Hewitt et al. (1960). "Clinical use of vancomycin." *Antimicrobial agents Annual:* 428-438

Downs, N.J., R. E. Neihart RE, et al. (1989). "Mild nephrotoxicity associated with vancomycin use." *Arch Intern Med* 149: 1777-1781.

Dutton, A. A. and P. C. Elmes (1959). "Vancomycin: report on treatment of patients with severe staphylococcal infections." *Br Med J* 1(5130): 1144-1149.

Farber, B., F. Moellering et al. (1983). " Retrospective study of the toxicity of preparations of vancomycin from 1974 to 1981." *Antimicrobial agents and chemotherapy*: 138-141.

Fowler, V. G., Jr., H. W. Boucher, et al. (2006). "Daptomycin versus standard therapy for bacteremia and endocarditis caused by Staphylococcus aureus." *N Engl J Med* 355(7): 653-665.

Frimat, L., D. Hestin, et al. (1995). "Acute renal failure due to vancomycin alone." *Nephrol Dial Transplant* 10(4): 550-551.

Ge, Y., D. Biek, et al. (2008). "In vitro profiling of ceftaroline against a collection of recent bacterial clinical isolates from across the United States." *Antimicrob Agents Chemother* 52(9): 3398-3407.

Goetz, M. B. and J. Sayers (1993). "Nephrotoxicity of vancomycin and aminoglycoside therapy separately and in combination." *J Antimicrob Chemother* 32(2): 325-334.

Hermsen, E. D., M. Hanson, et al. (2010). "Clinical outcomes and nephrotoxicity associated with vancomycin trough concentrations during treatment of deep-seated infections." *Expert Opin Drug Saf* 9(1): 9-14.

Hidayat, L. K., D. I. Hsu, et al. (2006). "High-dose vancomycin therapy for methicillin-resistant Staphylococcus aureus infections: efficacy and toxicity." *Arch Intern Med* 166(19): 2138-2144.

Iizawa, Y., J. Nagai, et al. (2004). "In vitro antimicrobial activity of T-91825, a novel anti-MRSA cephalosporin, and in vivo anti-MRSA activity of its prodrug, TAK-599." *J Infect Chemother* 10(3): 146-156.

Ingram, P. R., D. C. Lye, et al. (2008). "Risk factors for nephrotoxicity associated with continuous vancomycin infusion in outpatient parenteral antibiotic therapy." *J Antimicrob Chemother* 62(1): 168-171.

Kalil, A.C., M.H. Murthy, et al. (2010). "Linezolid versus vancomycin or teicoplanin for nosocomial pneumonia: a systematic review and meta-analysis." *Crit Care Med* 38: 1802-1808.

Ladino, M., M. Alex et al. (2008). "Acute and reversible nephrotoxicity: case reports" *Nephrol Dial Transplant* 1(1): 4-10.

Lodise, T. P., B. Lomaestro, et al. (2008). "Larger vancomycin doses (at least four grams per day) are associated with an increased incidence of nephrotoxicity." *Antimicrob Agents Chemother* 52(4): 1330-1336.

Van Laethem, Y., P. Hermans P, et al. (1988). "Teicoplanin compared with vancomycin in methicillin-resistant Staphylococcus aureus infections: preliminary results." *J Antimicrob Chemother* 21 Suppl A: 81-87.

Mellor, J.A., J. Kingdom, et al. (1985). "Vancomycin toxicity: a prospective study." *J Antimicrob Chemother* 15: 773-780.

Moellering, R.T., D.J. Krogstat and D.J. Greenblatt (1981). "Vancomycin theray in patients with impaired renal function: A nomogram for dosage." *Ann Intern Med* 94:343-347.

Noel, G. J., K. Bush, et al. (2008 a). "A randomized, double-blind trial comparing ceftobiprole medocaril with vancomycin plus ceftazidime for the treatment of patients with complicated skin and skin-structure infections." *Clin Infect Dis* 46(5): 647-655.

Noel, G. J., R. S. Strauss, et al. (2008 b). "Results of a double-blind, randomized trial of ceftobiprole treatment of complicated skin and skin structure infections caused by gram-positive bacteria." *Antimicrob Agents Chemother* 52(1): 37-44.

Odio, C., G.H. McCracken Jr. and J.D. Nelson (1984). "Nephrotoxicity associated with vancomycin-aminoglycoside therapy in four children." *J Pediatr* 105: 491-493.

Pertel, P. E., B. I. Eisenstein, et al. (2009). "The efficacy and safety of daptomycin vs. vancomycin for the treatment of cellulitis and erysipelas." *Int J Clin Pract* 63(3): 368-375.

Pritchard, L., C. Baker, et al. (2010). "Increasing vancomycin serum trough concentrations and incidence of nephrotoxicity." *Am J Med* 123(12): 1143-1149.

Psevdos, G., Jr., E. Gonzalez, et al. (2009). "Acute renal failure in patients with AIDS on tenofovir while receiving prolonged vancomycin course for osteomyelitis." *AIDS Read* 19(6): 245-248.

Rodriguez Colomo, O., F. Alvarez Lerma, et al. (2011). "Impact of administration of vancomycin or linezolid to critically ill patients with impaired renal function." *Eur J Clin Microbiol Infect Dis* 30(5): 635-643.

Rubinstein, E., S. Cammarata, et al. (2001). "Linezolid (PNU-100766) versus vancomycin in the treatment of hospitalized patients with nosocomial pneumonia: a randomized, double-blind, multicenter study." *Clin Infect Dis* 32(3): 402-412.

Rybak, M. J., L. M. Albrecht, et al. (1990). "Nephrotoxicity of vancomycin, alone and with an aminoglycoside." *J Antimicrob Chemother* 25(4): 679-687.

Rybak, M. J., B. M. Lomaestro, et al. (2009). "Vancomycin therapeutic guidelines: a summary of consensus recommendations from the infectious diseases Society of America, the American Society of Health-System Pharmacists, and the Society of Infectious Diseases Pharmacists." *Clin Infect Dis* 49(3): 325-327.

Shah-Khan, F., M. H. Scheetz, et al. (2011). "Biopsy-Proven Acute Tubular Necrosis due to Vancomycin Toxicity." *Int J Nephrol* 2011: 436856.

Sokol, H., C. Vigneau, et al. (2004). "Biopsy-proven anuric acute tubular necrosis associated with vancomycin and one dose of aminoside." *Nephrol Dial Transplant* 19(7): 1921-1922.

Sokol, H., C. Vigneau, et al. (2004). "Biopsy-proven anuric acute tubular necrosis associated with vancomycin and one dose of aminoside." *Nephrol Dial Transplant* 19(7): 1921-1922.

Sorrell, T.C. and P.J. Collignon. "A prospective study of adverse reactions associated with vancomycin therapy." *J Antimicrob Chemother* 16: 235-241.

Vance-Bryan, K., J. C. Rotschafer, et al. (1994). "A comparative assessment of vancomycin-associated nephrotoxicity in the young versus the elderly hospitalized patient." *J Antimicrob Chemother* 33(4): 811-821.

Walraven, C. J., M. S. North, et al. (2011). "Site of infection rather than vancomycin MIC predicts vancomycin treatment failure in methicillin-resistant Staphylococcus aureus bacteraemia." *J Antimicrob Chemother* 66(10): 2386-2392.

Wilson, S. E., W. O'Riordan, et al. (2009). "Telavancin versus vancomycin for the treatment of complicated skin and skin-structure infections associated with surgical procedures." *Am J Surg* 197(6): 791-796.